SBAs and MCQs for the Final FRCA

SBAs and MCQs for the Final FRCA

Edited by

Rakesh Tandon

Consultant Anaesthetist, Addenbrooke's Hospital,
Cambridge University Hospitals, Cambridge, UK

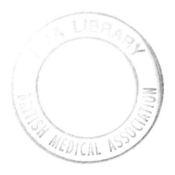

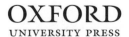

OXFORD
UNIVERSITY PRESS

OXFORD
UNIVERSITY PRESS

Great Clarendon Street, Oxford, OX2 6DP,
United Kingdom

Oxford University Press is a department of the University of Oxford.
It furthers the University's objective of excellence in research, scholarship,
and education by publishing worldwide. Oxford is a registered trade mark of
Oxford University Press in the UK and in certain other countries

© Oxford University Press 2012

The moral rights of the authors have been asserted

First Edition published 2012

Impression: 1

British Library Cataloguing in Publication Data
Data available

Library of Congress Cataloging in Publication Data
Data available

ISBN 978–0–19–966133–6

Printed and bound by
CPI Group (UK) Ltd, Croydon, CR0 4YY

Oxford University Press makes no representation, express or implied, that the
drug dosages in this book are correct. Readers must therefore always check
the product information and clinical procedures with the most up-to-date
published product information and data sheets provided by the manufacturers
and the most recent codes of conduct and safety regulations. The authors and
the publishers do not accept responsibility or legal liability for any errors in the
text or for the misuse or misapplication of material in this work. Except where
otherwise stated, drug dosages and recommendations are for the non-pregnant
adult who is not breast-feeding.

Links to third party websites are provided by Oxford in good faith and for
information only. Oxford disclaims any responsibility for the materials contained
in any third party website referenced in this work.

DEDICATION

*I dedicate this book to my amazing parents for making me what I am today,
along with the all the teachers in anaesthesia.
And to my lovely wife Kavita and lovely kids Aman, Devika, and Ansh
for being so supportive and understanding.*

Rakesh Tandon

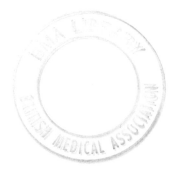

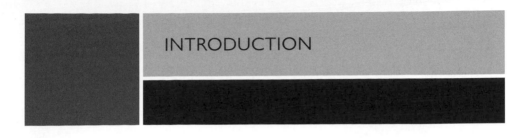

INTRODUCTION

The Royal College of Anaesthetists has set out a new curriculum for the Certificate of Completion of Training. The FRCA examination is an important tool for assessing the progress of trainees through the Certificate of Completion of Training. The college has changed the examination to produce a fair, reliable, and robust examination that reflects best contemporary assessment practice. In 2011 the FRCA multiple-choice examination was changed, with the removal of negative marking and the addition of single best answer multiple-choice questions (MCQs), but there is little published material available for prospective examination candidates in terms of targeted examination guidance combined with complete MCQ practice. Our aim was to fill this gap.

This new book, *SBAs and MCQs for the Final FRCA*, is intended for trainee anaesthetists as well as trainers, and offers well-researched, relevant, and carefully constructed questions with evidence-based answers. The book specifically addresses the new emphasis in the FRCA examination, giving candidates an insight into the way the examination works, with general guidance on examination techniques and providing readily accessible information relating to a wide range of potential questions.

There are other books available that are aimed at single best answer MCQs only, but the recent changes in the examinations set by the Royal College of Anaesthetists have created the need for a book which combines TAF questions with SBA questions, which is what this book does.

The final FRCA examination syllabus is large in both depth and breadth, which makes it difficult to cover in a single volume. While there are some excellent materials from different sources available to trainees who are revising, this book offers the advantage of covering the wide variety of topics specific to the examination within a single volume. A further advantage is that this book can be used by examination candidates to set up mock examinations. It will also be a useful resource for consultants or trainers in various departments who help to set up mock examinations for their trainees.

The book is written with the sole aim of covering the final FRCA examination, as well as the syllabus, and contains conventional TAF and SBA questions. This allows the candidates approaching the final FRCA to practice questions as they will appear in the real examination.

We aim to cover all aspects of the syllabus along the lines laid out by the Royal College of Anaesthetists. The explanations written in response to the questions are well referenced and provide useful information.

The book has five chapters, which cover all aspects of anaesthesia as prescribed by the Royal College of Anaesthetists. The Final Examination MCQ paper comprises 90 questions to be completed in 3 hours. This is divided into two sections: 60 MCQs and 30 SBA questions. Each chapter in this book has this same structure. There is also a final chapter consisting of three 30 SBA questions set out as a mini-examination in order to provide more SBA practice.

The MCQs are divided as follows:

- 20 questions in medicine and surgery
- 20 questions in applied basic science
- 15 questions in intensive care medicine
- 5 questions in pain management.

The MCQs are aimed to test factual knowledge. Each question has five possible stems. Each stem is to be marked True or False. All the questions are marked equally, with the correct answer scoring +1 and the wrong answer 0, with no negative marking.

The SBA questions are divided into:

- 20 questions in clinical anaesthesia
- 5 questions in intensive care medicine
- 5 questions in pain management.

The SBA questions aim to test the application of knowledge and problem solving that is essential in the clinical practice. They also test that candidates have an understanding that is more than a simple recall of the fact. The SBA questions test the application of knowledge to an evolving clinical scenario.

The scenario is followed by a lead question, which is precise and specific. The answer to the lead question is one of five possible solutions or responses, but only one of the five options is the best answer. The correct approach is to read the stem and the lead question carefully without looking at the options. The best answer should be quite clear to the well-prepared candidate at this stage. Four marks are scored for each correct answer. As there is no negative marking in the MCQ examination candidates are advised to attempt all the questions.

To pass the examination a broad-based knowledge of the curriculum is required along with practical experience of clinical anaesthesia, critical care, and pain management. It is advisable to use MCQ and SBA practice papers, which will help candidates to assess their knowledge as well as become familiar with the style of the examination and the level of knowledge expected. This book provides perfect revision as it follows the pattern used by the college.

ACKNOWLEDGEMENTS

The Royal College of Anaesthetists has recently changed the format of the Final FRCA Examination multiple-choice paper. This is now divided into two sections, the first with 60 multiple-choice true–false (TAF) questions and the second with 30 questions with a single best answer (SBA). The examination is intended to test the application of knowledge and problem solving for safe practice of anaesthesia. This book is based on the TAF and SBA questions as set out by the most recent requirements and guidance from Royal College of Anaesthetists.

The Commissioning Editor and Publishing Strategist for Medicine at Oxford University Press, Chris Reid, had the foresight to see that a new book was needed to help the trainees prepare for the new examination. We are very grateful to him for his confidence in our team. Once the proposal was accepted a team of enthusiastic writers willing to take on the challenge was assembled, and the task was steered to completion. We are all grateful to him for this initiative.

I wish to express my personal gratitude to the individual contributors with their massive wealth of experience and expertise. To all of them I record my thanks, not only for their thoughtful contributions, but also for their promptness when manuscripts have been returned for amendments. I would particularly like to thank Dr Ashish Shetty and Dr JLC Wheble, Sqn Ldr for their assistance in contributing in reviewing the additional chapters and providing the extra questions.

We are grateful for the efficient copy-editing by Anglosphere Editing Limited.

Finally, to Sarah Stephenson, Production Editor, who has put in the extra effort to produce the book in record time. We are grateful for her overseeing the project through to publication.

We extend our thanks to all the consultants and trainees who have attended the Cambridge Final FRCA course and provided us with the suggestions and feedback which are incorporated into this book.

Rakesh Tandon

CONTENTS

CONTRIBUTORS

Ajit Bhat Anaesthesia Registrar, Addenbrooke's Hospital, Cambridge, UK

Ben Fox Anaesthesia Registrar, Addenbrooke's Cambridge University Hospital, Cambridge, UK

Thomas Kriz Anaesthesia Registrar, Addenbrooke's Cambridge University Hospital, Cambridge, UK

Maria Ochoa-Ferraro Anaesthesia Registrar, Addenbrooke's Hospital, Cambridge, UK

Anand Sharma Anaesthesia Registrar, Addenbrooke's Hospital, Cambridge, UK

Ashish Shetty Anaesthesia Registrar, Addenbrooke's Hospital, Cambridge, UK

Joanna Wheble Anaesthesia Registrar, Addenbrooke's Hospital, Cambridge, UK

ABBREVIATIONS

3OH PTM	3-hydroxy phenyl trimethyl ammonium
5HT	5-hydroxytryptamine
AAA	abdominal aortic aneurysm
AAS	atlanto-axial subluxation
AC	activated charcoal
ACTH	adrenocorticotropic hormone
AD	autonomic dysreflexia
ADH	anti-diuretic hormone
ADT	accidental dural tap
AES	anti-embolism stockings
AF	atrial fibrillation
AFE	amniotic fluid metabolism
AHE	acute hyponatraemic encephalopathy
AICD	implantable cardioverter-defibrillator
AIP	acute intermittent porphyria
AKI	acute kidney injury
ALI	acute lung injury
ARDS	adult respiratory distress syndrome
ARF	acute renal failure
AS	aortic stenosis
AUC	area under curve
BGPC	blood gas partition coefficient
BMI	body mass index
BP	blood pressure
CABG	coronary artery bypass graft
CDH	congenital diaphragmatic hernia
CICV	'can't intubate can't ventilate'
CIM	critical illness myopathy
CIP	critical illness polyneuropathy
CNB	central neuraxial blocks
CNS	central nervous system
CO	cardiac output

COHb	carboxyhaemoglobin
COPD	chronic obstructive pulmonary disease
CPAP	continuous positive airway pressure
CPB	cardiopulmonary bypass
CPD	cephalo-pelvic disproportion
CPSP	central post-stroke pain
CPSP	chronic post-surgical pain
CRF	chronic renal failure
CRPS	chronic regional pain syndrome
CRPS	complex regional pain syndrome i
CS	compartment syndrome
CSF	cerebrospinal fluid
CSWS	cerebral salt wasting syndrome
CVP	central venous pressure
CVST	central venous sinus thrombosis
DDAVP	desmopressin
DHPR	dihydropyridine receptor
DI	diabetes insipidus
DIC	disseminated intravascular coagulation
DKA	diabetic ketoacidosis
DN	dibucaine number
DNAR	do not attempt resuscitation
DVT	deep vein thrombosis
ECMO	extracorporeal membrane oxygenation
ECT	electroconvulsive therapy
EGDT	early goal-directed therapy
EN	enteral nutrition
ESRD	end-stage renal disease
ETT	endotracheal tube
FBC	full blood count
FDP	flexor digitorum profundus
FFP	fresh frozen plasma
FGF	fresh gas flow
FN	fluoride number
FRC	functional residual capacity
FVC	forced vital capacity
GABA	γ-aminobutyric acid
GAS	group a streptococcal infection
GCS	Glasgow Coma Scale
GFR	glomerular filtration rate

GH	growth hormone
GHRH	growth hormone-releasing hormone
HAART	highly active antiretroviral therapy
HbF	haemoglobin foetal
HBOT	hyperbaric oxygen therapy
HbS	haemoglobin s
HCP	hereditary coproporphyria
HD	haemodialysis
HERG	human ether-a-go-go-related gene
HF	haemofiltration
HPO	hypertrophic pulmonary osteopathy
HPV	hypoxic pulmonary vasoconstriction
HS	hereditary spherocytosis
HTIG	human tetanus immunoglobulin
IABP	intra-aortic balloon pump
IBV	ideal body weight
ICP	intracranial pressure
IHD	intermittent haemodialysis
IIM	internal intercostal membrane
INR	international normalized ratio
IPPV	intermittent positive pressure ventilation
IQR	interquartile range
ITP	immune thrombocytopenic purpura
IV	intravenous
IVC	inferior vena cava
JVP	jugular venous pressure
LA	local anaesthetic
LCNT	lateral cutaneous nerve of the thigh
LDF	leucocyte-depleted filters
LDL	low-density lipoprotein
LMA	laryngeal mask airway
LMA	laryngeal mask airway
LMWH	low molecular weight heparin
LSCS	lower segment caesarian section
LV	left ventricular
LVEF	left ventricular ejection fraction
MAC	minimum alveolar concentration
MAOI	monoamine oxidase inhibitors
MAP	mean arterial pressure
MEN	multiple endocrine neoplasia

MIGB	meta-iodobenzyl guanidine
MG	myasthenia gravis
MH	malignant hyperthermia
MR	mitral regurgitation
MVD	microvascular decompression
NG	nasogastric
NICE	national institute for clinical excellence
NIRS	near-infrared spectroscopy
NM	neuromuscular
NMDA	N-methyl-D-aspartate
NMJ	neuromuscular junction
NNRTIs	non-nucleoside reverse transcriptase inhibitors
NO	nitric oxide
NOS	NO synthase
NRTIs	nucleoside reverse transcriptase inhibitors
NSAIDs	non-steroidal anti-inflammatory drugs
OCR	oculo-cardiac reflex
OLV	one lung ventilation
OSA	obstructive sleep apnoea
PAFC	pulmonary artery flotation catheters
PAOP	pulmonary artery occlusion pressure
PCC	prothrombin complex concentrate
PCWP	pulmonary capillary wedge pressure
PDE	phosphodiesterase
PDPH	post-dural puncture headache
PE	pulmonary embolism
PEEP	positive end-expiratory pressure
PEFR	peak expiratory flow rates
PEG	percutaneous endoscopic gastrostomy
PET	pre-eclamptic toxemia
PHP	primary hyperparathyroidism
PHT	pulmonary hypertension
PIs	protease inhibitors
PN	parenteral nutrition
PNS	peripheral nervous system
POCD	postoperative cognitive dysfunction
PP	plumboporphyria
PPM	pre-existing permanent pacemaker
PSG	polysomnography
PSI	pneumonia severity index

PTH	parathyroid hormone
PTR	prothrombin time ratio
PVB	paravertebral blockade
PVL	panton-valentine leukocidin
PVS	paravertebral space
RBC	red blood cell
RF	radiofrequency
rFVIIa	recombinant factor VIIa
RLN	recurrent laryngeal nerve
RPP	rate–pressure product
rSO_2	regional cerebral tissue oxygen saturation
SAH	subarachnoid haemorrhage
SCD	sickle cell disease
SCI	spinal cord injury
SCTL	superior costotransverse ligament
SIADH	syndrome of inappropriate ADH secretion
SR	sarcoplasmic reticulum
SSRIs	selective serotonin reuptake inhibitors
SVR	systemic vascular resistance
TBI	traumatic brain injury
TCA	tricyclic antidepressant
TEG	thromboelastography
TENS	transcutaneous electrical nerve stimulation
TGN	trigeminal neuralgia
THR	total hip replacement
TIPSS	transjugular intrahepatic portosystemic stented shunt
TOE	transoesophageal echocardiogram
TRALI	transfusion-related acute lung injury
TSH	thyroid-stimulating hormone
TTE	transthoracic echocardiography
URTI	upper respiratory tract infection
VAP	ventilator associated pneumonia
V_D	volume of distribution
VF	ventricular fibrillation
VGCC	membrane voltage-gated calcium currents
VP	variegate porphyria
VTE	venous thromboembolism
vWD	von Willebrand's disease
vWF	von Willebrand factor

True/False

1. **Tissue oxygenation can be determined by:**
   A. Gastric tonometry.
   B. Tissue *oxygen* electrodes.
   C. Functional MRI.
   D. Positron emission tomography.
   E. Ultraviolet spectroscopy.

2. **The suggested cause for prothrombin complex concentrate's thrombotic risk is its high content of:**
   A. Calcium.
   B. Factor VII.
   C. Factor II.
   D. Factor X.
   E. Factor IX.

3. **Which patient factors are associated with large-scale fluid absorption during transurethral resection of the prostate (TURP)?**
   A. Hypertension.
   B. Weight.
   C. Varicose veins.
   D. Hydration.
   E. Smoking.

4. **Regarding laser surgery:**
   A. The laser light which is absorbed by a tissue surface exerts the clinical effect.
   B. The light produced from a laser tube is polychromatic.
   C. Medical instruments used with lasers should have matted surfaces.
   D. Eyes should be taped closed with plastic tape during laser surgery.
   E. Pulsed dye laser uses light at a wavelength that targets red blood cells within blood vessels.

5. **Factors associated with an increased risk of diastolic heart failure are:**
    A. Male gender.
    B. Renal disease.
    C. Well-controlled hypertension.
    D. Diabetes mellitus.
    E. Age more than 60.

6. **Effects of lithium include:**
    A. Increased norepinephrine uptake by post-synaptic membrane.
    B. Disruption of thyroid hormone homeostasis.
    C. Nephrogenic diabetes insipidus.
    D. Weight loss.
    E. Extrapyramidal side effects.

7. **The following statements are true of lithium.**
    A. It cannot cross the placenta.
    B. It mimics hypokalaemia in the heart.
    C. Its hyperexcitablility is due to sodium mimicry.
    D. It prolongs non-depolarizing but not depolarizing blockade.
    E. Management of its toxicity includes forced diuresis.

8. **Which of the following is not a postulated mechanism of action of conjugated oestrogens in reducing bleeding in uraemia?**
    A. Vasoconstriction.
    B. Increased von Willebrand factor.
    C. Increased factor VII.
    D. Increased factor XII.
    E. Increased antithrombin.

9. **With regards to smoking, which of the following statements is true?**
    A. There is an increase in the circulating catecholamine concentration due to smoking.
    B. Abstinence for more than 3 months decreases overall perioperative cardiovascular risk by 33%.
    C. Sustained postoperative abstinence decreases long-term mortality after CABG.
    D. It increases airway reactivity and decrease in FEV_1.
    E. It has minimal effects on wound healing.

10. **For orally acting factor Xa inhibitors, which of the following statements is true?**
    A. They reduce platelet function.
    B. Their effect can be monitored by PT.
    C. There is an increased bleeding risk compared to low molecular weight heparin.
    D. They are licensed for prevention of venous thromboembolism in hip but not knee arthroplasty.
    E. Regular monitoring of coagulation is required.

11. Regarding renal physiology:

A. The osmotic gradient increases from the corticomedullary boundary to the tip of the medulla.
B. The osmotic gradient disappears in diuresis.
C. NaCl and urea are the major constituents of the osmotic gradient in the inner medulla.
D. The inner medullary tip has osmolality greater than urine during antidiuresis.
E. Sodium, potassium, and urea are major urinary solutes.

12. Risk factors increasing chances of stent thrombosis include:

A. Diabetes.
B. Renal impairment.
C. Stent length <18 mm.
D. Low ejection fraction.
E. Young age.

13. Which of the following are not criteria for identifying pregnant women suffering from H1N1 infection who may benefit from intensive care?

A. Dyspnoea with PaO_2 of 10 kPa.
B. Influenza-related pneumonia.
C. Confirmed/suspected swine flu.
D. Severe acidosis with pH < 7.26.
E. Progressive hypercapnia.

14. The sensation of dyspnoea in chronic obstructive pulmonary disease:

A. Is improved by opiates.
B. Is improved in both affective and sensory dimensions by attention distraction.
C. Is improved by bronchodilators, especially in reversible broncho-constriction.
D. Is improved during exercise by inhaled furosemide via sympathetic mechanisms.
E. Is relieved at rest by in-phase chest wall vibration.

15. Regarding cell salvage in obstetrics:

A. There is a risk of amniotic fluid embolism.
B. Cell savers with leucocyte depletion filters significantly reduce both amniotic fluid and foetal red-cell levels in salvaged blood.
C. Any risk of allo-immunization from foetal red cells in cell salvage is significantly higher than a normal vaginal delivery.
D. The use of one suction device is unsafe, and at least two are needed.
E. Cell salvage in obstetrics is limited due to the high incidence of haemorrhage outside the operating theatre.

16. The new anaesthetic agent PFO713:

A. Is similar to propofol, but with 2,6 optically active groups on the phenol ring.
B. Is a GABAA agonist.
C. Is soluble in water and does not produce pain on injection.
D. Has slower onset of action and longer duration than propofol.
E. Has been evaluated in humans only in the R,R form.

17. Hypothermia can cause:
   A. Increased plasma viscosity.
   B. Increased platelet count.
   C. Hyperglycaemia.
   D. Reduced glomerular filtration rate.
   E. Arrhythmia.

18. Which of the following neuromuscular conditions is not associated with malignant hyperthermia?
   A. Duchene's muscular dystrophy.
   B. King Denborough syndrome.
   C. Central core disease.
   D. Becker muscular dystrophy.
   E. Evans myopathy.

19. Complications of obstructive sleep apnoea are:
   A. Decrease in brain white matter.
   B. Failure of cerebral autoregulation.
   C. Dyslipidemia.
   D. Impaired glucose tolerance.
   E. Increased platelet aggregation.

20. Boundaries of the paravertebral space are:
   A. Superiorly by the angle of the ribs.
   B. Inferiorly by the crurae of the diaphragm.
   C. Anteriorly by the visceral pleura.
   D. Posteriorly by the costotransverse ligament and the posterior intercostal membrane.
   E. Laterally by the ligamentum flavum.

21. The common ECG abnormalities associated with morbid obesity are:
   A. High voltage complexes.
   B. LV hypertrophy or strain.
   C. Prolonged QT/QTc.
   D. Inferolateral T-wave abnormalities.
   E. Right-axis deviation or RBBB with P pulmonale.

22. In obese patients, which of the following drugs need to be administered based on actual body weight?
   A. Weak or moderately lipophilic drugs.
   B. Non-depolarizing muscle relaxants.
   C. Suxamethonium.
   D. Remifentanil.
   E. Induction agents.

23. Hypoxic pulmonary vasoconstriction is impaired by:

A. Supine position.
B. Vasoconstrictors.
C. Failure of lung collapse by a double lumen tube.
D. Inhalational anaesthetic agents.
E. Nitrates.

24. Endobronchial blockers are preferred:

A. In tall patients.
B. In patients already intubated.
C. Where intubation is difficult.
D. Where there is a need to avoid airway injury.
E. Where lung resection is not required.

25. Regarding diffusion of gas, the rate of diffusion of a gas across a membrane is:

A. Directly proportional to the surface area of the membrane.
B. Inversely proportional to the partial pressure gradient.
C. Directly proportional to thickness of the membrane.
D. Directly proportional to the molecular weight of the gas.
E. Inversely proportional to the density of the gas.

26. Which of the following statements are true for sickle cell anaemia?

A. Cardiomegaly is usually due to anaemia.
B. Eye changes include cataract.
C. Penicillin can precipitate haemolysis.
D. There is an increased incidence of TIAs.
E. Homozygous (SS) sickle at PaO_2 of 6.5–8.0 kPa.

27. Activated charcoal is useful for which of these poisons?

A. Digoxin.
B. Lithium.
C. Alcohol.
D. Petroleum distillates.
E. Acetaminophen.

28. Regarding gas flow:

A. Critical flow of anaesthetic gas in an airway in L/min is the same as the numerical value of the diameter of the airway in mm.
B. Turbulence in the circulatory system is often heard as a bruit.
C. Smaller air passages have laminar flow due to the low speed of gas.
D. In cyclical breathing, turbulent flow occurs during peak flow.
E. Critical flow in humidified, warm anaesthetic gas can be 10% lower than in dry gas at 20°C.

29. A man presents to accident and emergency (A&E) with ethylene glycol poisoning. The following are expected:

A. Decreased anion gap.

B. Increased osmolar gap.

C. Type B lactic acidosis.

D. Administration of enteral charcoal.

E. Urate crystals in the urine.

30. Regarding albumin, which of the following statements are true?

A. Albumin transports steroid hormones.

B. Albumin has a positive charge.

C. Low albumin in sepsis is predominantly due to sepsis-induced depression of synthesis.

D. Replacement of albumin in nephrotic syndrome is not beneficial.

E. The only established contraindication for albumin use is allergy.

31. Regarding helium:

A. Greater flow of helium/oxygen mixture will occur in turbulence, due to the latter's dependence on viscosity.

B. It use in asthma is limited, as peripheral airflow is laminar.

C. It is supplied in brown cylinders at 147 bar.

D. It is denser than nitrogen.

E. It is available with 30% oxygen.

32. Regarding carcinoid syndrome and the heart:

A. Symptoms may suggest biventricular involvement.

B. Mixed tricuspid and pulmonary valve disease are well recognized.

C. Classical presentation of the disease involves peripheral oedema.

D. Fibrous thickening of endocardium causes fragile valve leaflets.

E. The changes are unrelated to duration.

33. Which of the following statements on cardiac output monitoring are untrue?

A. 2D aortic valve measurement is associated with significant error in transoesophageal echo.

B. Pulse pressure analysis is of limited use in arrthymias.

C. Oesophageal Doppler is not influenced by non-linear changes in systemic vascular resistance.

D. Thermodilution can provide an erroneous result in valvular heart disease.

E. Pulse pressure methods provide the means for continuous cardiac output measurement.

34. Regarding Neostigmine which statements are true?

A. Can be used intrathecally for analgesia.

B. It is excreted hepatically.

C. Only parental preparations are available.

D. It affects autonomic ganglion in doses used in anaesthesia.

E. In large doses, it can cause depolarizing blockade.

35. **Regarding temperature measurement, choose which of the following statements are true:**
    A. Nasal temperature is constant and reliable.
    B. Rectal temperature measurement in adults is inaccurate, but quick to respond to changes.
    C. Lower oesophageal temperature may fluctuate due to air in the trachea.
    D. Ear temperature probes are designed to measure aural cavity temperatures.
    E. Nasopharyngeal temperature measurement is less effective in intubated patients.

36. **Aspirin causes:**
    A. Increase in CO_2 production.
    B. Respiratory acidosis.
    C. Hypothermia.
    D. Bleeding secondary to hypofibrinogenaemia.
    E. High-output renal failure.

37. **Propranolol:**
    A. Reduces inotropic effect of digoxin.
    B. Causes hyperglycaemia.
    C. Lowers airway resistance.
    D. Is the treatment of choice for ventricular ectopics in myocardial infarction.
    E. Possesses intrinsic antiarrhythmic properties.

38. **Pericarditis may occur with:**
    A. Uraemia.
    B. Coxsackie B virus.
    C. Tuberculosis.
    D. Staphylococcal infections.
    E. Myocardial infarction.

39. **The Fick principle can be used to measure:**
    A. Renal output.
    B. Respiratory rate.
    C. Cerebral blood flow.
    D. Cardiac output.
    E. Peripheral-limb blood flow.

40. **The critical temperature of a gas is the temperature:**
    A. Below which it solidifies.
    B. Above which it will not liquefy despite increased pressure.
    C. At which it sublimes.
    D. At which it liquefies if pressure is decreased.
    E. At which kinetic energy is zero.

41. **The laminar flow of gas through a tube is:**

   A. Proportional to the square root of the pressure drop along the tube.

   B. Proportional to the length of the tube.

   C. Proportional to the fourth power of the diameter.

   D. Inversely proportional to the square of the viscosity of the gas.

   E. Inversely proportional to the square root of the density of the gas.

42. **A thermistor:**

   A. Is a type of transducer.

   B. Comprises a junction of dissimilar metals.

   C. Is used for electrical measurements of temperature.

   D. Is conveniently used in a Wheatstone bridge circuit.

   E. Is very delicate.

43. **For cricoid pressure to be effective the following are required:**

   A. A complete cricoid ring.

   B. Nasogastric tube must be removed.

   C. Neck extension.

   D. Pre-oxygenation for 5 min.

   E. Pressure on the oesophagus against the vertebral body.

44. **Complications of supraclavicular brachial plexus block include:**

   A. Horner's syndrome.

   B. Phrenic nerve palsy.

   C. Subclavian artery puncture.

   D. Recurrent laryngeal nerve palsy.

   E. Subarachnoid injection of local anaesthetic.

45. **Blocking the ulnar nerve at the wrist causes:**

   A. Paralysis of adductor pollicis.

   B. Analgesia in the C8 dermatome.

   C. Analgesia of the palmar aspect of the ulnar 1½ fingers.

   D. Analgesia of the dorsal aspect of the ulnar 1½ fingers.

   E. Vasoconstriction in the medial 1½ fingers.

46. **The pudendal nerve:**

   A. Has anterior primary rami S2/3/4.

   B. Passes through the lesser sciatic foramen.

   C. Gives sensation to the perineum.

   D. Provides motor function to the urethral sphincter.

   E. Descends onto the piriformis muscle.

47. The following condition will decrease lung compliance:

A. Pulmonary oedema.
B. Emphysema.
C. Pulmonary vascular engorgement.
D. 80-year-old male.
E. Pulmonary fibrosis.

48. A recent massive pulmonary embolus is suggested by the following:

A. Rise in central venous pressure.
B. Haemoptysis.
C. Deep Q-wave and inverted T-wave in V3.
D. Fall in left atrial pressure.
E. Increased pulmonary arterial occlusion pressure.

49. A constant pulse rate during and immediately after a Valsalva manoeuvre is found in:

A. Uncomplicated aortic regurgitation.
B. Horner's syndrome.
C. Diabetes mellitus.
D. Heart failure.
E. Cervical spondylosis.

50. A patient with a low fixed cardiac output may be suffering from:

A. Mitral stenosis.
B. Ventricular septal defect.
C. Aortic stenosis.
D. Myocardial infarction.
E. Pulmonary stenosis.

51. In primary thyrotoxicosis:

A. Atrial fibrillation is common.
B. Carbimazole increases the size of the gland.
C. The cause is commonly an adenoma.
D. Myopathy is a common problem.
E. Thyroid-stimulating hormone levels are normal or high.

52. In hyperparathyroidism one sees:

A. Hyperchloraemia.
B. Increased serum calcium and a raised urinary calcium.
C. Raised serum alkaline phosphatase activity.
D. Phosphaturia.
E. Hypotension.

53. **VitamIn B12 is the appropriate treatment for anaemia caused by:**
    A. Pregnancy.
    B. Crohn's disease of the terminal ileum.
    C. Phenytoin treatment of epilepsy.
    D. Vegetarian diet.
    E. Total gastrectomy.

54. **A young man presents with haemoglobin of 8 g/dL and a reticulocyte count of 10%. He may have:**
    A. Acute leukaemia.
    B. Aplastic anaemia.
    C. Had chronic haemorrhage.
    D. Had acute haemorrhage.
    E. Untreated pernicious anaemia.

55. **Dystrophia myotonica is associated with:**
    A. Abnormal oesophageal motility.
    B. Cardiomyopathy.
    C. Optic atrophy.
    D. Ptosis.
    E. Diabetes mellitus.

56. **The following are true about the foetal circulation:**
    A. The pO_2 in the descending aorta is lower than that in the aortic arch.
    B. The ductus venosus contains mixed venous blood.
    C. The ductus arteriosus closes due to the rise in systemic pressure.
    D. The closure of the foramen ovale is due to changes in left and right atrial pressures.
    E. Blood from the inferior vena cava can reach the systemic circulation without passing through the left side of the heart.

57. **In a patient on a monoamine oxidase inhibitor, the following drugs may interact:**
    A. Pethidine.
    B. Amphetamine.
    C. Tricyclic antidepressant.
    D. Adrenaline.
    E. Midazolam.

58. **Amiodarone can cause the following:**
    A. Corneal microdeposits.
    B. Hyperthyroidism.
    C. Photosensitivity.
    D. Peripheral neuritis.
    E. Bigeminy.

59. Ritodrine may cause:

  A. Pulmonary oedema.
  B. Bradycardia.
  C. Heart block.
  D. Increased peripheral vascular resistance.
  E. Increased force of contraction of uterine muscle.

60. Skin pigmentation occurs in the following conditions:

  A. Vitiligo.
  B. Melasma.
  C. Infective endocarditis.
  D. Haemochromatosis.
  E. Sheehan's syndrome.

Single Best Answers

1. **A young cyclist had a road traffic accident and fractured his tibia. He is having open reduction and internal fixation. During the operation there is sudden loss of end tidal carbon dioxide. This was followed by fall in blood pressure. What is the most likely diagnosis?**
    A. Pneumothorax.
    B. Haemorrhage.
    C. Fat embolism.
    D. Hyponatriemia.
    E. Myocardial ischemia.

2. **A 72-year-old male is undergoing oesophagectomy with one lung anaesthesia. Half-way through the operation, the oxygen saturation drops from 95% to 84%. What will be the most appropriate step?**
    A. Check pipeline pressure and gas analyser, and anaesthetic flow meter.
    B. Check breathing circuit for disconnection.
    C. Increase the FiO_2 to 1.
    D. Stop surgery and re-inflate lungs.
    E. Check the position of the tube.

3. **A patient with a psychiatric disorder is scheduled for an endoscopic repair of his abdominal aortic aneurysm. He has been known to be uncontrollable, but with his medications is now well adjusted. Which of the following psychoactive drugs will you not continue until the day of the surgery?**
    A. SSRIs.
    B. Lithium.
    C. Benzodiazepines.
    D. Prochloeperazine.
    E. Risperidone.

4. **An 85-year-old patient with history of heart disease is undergoing a laprotomy for caecal perforation and septicaemic shock. You think he has adequately fluid resuscitated. Which of the following is the best indicator of adequate filling in the presence of IPPV and anaesthesia?**
    A. CVP of 12 mmHg.
    B. Systolic blood pressure 120 mmHg.
    C. Heart rate <100 bpm.
    D. Systolic pressure variation less than 10 mmHg.
    E. Capillary refill time <3 s.

5. **A 44-year-old woman is diagnosed with breast cancer and is scheduled for mastectomy. On pre-assessment there is no other medical issue and she has a mild scoliosis. You are planning a paravertebral block for postoperative pain relief. Regarding paravertebral block, which of the following is correct?**

    A. Chest deformity is a relative contraindication.
    B. Opiates may help in block quality and duration.
    C. Hypotension is the most common serious complication.
    D. Paravertebral block, given below the umbilicus, may inhibit the stress response.
    E. Additional nursing training may be required to look after the patient post operatively.

6. **You are going to anaesthetize a child with cerebral palsy for tonsillectomy. The child has a history of difficult intubation. Which of the following is the most important thing you will note?**

    A. There is an increased sensitivity to non-depolarizing agents.
    B. Suxamethonium is not contraindicated.
    C. There is a small risk of malignant hyperthermia.
    D. Co-existent anticonvulsant therapy can increase resistance to volatile anaesthetics, increasing MAC values.
    E. Thiopentone is the preferred induction agent.

7. **A 20-year-old is undergoing emergency laparoscopic appendicectomy. He had rapid sequence induction for general anaesthesia. During the procedure the heart rate increases from 80 to 130/min, blood pressure 120/60 to 150/80 mmHg and entidal carbon dioxide is increasing 6.5 to 8.5 while on an inhalational agent. The patient is sweating and his temperature is 39.5°C. What would be the most appropriate initial step?**

    A. Change the anaesthetic machine to a vapour-free machine.
    B. Disconnect the vaporizer and ventilate with 100% oxygen.
    C. Intravenous Dantrolene 2 mg/kg IV to a maximum of 10 mg/kg.
    D. Surgery should be stopped and the patient transferred to critical care.
    E. Check for signs of compartment syndrome.

8. **You are about to anaesthetize a patient with a large goitre compressing the airway. During the team briefing which of the following equipment you would ask to be readily available?**

    A. McCoy laryngoscope.
    B. Bougie.
    C. Fibre optic laryngoscope.
    D. Emergency tracheostomy kit.
    E. Rigid bronchoscope.

9. You have anaesthetized a 54-year-old male for laryngoscopy and oseophagoscopy. The ENT surgeon finishes the procedure within 10 min of the intubating dose of atracurium. At the end of the anaesthesia, what will be most appropriate clinical indicator for adequate neuromuscular function after reversal of non-depolarizing blockade?
    A. Tongue protrusion when asked.
    B. Good cough.
    C. Sustained head lift >5 s.
    D. Maintain sustained hand grip.
    E. Inspiratory pressure −20 cmH$_2$O.

10. A patient is scheduled for a radical prostatectomy; he has bicuspid aortic stenosis. Which of the following options will you choose in his management?
    A. Antibiotic prophylaxis.
    B. Reduced afterload after a spinal anaesthetic to reduce cardiac strain.
    C. Avoid tachycardia to ensure ventricular filling.
    D. No antibiotic prophylaxis is required.
    E. Promote peripheral vasoconstriction.

11. A 35-year-old woman with cervical spinal cord injury sustained 2 years ago is scheduled for a laprotomy. She has large intestinal mass with associated shortness of breath. There is history of autonomic dysreflexia. Pick the best statement regarding her management:
    A. β-blockers are indicated for autonomic dysreflexia.
    B. Rapid sequence intubation is indicated for GA due to a risk of aspiration.
    C. Slight head-down position promotes an improvement in FVC.
    D. Fertility in affected females is reduced, so the abdominal mass is unlikely to be her uterus.
    E. Clinically significant hyperkalaemia after suxamethonium can persist until 18 months.

12. You are setting up an ENT theatre for a laser ablation of vocal-cord nodules. In order to prepare for airway fire:
    A. Canvas tapes should be avoided.
    B. The best airway is a modified laser tube with saline-filled cuffs.
    C. The first step in an airway fire is to stop ventilating the patient.
    D. Since oxygen supports combustion, gas mixtures of 21% oxygen in nitrous oxide are suitable.
    E. Protective reflective eye covers are needed.

13. **A patient suffered dural puncture during a labour epidural. She develops a headache and nausea after a day. Choose the incorrect statement regarding her management:**

A. Prophylaxis of her headache includes bed rest.
B. ACTH can alleviate symptoms.
C. Expect her to be nauseous, as nausea accompanies headache in 60% of patients.
D. Epidural saline infusions are dangerous as they can cause lower-limb radicular pain.
E. There is no evidence hydration reduces the incidence of headache.

14. **A 27-year-old man has made a complaint to the hospital regarding ulnar neuropathy. He says he developed ulnar nerve injury due to inadequate care during his long anaesthetic for a lower-limb free flap. The operation was conducted under a combine spinal–epidural, and you think he was comfortable during the operation. Pick the best statement regarding his condition:**

A. This condition is more common in female patients due to fat compressing nerve in the ulnar groove.
B. 85% of cases occur under general anaesthetic.
C. Prevention includes additional padding and abduction of neutral arm as it reduces ulnar compression.
D. Common in young patients due to increased muscle bulk.
E. A difference in nerve conduction from the contralateral unaffected arm is diagnostic.

15. **A medical registrar has referred an 18-year-old patient with bilateral progressive leg weakness. The leg weakness followed flu-like symptoms a week ago. Which of the following management approaches is most appropriate for the patient?**

A. Diagnosis is Guillain–Barré syndrome; requires ICU admission and physiotherapy.
B. Diagnosis is Guillain–Barré syndrome; requires ICU admission for non-invasive ventilation.
C. Diagnosis is Guillain–Barré syndrome; requires ICU admission and corticosteroid therapy.
D. Diagnosis is Guillain–Barré syndrome; requires ICU admission and CSF filtration.
E. Diagnosis is Guillain–Barré syndrome; requires ICU admission and immunoglobin therapy.

16. **A 38-year-old man has been retrieved from a house fire with 30% burns. He was admitted to the high-dependency unit 24 h ago. He is stable, with normal blood gases, and is on patient-controlled morphine. The nurse responsible for his care requests you to review the patient and possibly discharge him to the ward. What is the most appropriate explanation to keep him in HDU?**

A. Burn patients require multiple surgical procedures.
B. Patients with partial thickness burns have higher analgesic requirements.
C. Burn patients with >25% BSA require monitoring of COHb and cyanide levels.
D. Burns patients with >25% BSA produce systemic inflammatory responses.
E. Fluid resuscitation is still required.

17. **A patient with a heart–lung transplant is scheduled for elective inguinal hernia repair. With respect to anaesthetic management, which of the following statements is appropriate?**
    A. The resting heart rate is 100–110/min due to sympathetic upregulation following denervation.
    B. Nitric oxide responsiveness and coronary blood flow are increased.
    C. Patients are susceptible to pulmonary oedema due to a high risk of diastolic dysfunction.
    D. Regional anaesthesia will be best in view of the altered physiology of the heart.
    E. Due to immunosuppression, denervation, and a high risk of pulmonary dysfunction, patients with heart–lung transplants should ideally be intubated.

18. **A 56-year-old man with acute bowel obstruction is on the emergency list for laprotomy. He has a significant history of hypertension and depression. He is on bendroflumethiazide, enalapril, and phenelzine. During the operation his blood pressure went down to 65/30 from 140/90 and his heart rate was 120/min. Fluid resuscitation continued, but the blood pressure rose to 70/40. What would be the most appropriate treatment at this stage?**
    A. Intravenous bolus of ephedrine 6 mg/ml, monitoring the response.
    B. Intravenous bolus of metaraminol 500 mcg/ml, monitoring the response.
    C. Noradrenaline infusion with arterial monitoring.
    D. Vasopressin infusion with arterial monitoring.
    E. Phenylephrine bolus.

19. **You are assessing a 10-year-old boy with Down's syndrome for a laproscopic appendectomy. He has a pansystolic murmur, high lymphocytic count, and is septic. Which of the following statements would you consider inappropriate?**
    A. Endocardial cushion and ventricular septal defects are common cardiac problems.
    B. High risk of atlantioaxial instability necessitates screening lateral radiographs.
    C. No abnormal responsiveness to anaesthetics is documented.
    D. Incidence of leukaemia and polycythemia is common.
    E. Eisenmenger's syndrome may complicate obstructive sleep apnea.

20. **A 55-year-old male is on an elective list for removal of the thymus gland. He has recently been diagnosed with myasthenia gravis, and is on cholinesterase inhibitors and prednisolone. He denies any respiratory problems but suffers from chronic fatigue syndrome. His preoperative investigations are all normal. The best anaesthetic management for this patient would be:**
    A. RSI using suxamethonium.
    B. A reduced dose of non-depolarizing neuromuscular blocking agents should be used for intubation.
    C. Neuromuscular block must be reversed using cholinesterase inhibitors.
    D. Postoperative ventilation.
    E. An intensive care bed postoperatively.

21. **A 95-year-old ASA 2 is scheduled to have his hip fracture fixed. You discuss the anaesthetic options with the patient and decide to avoid a general anaesthetic and offer the patient spinal anaesthesia. Which of the following reasons would you give?**
    A. Spinal anaesthesia for hip surgery reduces one-month mortality.
    B. There is reduced autoregulation in the brain and kidneys.
    C. Due to a smaller muscle mass, a moderate increase in serum creatinine is indicative of severe renal impairment.
    D. FVC, FEV1, FRC, VC, and CC are all reduced.
    E. Reduced total body water and plasma proteins.

22. **A 23-year-old Afro-Caribbean patient has an open tibial fracture and is on the emergency list for open reduction and internal fixation of tibia. The surgeon is concerned about the compartment pressure. The normal pressure in the lower limb muscle compartment is:**
    A. 10–12 mmHg.
    B. 6–12 mmHg.
    C. 10–20 mmHg.
    D. 0–5 mmHg.
    E. 15–20 mmHg.

23. **A young university student slipped on an icy road and suffered a humeral bone fracture. As the fracture is open it requires an emergency procedure for open reduction and internal fixation. She has a very low pain threshold and morphine makes her very sick. She is happy to have a nerve block. Which nerve block is most suitable for her?**
    A. Axillary brachial plexus block.
    B. Axillary brachial plexus block with fentanyl PCA.
    C. Interscalene brachial plexus block.
    D. Supraclavicular brachial plexus block.
    E. Infraclavicular brachial plexus block.

24. **A 65-year-old woman with community-acquired pneumonia is admitted with a chest infection. She has fever, tachyardia, hypotension, and hypoxia. A provisional diagnosis of septicemic shock is made and she is admitted to the HDU for critical care. When you resuscitate her, which of the following is not a clinical target for goal-directed therapy for severe sepsis?**
    A. Central venous pressure ≥12 mmHg in ventilated patients.
    B. Mean arterial pressure 65–90 mmHg.
    C. Urine output ≥0.5 mL/kg/h.
    D. Haemoglobin ≥8 g/dL.
    E. Central venous oxygen saturation ≥70 mmHg.

25. **A 60-year-old man underwent a scheduled Hartmann's procedure for a gastrointestinal tract malignancy. Postoperative pain was well controlled using an epidural infusion containing 0.1% bupivacaine with 2 mcg/ mL of fentanyl. Twenty-four hours after the operation, he developed a temperature of 39.5°C, severe backache, and heaviness and weakness of the right leg for the previous 2 h. The most appropriate step in this case would be:**

   A. Stop the epidural infusion and observe for recovery of motor power.
   B. Withdraw the epidural catheter by 1 cm and monitor for return of motor power.
   C. Remove the epidural catheter and send the tip for culture.
   D. Discontinue the epidural, do a full septic screen, and start broad-spectrum antibiotics pending culture results.
   E. Perform an urgent MRI and refer to a neurosurgeon.

26. **A 75-year-old woman presents to the pain clinic with an 8-week history of severe pain in the right eye. This pain is continuous with a burning sensation. She was treated with intermittent steroids for a painful rash which she developed a few weeks ago. The most likely cause for her pain is:**

   A. Atypical facial pain.
   B. Late signs and symptoms of polymyalgia rheumatica.
   C. Post-herpetic neuralgia.
   D. Trigeminal neuralgia.
   E. Atypical presentation of trigeminal neuralgia.

27. **A 55-year-old patient is on your list for elective thyroidectomy for a large goitre. She is on medications for hypertension. During preoperative assessment she informs you that over the last couple of weeks she has noticed that on extending her neck, her arms feel weak and slightly numb. She has not mentioned this to her doctors earlier. The next appropriate step in planning her airway management during anaesthesia would be:**

   A. Plan a careful conventional laryngoscopy and intubation, taking care to minimize neck movement.
   B. Plan the use of a flexible laryngeal mask airway and intermittent positive pressure ventilation.
   C. Plan an awake fibreoptic technique for intubation.
   D. Obtain an MRI of the neck to look for posterior atlanto-axial subluxation.
   E. Plan an elective tracheostomy prior to induction of anaesthesia.

28. **A 30-year-old man underwent a nailing of the tibia following a compound fracture sustained in a road traffic accident. Postoperatively he was comfortable on PCA morphine. Six hours postoperatively you are called by the nurse to review the patient as he is complaining of severe pain in the leg and paraesthesia. Examination reveals a tense, swollen leg, with reduced sensation and severe pain on passive stretching of the calf muscle, and with distal pulse palpable. The most appropriate management would be:**

   A. A bolus of 5 mg intraveous morphine followed by PCA morphine.
   B. Urgent referral to the trauma surgeon for suspected compartment syndrome.
   C. A postoperative femoral nerve block to augment the effect of morphine analgesia.
   D. Arrange postoperative placement of epidural catheter with a continuous epidural infusion, as the PCA is not adequately controlling the pain.
   E. Full septic screen to check inflammatory markers and start antibiotics for suspected postoperative sepsis.

29. **A 40-year-old patient has sustained a fall from height and has broken his right femoral shaft. He undergoes a femoral nailing the next day but develops confusion and becomes hypoxic in the recovery. You suspect fat embolism. Which of the following is a major Gurd's criteria for the diagnosis of fat embolism?**

   A. Fat in urine and sputum.
   B. Emboli in the retina on fundoscopy.
   C. Axillary petechiae.
   D. Tachypnoea.
   E. $PaO_2 < 8.0$ kPa on room air.

30. **A 77-year-old lady is admitted to A&E following a fall at home. She is brought to the department by ambulance technicians without spinal immobilization. She has bilateral head of humerus fractures, a nasal fracture, and multiple lacerations to her face. She suffers from severe rheumatoid arthritis. What should be done urgently before she is referred to the orthopedic team?**

   A. Call the maxillo-facial team to suture the lacerations.
   B. Spinal immobilization and CT scan of the cervical spine.
   C. Reduce displaced humeral fracture.
   D. Give her antibiotics.
   E. Tetanus vaccination.

True/False

1. Answers: T T T T F

Body tissue requires a continuous supply of oxygen for production of ATP. Oxygen supply is considered adequate when it can sustain aerobic metabolism. Conditions like non-healing wounds, necrotizing infections, and crush injury are all examples where there is impaired tissue oxygenation.

The methods available, and being developed, to measure tissue oxygenation include:

- blood gas analysis
- pulse oximetry
- gastric tonometry
- near-infrared spectroscopy (NIRS)
- transcutaneous oxygen measurement
- magnetic resonance imaging (functional MR imaging, MR spectroscopy)
- electron paramagnetic resonance
- positron emission tomography.

Continuous real-time monitoring of the adequacy of cerebral perfusion can provide important therapeutic information in a variety of clinical settings. The current clinical availability of several NIRS-based cerebral oximetry devices represents a potentially important development for the detection of cerebral ischaemia.

NIR light can be used to measure regional cerebral tissue oxygen saturation (rSO_2). This technique uses principles of optical spectrophotometry that make use of the fact that biological material, including the skull, is relatively transparent in the NIR range. Oxygen can be measured by IR spectroscopy. Oxygen does not absorb or reflect ultraviolet light.

Yentis SM, Hirsch NP, Smith GB. *A–Z of Anaesthesia and Intensive Care*. Butterworth Heinemann, 2004: p. 501.

Robertson PW, Hart BB. Assessment of tissue oxygenation, *Respir Care Clin N Am*, 1999; 5(2): 221–63.

2. Answers: F F T F F

Factor II in prothrombin complex can cause aggressive thrombosis. None of the other factors have been implicated in uncontrolled clot formation.

Patients receiving oral anticoagulation therapy require correction of coagulopathy. Before elective surgery, anticoagulation reversal may be undertaken over several days by discontinuing warfarin or vitamin K treatment, but rapid correction is required in an emergency. European and American guidelines recommend prothrombin complex concentrates (PCCs) for anticoagulation reversal in patients with life-threatening bleeding and an increased international normalized ratio. Compared with human fresh frozen plasma, PCCs provide quicker correction of the international normalized ratio and improved bleeding control. Recombinant activated factor VII is a potential alternative to PCCs, but preclinical comparisons suggest that PCCs are more effective in correcting coagulopathy. Although many patients who require rapid reversal of warfarin are currently treated with fresh frozen plasma, PCCs should be considered as an alternative therapy.

Levy J, Tanaka K, Dietrich W. Perioperative hemostatic management of patients treated with Vitamin K antagonists. *Anesthesiology* 2009; 5: 918–26.

3. Answers: F F F F T

The length of surgery, prostate mass, venous plexus, and overhydration are theorized to increase bleeding. Only smoking has been consistently shown to be related to increases in fluid absorption.

The factors that affect the higher rate of absorption are:

- high pressure of the irrigation fluid—the height of the bag should be kept at 70 cm to achieve adequate flow of fluid
- low venous pressure, e.g. if the patient is hypovolaemic or hypotensive
- prolonged surgery, especially >1 h
- large blood loss, implying a large number of open veins
- capsular perforation or bladder perforation, allowing a large volume of irrigation fluid into the peritoneal cavity, where it is rapidly absorbed.

The transurethral resection of the prostate (TURP) syndrome clinical symptoms are:

- mild: anorexia, headache, nausea, vomiting, lethargy
- moderate: personality change, muscle cramps and weakness, confusion, ataxia
- severe: drowsiness.

Signs are again highly variable and depend on the level and rate of fall of serum sodium. They may include:

- neurological signs
  - decreased level of consciousness
  - cognitive impairment (e.g. short-term memory loss, disorientation, confusion depression)
  - focal or generalized seizures
  - brain stem herniation (seen in severe acute hyponatraemia); signs include coma, fixed, unilateral, dilated pupil, decorticate or decerebrate posturing, respiratory arrest
- signs of hypovolaemia
  - dry mucous membranes
  - tachycardia
  - diminished skin turgor
- signs of hypervolaemia
  - pulmonary rales
  - S3 gallop (third heart sound)
  - jugular venous distension
  - peripheral oedema
  - ascites.

The common symptoms are headache, restlessness, nausea and vomiting, convulsions, coma, tachypnoea, hypertension, and dyspnoea secondary to pulmonary oedema. Haematological symptoms are hyperglycinemia, hyperammonemia, hyponatremia, hypo-osmolality haemolysis, and acute renal failure.

Hahn RG. Fluid absorption in endoscopic surgery. *Br J Anaesth* 2006; 96: 8.

O'Donnell AM, Foo ITH. Anaesthesia for transurethral resection of the prostate. *Contin Educ Anaesth Crit Care Pain*, 2009; 9(3): 92–96.

4. Answers: T F T F T

Energy applied in a laser tube creates stimulated emissions of photons, which are aligned by mirrors into a focused high-intensity beam. The high energy density of a laser is the result of following characteristics:

- There is high a high degree of mono-chromaticity.
- The electromagnetic field of all photons in the laser beam oscillates synchronously in the same phase.
- Laser light remains in a narrow collimated beam.

These characteristics of monochromatic light (all waves of same wavelength)—parallel, coherent, and in phase—allow for a very concentrated energy delivery, often producing heat.

Laser light absorbed by tissues and converted to heat exerts its clinical effect. Medical instruments used with lasers should have matt rather than shiny surfaces, as laser light can be reflected off mirror-like surfaces. Plastic tapes should be avoided as they are combustible. Pulsed dye lasers use light at a wavelength that targets red blood cells within blood vessels and is used for treating port wine skin lesions.

Saddler J. Laser surgery. In: Allman KG, Wilson IH (eds), *Oxford Handbook of Anaesthesia*. Oxford University Press, 2004: pp. 673–77.

Ramphil IJ. Anaesthesia for laser surgery. In: Miller RD. *Millers's Anaesthesia*, 6th edn. Elsevier, 2005: pp. 2573–88.

5. Answers: F F F T T

Diastolic heart failure, a major cause of morbidity and mortality, is defined as symptoms of heart failure in a patient with preserved left ventricular function. It is characterized by a stiff left ventricle with decreased compliance and impaired relaxation, which leads to increased end diastolic pressure. Signs and symptoms are similar to those of heart failure with systolic dysfunction. The diagnosis of diastolic heart failure is best made with Doppler echocardiography. The focus of pharmacologic treatment of diastolic heart failure is on normalizing blood pressure, promoting regression of left ventricular hypertrophy, avoiding tachycardia, treating symptoms of congestion, and maintaining normal atrial contraction. Diuretic therapy is the mainstay of treatment for preventing pulmonary congestion, while β-blockers appear to be useful in preventing tachycardia and thereby prolonging left ventricular diastolic filling time.

Diabetes disease, along with peripheral arteriopathy and autonomic imbalance, increases the risk of diastolic dysfunction. Gender, hypertension, and renal-disease-associated fluid shifts have no bearing on diastolic heart failure.

Diastolic dysfunction is more common in the elderly, partly because of increased collagen cross-linking, increased smooth muscle content, and loss of elastic fibres. These changes tend to decrease ventricular compliance, making patients with diastolic dysfunction more susceptible to the adverse effects of hypertension, tachycardia, and atrial fibrillation.

Pirracchio R, Cholley B, De Hert S, Solal A, Mebazaa A. Diastolic heart failure in anaesthesia and critical care. *Brit J Anaesth* 2007; 98: 707–21.

6. Answers: F T T F T

Lithium is used to treat the manic episodes of manic depression. Manic symptoms include hyperactivity, rushed speech, poor judgment, reduced need for sleep, aggression, and anger. It also helps to prevent or lessen the intensity of manic episodes.

Lithium mimics sodium, and hence in the cellular phase enters the cell via fast voltage-gated channels but is not removed by the Na-K-ATPase. This leads to the intracellular accumulation.

Mechanism of action

The mechanism by which lithium has its therapeutic effect is complex and not fully elucidated, but includes:

- increase in the uptake of norepinephrine by the presynaptic membrane
- increase in its subsequent metabolism by monoamine oxidases.

Second messenger systems may be another target, and lithium can inhibit adenylate cyclase-reducing cAMP signalling.

When the serum level is above 1.5 mmol/L, lithium is toxic. The signs and symptoms of lithium toxicity are nausea, vomiting, abdominal pain, diarrhoea, blurred vision, ataxia and tremor, arrhythmias, nystagmus, hyperreflexia, convulsions, coma, and death (0.3 mmol/L).

Lithium can cause weight gain and periorbital oedema. Increased norepinephrine uptake explains its clinical role in bipolar disorders. Thyroid function and electrolytes should be monitored in patients on lithium.

Flood S, Bodenham A. Lithium: mimicry, mania, and muscle relaxants. *Contin Educ Anaesth Crit Care Pain* 2010, 10(3): 77–80.

7. Answers: F T T F F

Lithium crosses the placenta and can cause foetal morbidity. It prolongs both depolarizing and non-depolarizing blockade by blocking the sodium channel. Forced diuresis and thiazides are contraindicated in the management of toxicity, as they promote salt and water retention, with lithium reabsorption.

Features of lithium pharmacology include:

- oral lithium is rapidly absorbed, with 100% bioavailability
- lithium mimics Na^+ and decreases the release of neurotransmitters
- peak plasma levels usually occur 1–4 h after a single dose
- volume of distribution approximates to total body water
- lithium is not bound to plasma proteins and tends to accumulate in bone and thyroid tissue; patients on lithium may present with an enlarged and underactive thyroid gland.

Lithium is excreted via the kidneys and exhibits rapid and delayed phases of excretion. Approximately half of an oral dose is excreted within 12 h of administration. The remainder takes 7–14 days to be eliminated. The ion is freely filtered at the glomerulus, following which 80% is reabsorbed via the proximal tubule. The proximal tubule is the only site of lithium reabsorption in the kidney and the process is competitive with sodium reabsorption.

Flood S, Bodenham A. Lithium: mimicry, mania, and muscle relaxants. *Contin Educ Anaesth Crit Care Pain* 2010, 10(3): 77–80.

8. Answers: T F F F F

Oestrogens can cause vasodilation. This accounts for the hypotension and reflex tachycardia seen when used after delivery.

Nitric oxide (NO), a potent vasodilator, has cardio-protective effects, including regulation of blood flow and inhibition of platelet aggregation. In vascular endothelium, oestrogens increase synthesis of NO and expression of NO synthase (NOS). After the menopause there is a profound increase in cardiovascular diseases, which is mainly caused by an enhanced development of atherosclerosis caused by an estrogen deficiency. The most important pathomechanisms are the rise in low-density lipoprotein (LDL)-cholesterol and triglycerides, as a result of an impaired elimination of LDL and remnants in the liver, and an enhancement of LDL oxidation in the arterial intima. Moreover, at the site of endothelial lesions, the occurrence of vasospasms and platelet aggregation is facilitated in estrogen-deficient women, leading to ischemia.

Mahdy AM, Webster NR. Perioperative systemic haemostatic agents. *Brit J Anaesth* 2004; 93: 842–58.

9. Answers: T T T T F

Nicotine increases sympathetic activity, as there is a rise in circulating catecholamines. It has a half-life of about 1 h. Carboxyhemoglobin has a half-life of about 4 h, which impedes the release of oxygen to tissues, hence impairing the oxygen supply/demand ratio and also impeding release of oxygen to tissues, leading to increased frequency of cardiac arrhythmias. Carboxyhemoglobin increases airway reactivity, increases the risk of laryngospasm in recovery, and accelerates age-related decline in the forced expiratory volume in 1 sec (FEV_1). Abstinence from smoking for more than 3 months decreases overall perioperative cardiovascular risk by 33%. Preoperative abstinence for even 12 h should theoretically decrease perioperative ischaemia risk. Sustained postoperative abstinence decreases long-term mortality after coronary artery bypass graft (CABG). Cough and wheezing takes several months to resolve and at least 12 weeks of abstinence is needed to ensure that the risk of postoperative respiratory problems requiring intervention is reduced to normal. The incidence of wound complications is normalized after 4 weeks of preoperative abstinence. Smoking also increases the incidence of wound dehiscence and infection.

Wound and bone healing

Nicotine causes:

- increased incidence of wound dehiscence and infection (especially in face-lifts)
- increased incidence of non-union of fusions and delayed healing of fractures—the mechanisms are unknown but may include impaired nitric-oxide release in microvessels.

Postoperative abstinence is more important than preoperative abstinence for effects on bone healing (unaffected by nicotine replacement therapy (NRT)). The incidence of wound complications is normalized if there is a 4-week preoperative abstinence.

Abstinence from smoking

Abstinence for >3 months decreases overall perioperative cardiovascular risk by 33%. Acute preoperative abstinence (e.g. 12 h) theoretically should decrease perioperative ischemia risk (unproven). Sustained postoperative abstinence decreases long-term mortality after CABG.

Werner DO et al. Perioperative abstinence from smoking. *Anesthesiol* 2006; 104: 356–67.

Tønnesen, H. Smoking and alcohol intervention before surgery: evidence for best practice. *Brit J Anaesth* 2009; 102(3): 297–306.

10. Answers: F T F F F

Orally acting Xa inhibitors are used for thrombo prophylaxis, particularly after joint replacement, and are clinically easier and safer to use than heparin and its analogues. There is no increased risk of bleeding compared to heparin and its analogues.

Rivaroxaban is a new oral anticoagulant approved by NICE for thromboprophylaxis after hip- or knee-joint replacement surgery. The usual dose is 10 mg once a day. It works by inhibiting activated Factor X.

The real advantage of the drug is it does not need routine coagulation monitoring. It does not have a specific antidote. It has dose-proportional increases in plasma concentrations, and effects on activated partial thromboplastin time (APTT), prothrombin time (PT), international normalized ratio (INR), and thrombin time (TT).

Barker R, Marval P. Venous thromboembolism: risks and prevention. *Contin Educ Anaesth Crit Care Pain* 2011; 11: 18–23.

11. Answers: T F T F T

Osmotic gradients in mammalian kidneys increase from the cortico-medullary boundary to the tip of the medulla. The osmotic gradient is maintained in diuresis, although its magnitude is diminished. NaCl and urea are major constituents of the gradient in the inner medulla, while NaCl is a major constituent in the outer medulla. The inner medullary tip has an osmolalty similar to urine during antidiuresis. Sodium, potassium, major univariate anions, and urea are the major urinary solutes, while urea is the predominant urinary solute during antidiuresis.

Sands JM, Layton, HE. The physiology of urinary concentration: an update. *Semin Nephrol* 2009; 29, 178–95.

12. Answers: T T F T F

Risk factors for stent thrombosis include:

- premature discontinuation of antiplatelet therapy—found to be the most important predictor of stent thrombosis
- renal impairment—linked with microvascular and metabolic abnormalities that predispose to thrombus formation
- diabetes mellitus
- old age
- low ejection fraction
- prior brachytherapy
- stent insertion for acute coronary syndrome
- long (>18 mm) stents
- ostial stenting, overlapping and multiple stents, bifurcation stenting, duration <1 year, and suboptimal results with stents.

The stent type itself is not considered to be an independent predictor of thrombosis.

Hall R, Mazer CD. Antiplatelet drugs: a review of their pharmacology and management in the peri operative period. *Anaesth Analg* 2011; 112: 292–318.

13. Answers: F T F T T

Department of Health guidelines (2009) state the criteria for identifying pregnant women suffering from H1N1 infection who may benefit from intensive care:

- severe dyspnoea and hypoxemia with PaO_2 <8 kPa,
- influenza-related pneumonia
- progressive hypercapnia
- refractory hypotension
- septic shock
- severe acidosis with pH < 7.26
- deteriorating conscious level or Glasgow Coma Scale (GCS) < 10.

Pregnant women with confirmed/suspected swine flu who require hospital admission should be isolated whenever possible and cared for in a single room with barrier nursing (gloves, plastic aprons, surgical face masks, attention to hand washing and hygiene, etc.). At delivery, the use of surgical masks and eye protection in addition to plastic aprons is recommended as there is splash risk with Caesarean sections and instrumental deliveries.

Patel M, Dennis A, Flutter C, Khan Z. Pandemic (H1N1) 2009 influenza. *Brit J Anaesth* 2010; 104: 128–42.

14. Answers: T F T F T

Dyspnoea in COPD is improved with opiates, possibly by reducing central ventilatory drive. Bronchodilation reduces airway resistance. Attention distraction reduces the affective dimension, not the sensory, of dyspnoea in both healthy subjects and those with COPD. In-phase chest wall vibration relieves the sensation of dyspnoea at rest, although not of effort, in COPD. Inhaled furosemide is hypothesized to improve dyspnoea via vagal blockade, and is ineffective in cancer, possibly due to damaged nerve endings.

Nishino T. Dyspnoea: underlying mechanisms and treatment. *Brit J Anaesth* 2011; 106(4): 463–74.

15. Answers: T F F F T

The three phases of cell salvage process are collection, washing, and re-infusion.

- *Collection*. Blood from the operative field is collected by a dedicated suction device and a predetermined amount of heparinized saline is added and filtered during the process of collection. This blood is centrifuged to separate the RBCs, which are then washed.
- *Washing of RBCs*. This is performed (across a semipermeable membrane) to filter out free Hb, plasma, white cells, platelets, and heparin.
- *Retransfusion*. Washed RBCs are suspended in saline (to achieve a haematocrit of 60–70%) and then transfused back to the patient (within 6 h).

In obstetrics, cell salvage has been controversial due to the potential risk of amniotic fluid metabolism (AFE). However, two recent systematic reviews suggest that use of cell salvage is safe in an obstetric setting. NICE guidelines (2005) concluded that cell salvage with leucocyte-depleted filters (LDF) is safe. Cell savers with LDF are effective for amniotic fluid, but not foetal RBCs.

Any allo immunization risk from foetal RBCs transfused, but is unlikely to be greater than for normal vaginal deliveries.

The use of one suction device may be as safe and increase the efficacy of RBC recovery.

Ashworth A, Klein AA. Cell salvage as part of a blood conservation strategy in anaesthesia. *Brit J Anaesth* 2010; 105(4): 401–16.

16. Answers: T T F T T

PFO713 is similar in structure to propofol, but with larger side groups. Only the *R,R* form has been studied in humans. It acts as a $GABA_A$ agonist, behaving similarly to propofol in brain-slice assays. It is minimally soluble in water and has been investigated as a 1% oil-in-water emulsion. Onset is slower and duration longer than propofol. Ferret models have confirmed its anti-emetic properties.

Sneyd JR, Rigby J, Ones AE. New drugs and technologies, intravenous anaesthesia is on the move again. *Brit J Anaesth* 2010; 105(3): 246–54.

17. Answers: T F T T T

The side effects of hypothermia can be:

- cardiovascular
  - ◆ arrhythmias secondary to potassium loss
  - ◆ increased plasma viscosity
  - ◆ vasoconstriction impairing microcirculation
- coagulatory
  - ◆ impaired coagulation
  - ◆ reduced platelet count

- renal and metabolic
  - reduced glomerular filtration rate
  - metabolic acidosis
  - hyperglycaemia secondary to impaired glucose metabolism
  - effects on pharmacodynamics and pharmacokinetics
- cerebral
  - vasoconstriction during cooling
  - brain injury from hyperthermia during rewarming.

Conolly S, Arrowsmith JE, Klein AK. Deep hypothermic circulatory arrest. *Contin Educ Anaesth Crit Care Pain* 2010; 5: 138–42.

18. Answers: T F F T F

Malignant hyperthermia (MH) has a definite linkage to King–Denborough syndrome, central core disease, and Evans myopathy. Patients with other neuromuscular disorders have shown MH-type symptoms under general anaesthesia, but the link between these symptoms and true MH remains unclear. There is no association between Duchenne muscular dystrophy and MH; previous reports of what was described as 'normothermic MH' were almost certainly rhabdomyolysis.

The muscular dystrophies are rare, genetically determined degenerative muscle diseases. Important disease entities are the myotonic dystrophies and the Duchenne and Becker muscular dystrophies. Myotonic dystrophy, the most common inherited myopathy in adults, is a multisystem disorder presenting as myotonia (incomplete muscle relaxation), wasting, cardiac conduction abnormalities, cardiomyopathy, septal and valvular defects, endocrine dysfunction, and intellectual impairment. The disease is autosomal-dominant, but non-mendelian inheritance patterns have led to the identification of disease-specific trinucleotide repeat sequences in the non-coding region of a protein kinase gene. Treatment is supportive, although small trials have shown some benefit with recombinant human insulin-like growth factor and dehydroepiandrosterone.

Ragoonanan V, Russell W. Anaesthesia for children with neuromuscular disease. *Contin Educ Anaesth Crit Care Pain* 2010; 10: 143–47.

19. Answers: F T T T T

Sleep apnoea, obesity hypoventilation syndrome, and pickwickian syndrome are related conditions resulting in disturbed night-time sleep and are described by the term 'sleep-disordered breathing'. Obstructive sleep apnea (OSA) is an independent risk factor for serious neuro-cognitive and endocrine conditions, and cardiovascular morbidity and mortality, in all age groups.

Some facts about the OSA are:

- Patients with OSA are at increased risk of cerebro-vascular accidents, with a poorer outcome.
- Patients with OSA have reduced quality of life, leading to psychosocial problems, decreased cognitive function, and depression. These findings may be directly linked to an irreversible decrease in brain grey matter, as MRI and oximetry studies have demonstrated morphological changes in brain grey matter and a failure of cerebral autoregulatory blood flow.
- Childhood OSA patients are comparatively disadvantaged, with reports of reduced IQ, memory, and learning skills.
- Endocrine defects include dyslipidemia and glucose intolerance, even after adjusting for BMI age and gender.
- Activation of the inflammatory system causes increased platelet aggregation and pro-inflammatory cytokines.
- The hypoxia (absence of oxygen supply) through OSA may cause changes in the neurons of the hippocampus and the right frontal cortex in the brain. Research using neuro-imaging has

revealed evidence of hippocampal atrophy in people suffering from OSA. Some OSA sufferers have been found to have problems in mentally manipulating non-verbal information and in executive function.

The diagnosis of OSA is based on clinical history and examination alone. Predisposing conditions combined with a history of snoring, restless sleep, headaches, and daytime sleepiness should alert to the possibility of OSA. Additional diagnostic screening tools include a range of questionnaires.

Martinez G, Faber P. Obstructive sleep apnoea. *Contin Educ Anaesth Crit Care Pain* 2011; 1: 5–8.

20. Answers: F T F T T

Paravertebral blockade (PVB) is a regional anaesthesia technique in which local anaesthetic is administered inside the paravertebral space (PVS).

The PVS is wedge shaped. The parietal pleura is the anterolateral boundary; the posterolateral aspect of the vertebral body, the intervertebral disc, and foramen are the base; the superior costotransverse ligament (SCTL)—located between the lower border of the transverse process above and the upper border of the transverse process below—and its lateral continuation, and the internal intercostal membrane (IIM) form the posterior boundary.

The PVS is divided into an anterior, extrapleural compartment and a posterior, subendothoracic compartment by the endothoracic fascia, which is closely applied to the ribs and fuses medial to the periost and the midpoints of the vertebral bodies.

The PVS contains fatty tissue, spinal nerves, dorsal rami, rami communicantes, the sympathetic chain, and intercostal vessels.

Richardshon J, Lonnqvist PA, Naja Z. Bilateral thoracic paravertebral block: potential and practice. *Brit J Anaesth* 2011; 106(2): 164–71.

21. Answers: F T T T T

A preoperative ECG in morbid obesity is essential to exclude factors such as significant rhythm disturbances and cor pulmonale, and as a guide to the need for more extensive cardiac investigation. Patients with evidence of right ventricular hypertrophy or cor pulmonale may benefit from a period of elective nocturnal non-invasive ventilation before elective surgery. This can be spectacularly effective in relieving right heart failure, day-time somnolence, and pulmonary hypertension. Echocardiography may estimate systolic and diastolic function and chamber dimensions, although good images may be difficult to obtain by the transthoracic technique. Chest X-ray may be used to assess cardiothoracic ratio and evidence of cardiac failure.

Sabharwal A, Christelis N. Anaesthesia for bariatric surgery. *Contin Educ Anaesth Crit Care Pain* 2010; 10(4): 9–13.

Tunga A, Rock P. Perioperative concerns in sleep apnea. *Curr Op Anaesth* 2001; 14: 671–78.

22. Answers: F F T T F

The following factors affect drug pharmacokinetics in obesity:

- volume of distribution
  - decreased fraction of total body water
  - increased adipose tissue
  - increased lean body mass
  - altered tissue protein binding
  - increased blood volume and cardiac output
  - increased concentration free fatty acids, cholesterol, a1 acid glycoprotein
  - organomegaly

- plasma protein binding
  - ◆ adsorption of lipophilic drugs to lipoproteins so increased free drug available
  - ◆ plasma albumin unchanged
  - ◆ increased a1-acid glycoprotein
- drug clearance
  - ◆ increased renal blood flow
  - ◆ increased glomerular filtration rate (GFR)
  - ◆ increased tubular secretion
  - ◆ decreased hepatic blood flow in congestive cardiac failure.

Drugs with weak or moderate lipophilicity can be administered according to ideal body weight (IBW), as their volume of distribution (V_D) remains relatively consistent between obese and normal-weight individuals. A more accurate calculation of the drug dosage uses the lean body mass, which requires addition of 20% to IBW. Drugs in this group include the non-depolarizing neuromuscular blocking agents.

An exception to the above rule is remifentanil, the V_D of which is not affected in this manner, despite its highly lipophilic properties. Succinylcholine should be administered based on actual body weight because of the increase activity of plasma cholinesterase in proportion to body weight. Intravenous induction agents are highly lipophilic, with large V_D, and this needs to be considered when dosing, as different formulas have been used to establish an appropriate dose, although no one method supersedes the other in terms of effectiveness of dose prediction.

Sabharwal A, Christelis N. Anaesthesia for bariatric surgery. *Contin Educ Anaesth Crit Care Pain* 2010; 10(4): 9–13.

23. Answers: **T T T T T**

In a supine position the blood flow is higher in unventilated lungs, which attenuates hypoxic pulmonary vasoconstriction (HPV). Vasoconstrictors like phenylephrine increase pulmonary pressures. Distension of extra-alveolar pulmonary vessels during increased trans-pulmonary pressure by uncollapsed lungs and open chest walls resists HPV. Inhalational anaesthetics and nitrates vasodilate, opposing HPV.

HPV in the extra-alveolar pulmonary arterioles supplying the unventilated lung is an essential physiological response to minimize shunt and hence hypoxaemia during one-lung ventilation (OLV). This occurs when there is a reduction in alveolar partial pressure of oxygen of between 4 and 8 kPa. Factors that impair HPV in the non-ventilated lung and hence promote hypoxaemia during OLV include the following.

Increase in pulmonary artery pressure

An increase in pulmonary artery pressure may occur when:

- there is atelectasis in the ventilated lung, leading to increase in pulmonary vascular resistance
- excessive positive end-expiratory pressure is applied or develops intrinsically in the ventilated lung, leading to diversion of blood to the non-ventilated lung
- vasoconstrictor drugs are used, for example phenylephrine and epinephrine.

Supine position

In a supine position, the vertical height of the lungs is less than in the lateral decubitus or erect position, which reduces the height and allows blood flow to unventilated collapsed lung, thus attenuating HPV.

Failure of lung collapse

The unventilated non-dependent lung should collapse when the chest wall is open to the atmosphere. If this unventilated lung is held partially open, then intrapleural pressure becomes increasingly negative during inspiration. This effect leads to an increase in transpulmonary pressure (i.e. the pressure difference between alveoli and pleura) and hence distension of extra-alveolar pulmonary vessels that oppose HPV in the non-ventilated lung.

Vasodilators

Vasodilators, for example calcium antagonists, sodium nitroprusside, nitrates, α-antagonists, inhalation anaesthetic agents, and endogenous prostaglandins, are released during lung handling.

Ng A, Swanevelder J. Hypoxemia during one lung anaesthesia. *Contin Educ Anaesth Crit Care Pain* 2010; 10(4): 9–13.

24. Answers: T T T T

Endobronchial blockers consist of a balloon and a central lumen for application of suction and lung deflation or administration of oxygen.

When lung resection is not required, or if there are no issues with cross-contamination (e.g. pleural surgery, lung biopsy, and oesophagectomy), either a double-lumen tube or an endobronchial blocker may be utilized for OLV. In this situation, endobronchial blockers may be the preferred device. These are used when:

- the patient is already intubated (with a single-lumen tracheal tube) before an operation in the critical care unit
- the patient is to be ventilated after operation with a single-lumen tracheal tube
- a double-lumen endobronchial tube is relatively short in very tall patients and thus easy lung isolation cannot be achieved
- there is difficulty with laryngoscopy and hence placement of a double-lumen endobronchial tube
- minor airway injuries associated with double-lumen tubes are to be obviated; it has been shown in a randomized controlled trial that postoperative hoarseness and vocal cord lesions occur significantly more frequently with double-lumen endobronchial tubes than with endobronchial blockers.

Endobronchial blockers have a natural tendency to dislodge and cause airway obstruction. Hypoxaemia and cardiac arrest associated with malpositioning and airway obstruction have been reported.

Ng A, Swanevelder J. Hypoxemia during one lung anaesthesia. *Contin Educ Anaesth Crit Care Pain* 2010; 10(4): 9–13.

25. Answers: T F F F T

Diffusion of a gas across a lipid bilayer is directly proportional to the partial pressure gradient across the membrane, lipid solubility, area of the membrane, and the diffusion coefficient, and inversely proportional to the square root of the molecular weight, thickness of the membrane, and density of the gas.

Ficks law states that the net diffusion rate of a gas across a fluid membrane is proportional to the difference in partial pressure and membrane area, and inversely proportional to membrane thickness.

Graham's law states that the diffusion rate of a gas across a fluid membrane is proportional to the lipid solubility and inversely proportional to the square root of molecular weight (diffusion coefficient, which measures how easily a gas diffuses across a membrane).

Rate of diffusion = $P \times A \times dC/dx$, where P is the diffusion coefficient, A is the membrane area, and dC/dx is the concentration gradient.

David PD, Kenny GNC. Fluid flow. *Basic Physics and Measurement in Anaesthesia*. Butterworth Heinemann, 2003.

26. Answers: T T T T F

Sickle cell disease (SCD) is a congenital haemoglobinopathy characterized by a mutation on chromosome 11, resulting in the production of the unstable and relatively insoluble haemoglobin S. Vaso-occlusion and haemolysis are the hallmarks of SCD, resulting in recurrent painful episodes and organ dysfunction. Progressive inflammatory vascular endothelial damage may play a role in the pathophysiology.

Desaturation of haemoglobin S (HbS) results in the polymerization of haemoglobin, forming large aggregates called tactoids, which deform the red cells into the typical sickle shape. Homozygous (SS) cells begin to sickle at a much higher oxygen saturation, typically 85% (PaO_2 5.2–6.5 kPa) than heterozygous (AS) cells, which usually do well below the saturation of venous blood 40% (PaO_2 3.2–4.0 kPa). Sickling with sickle cell trait is therefore rarely a problem without concomitant stasis.

The pathophysiological consequences of sickling are twofold:

- small-vessel obstruction by sickle cells (vaso-occlusive events which can be extremely painful)
- haemolytic anaemia due to the greatly reduced half-life of SS cells when compared with normal red blood cells (12 vs 120 days).

The presence of foetal haemoglobin confers protection against sickling, and some adults may be prescribed hydroxyurea to elevate haemoglobin foetal (HbF) levels.

In addition to hypoxia, sickling is also exacerbated by cold, stasis, dehydration, and infection.

Cardiomegaly is usually due to anaemia, rarely from failure.

Eye changes include retinopathy, vitreous haemorrhage, and retinal detachment. There is an association with hereditary cataracts.

Oxidant drugs, including penicillin, can precipitate haemolysis.

Prosser DP, Sharma N. Cerebral palsy and anaesthesia. *Contin Educ Anaesth Crit Care Pain* 2010; 10(3): 72–76.

Babalola OE, Danboyi P, Abiose AA. Hereditary congenital cataracts associated with sickle cell anaemia in a Nigerian family. *Trop Doct* 2000; 30(1): 12–14.

27. Answers: T F F F T

Activated charcoal (AC) creates weak van der Waals forces, which bind with the substance in the gastrointestinal tract. The charcoal particles increase the surface area, which stops further absorption. AC should be given within 60 min of ingestion of poison but may have an effect for up to 2 h or longer post ingestion. Most drugs and chemicals are absorbed by AC. It can be administered orally or nasogastrically via a 16 F tube in the intubated patient.

The charcoal-to-toxin ratio is 10:1, with a usual dose of 25–50 g or 1 g/kg in a child. This dose should be given within 1 h of poison ingestion. The efficacy is time-dependent, with nearly 90% reduction in absorption 30 min after drug ingestion, decreasing to 30% at 1 h.

AC:

- reduces absorption of acetaminophen up to 2 h after ingestion
- should be given in repeat doses of 25 g, 4–6 hourly
- is useful for poisoning of salicylate, barbiturates, theophylline, quinine, digoxin, carbamazepine, phenytoin, and dapsone.
- interrupts the enterohepatic circulation of the drug if given in multiple doses, thereby reducing the plasma levels, and there are data that suggest this reduces the duration of toxicity.

An adverse effect from repeat doses is acute bowel obstruction from charcoal concretions, especially in the presence of an anticholinergic ileus.

AC is not useful for alcohol, methanol, petroleum distillates, corrosive acids and alkalis, lithium, iron, ethylene glycol, or methanol.

Ward C, Sair M. Oral poisoning: an update. *Contin Educ Anaesth Crit Care Pain* 2010; 10(1): 6–11.

28. Answers: T T T T F

The flow is defined as the mass of a substance that passes a certain point in 1 s. The units are litres per second.

For laminar flow, flow is directly proportional to pressure drop, but for turbulent flow, flow is directly proportional to the square root of pressure drop.

The Hagen Poisseulle equation applies to laminar flow:

$$Q = \pi P r^4 / 8 \eta l$$

where Q is the flow in litres/second, η is the viscosity in Pascals/seconds, P is the pressure in Pascals, r is the radius of the tube in metres, and l is the length of the tube in question in metres.

For every fluid in a given tube, there is a critical velocity beyond which the flow shifts to turbulent from laminar. This change depends on the volume flow and diameter of the tubing or airway. Warm humidified gas reduces its density by causing an increase in critical flow by 10%, a change seen in airways.

The critical flow in airways has the same numerical value in litres per minute as the diameter of the airway in millimetres. As breathing is cyclical, turbulent flow appears during peak flow, while laminar flow is present at all other times. Although the bronchi and air passages are narrower than the trachea, airflow through them is laminar, as flow is slower than in the trachea.

David PD, Kenny GNC. *Fluid Flow. Basic Physics and Measurement in Anaesthesia.* Butterworth Heinemann, 2003.

29. Answers: F T T F F

Ethylene glycol is an important toxic alcohol, in addition to ethanol, methanol, and isopropanol. As it is a component of radiator fluid and anti-freeze solutions it forms the one of the frequent causes of toxicity seen in accident and emergency situations. Its mechanism of action is by altering the colligative properties of solutions to which it is added, decreasing the freezing point and increasing the boiling point. Toxicity results from its metabolites, which are glycoaldehyde, glycolate, and oxalate. Oxalate accumulates in the body and is deposited as crystals in tissues. This causes neurological damage, including in the renal cortex, where it leads to renal failure and death. Profound acidosis can occur and this is classically a type B lactic acidosis—due to poor tissue perfusion. A high anion gap and osmolar gap occur due to unmeasured anionic compounds, along with hyperkalaemia and a consumptive hypocalcaemia.

Blood levels above 500 mg/L are indicative of severe toxicity. Overdose with these agents can be treated with oral or nasogastric ethanol because of its greater affinity for alcohol dehydrogenase; other treatments include haemodialysis, thiamine, and pyridoxine. Fomepizole blocks the metabolism of methanol and ethanol, and it can be injected 12-hourly. It is expensive and not widely available. Folate deficiency in primates is predictive of poor outcome in methanol toxicity and it is suggested that folate be given in a dose of 1 mg/kg/day for 48 h.

Ward C, Sair M. Oral poisoning: an update. *Contin Educ Anaesth Crit Care Pain* 2010; 10(1): 6–11.

Singer M, Webb AR. Poisoning. In: *Oxford Handbook of Critical Care*, 3rd edn. Oxford University Press, 2009: Chapter 30.

30. Answers: T F F F F

Albumin is produced by the liver at a rate of 9–12 g/day and is released in the circulation. Albumin has a strong negative charge. There is no storage of albumin and neither is it metabolized, even during catabolic states. The rate of production depends on the colloid osmotic pressure and the osmolality of the extravascular space. The albumin is distributed in intravascular (40%) and extravascular spaces (50%). Extravascular albumin exceeds the total intravascular amount by 30%.

The major function of plasma proteins are:

- vascular
  - maintenance of oncotic pressure
  - microvascular integrity
- transport
  - hormones (steroids, thyroxine)
  - fatty acids
  - bile salts
  - bilirubin
  - Ca^{2+}, Mg^{2+}, and other metals (copper, zinc)
  - drugs (warfarin, diazepam)
- metabolic
  - acid–base balance
  - antioxidant
  - anticoagulant.

The main functions of albumin are maintenance of oncotic pressure and transport.

Low albumin in sepsis is partly due to a reduced synthesis, but predominantly due to increased redistribution and catabolism.

Boldt J. Use of albumin: an update. *Brit J Anaesth* 2010; 104(3): 276–84.

31. Answers: F T F F F

Helium is less dense than nitrogen, so mixed with oxygen will flow more past orifices in turbulent flows. Laminar flows in smaller airways in asthma depend on viscosity, hence helium is of less use. It is supplied in brown cylinders at 137 bar and is dispensed with 21% oxygen.

Heliox is available in 80/20 and 70/30 mixtures of helium and oxygen. Helium has a density of only 0.178 g/L, much lower than oxygen (1.4 g/L), or nitrogen (1.25 g/L). The low density results in a lower Reynolds number for the same viscosity, velocity, and orifice diameter, thus making laminar flow more likely.

Yentis SM, Hirsch NP, Smith GB. *A–Z of Anaesthesia and Intensive Care*, Butterworth Heinemann, 2004: p. 254.

32. Answers: F T F F F

Carcinoid tumours are found late and patients may describe vague upper or lower gastrointestinal symptoms, with the average time from symptom onset to diagnosis being 9 years. Carcinoid syndrome affects approximately 10% of patients with carcinoid tumours. Vasoactive substances secreted by tumours arising in the gut must pass through the liver via the hepatic portal vein before circulating more extensively. Consequently, these vasoactive hormones are metabolized before they can exert widespread systemic effects.

The release of serotonin and other vasoactive substances such as histamine is responsible for the 'carcinoid syndrome'. This is typically intermittent and is characterized by flushing, sometimes associated with exercise or the ingestion of alcohol or high tyramine content foods such as blue cheeses and chocolate. Diarrhoea, lacrymation, rhinorrhoea, and ultimately right-sided valvular heart disease may also occur. Carcinoid heart disease classically affects the right side of the heart, with fibrous thickening of the endocardium causing retraction and fixation of the tricuspid valve leaflets, and is related to the duration of exposure to high concentrations of 5-hydroxytryptamine (5HT). Mixed tricuspid and pulmonary valvular disease are more common. Left heart involvement is uncommon.

Powell B, al Mukhtar A, Hills GH. Carcinoid: the disease and its implications for anaesthesia. *Contin Educ Anaesth Crit Care Pain* 2011; 11: 9–13.

33. Answers: F F T F F

Two-dimensional aortic valve view measurements in transoesophageal echocardiogram (TOE) can be inaccurate. Pulse-pressure analysis relies on the regularity of the pulse for its calculations, hence produces inaccuracy in arrhythmias. However, in the right situations, it can be used to provide continuous cardiac output measurement. Thermodilution in the presence of valvular lesions can be erroneous due to improper circulation of blood.

Oesophageal Doppler only measures descending thoracic aortic flow, rather than direct cardiac output. This is influenced by non-linear changes in systemic vascular resistance (SVR) and cardiac output.

Casserly B, Read R, Mitchell M. Haemodynamic monitoring in sepsis. *Crit Care Clin* 2009; 25: 803–23.

34. Answers: F F F F T

Neostigmine is a white crystalline powder that is odourless and readily soluble in water. It is a synthetic quarternary ammonium compound, hence poorly absorbed by the oral route. It is given by subcutaneous, intramuscular, and intravenous routes. It is a quaternary ammonium structure that does not cross the placenta and is 15–25% bound to serum albumin. The volume of distribution is large due to extensive tissue localization.

Neostigmine undergoes hydrolysis by chloinesterases to 3-hydroxy phenyl trimethyl ammonium (3OH-PTM), which is inactive. Neostigmine is also metabolized by microsomal enzymes in liver. Neostigmine and 3OH-PTM are excreted by renal tubular excretion and the same proportion is destroyed by the liver. Renal failure delays plasma clearance of neostigmine. The plasma half-life of neostigmine is 30–50 min.

Intrathecal neostigmine inhibits metabolism of spinally released acetylcholine and produces analgesia in animals and humans. It increases blood pressure and heart rate by direct stimulation of preganglioninc sympathetic neurons in the spinal cord. It reduces the uterine activity by β-adrenergic effects and reduces the uterine blood flow by α-adrenergic action. The potency of intrathecal neostigmine is increased in the postoperative period because the descending noradrenergic or cholinergic antinociceptive spinal system is activated by ongoing pain, causing an increase in release of acetylcholine, which, in the presence of neostigmine, results in augmented selective analgesia.

Intrathecal neostigmine, while analgesic, causes nausea and vomiting. It is excreted renally, and is available in oral and intravenous preparations. Its effect on autonomic ganglion is mild.

Clinical uses of neostigmine are:

- reversal of residual non-depolarizing neuromuscular blockade
- in the treatment of myasthenia gravis
- in the treatment of glaucoma
- in the treatment of paralytic ileus and atony of urinary bladder.

Yentis SM, Hirsch NP, Smith GB. *A–Z of Anaesthesia and Intensive Care*. Butterworth Heinemann, 2004: p. 382.

35. Answers: F F T F F

Nasal temperature fluctuates widely due to the passage of inspired and expired air currents. This is utilized in the design of respiratory monitors. The nose, however, can be used to measure body temperature in an anaesthetized patient with a cuffed endotracheal tube because of the absence of air currents.

Lower oesophageal temperature may fluctuate due to the proximity of the trachea with its air currents.

Rectal temperature takes time to equilibrate with the core. There is a risk of perforation in babies.

Ear probes measure tympanic membrane temperature, with a risk of eardrum perforation.

Davis PD, Kenny GNC. *Temperature. Basic Physics and Measurement in Anaesthesia.* Butterworth Heinemann, 2003.

36. Answers: T F F F F

The common side effects of aspirin are vomiting, dehydration, tinnitus, vertigo, deafness, sweating, warm extremities with bounding pulses, increased respiratory rate, and hyperventilation. Some degree of acid–base disturbance is present in most cases.

A mixed respiratory alkalosis and metabolic acidosis with normal or high arterial pH (normal or reduced hydrogen ion concentration) is usual in adults and children over the age of 4 years.

Uncommon features include haematemesis, hyperpyrexia, hypoglycaemia, hypokalaemia, thrombocytopaenia, increased prothrombin time/international normalized ratio, intravascular coagulation, renal failure, and non-cardiac pulmonary oedema.

Central nervous system features include confusion, disorientation, coma, and convulsions, all of which are less common in adults than in children.

The toxic effects of salicylates are complex. Respiratory centres are directly stimulated. Salicylates cause an inhibition of the citric acid cycle and an uncoupling of oxidative phosphorylation. In addition, lipid metabolism is stimulated, while amino acid metabolism is inhibited. Catabolism can occur secondary to the inhibition of ATP-dependent reactions with the following results:

- increased oxygen consumption
- increased carbon dioxide production
- accelerated activity of the glycolytic and lipolytic pathways
- depletion of hepatic glycogen
- hyperpyrexia.

There are acid–base disturbances initially, and a respiratory alkalosis develops secondary to direct stimulation of the respiratory centres. This may be the only consequence of mild salicylism. The kidneys excrete potassium, sodium, and bicarbonate, resulting in alkaline urine.

British National Formulary, 61st edn. British Medical Association and Royal Pharmaceutical Society of Great Britain, 2011.

Sasada M, Smith S. *Drugs in Anaesthesia and Intensive Care.* Oxford University Press, 2003.

Ward C. Oral poisoning : an update. *Contin Educ Anaesth Crit Care Pain* 2010; 10(1): 6–11.

Penny L, Moriarty T. Poisoning in Children. *Contin Educ Anaesth Crit Care Pain* 2009; 9(4): 109–13.

37. Answers: F F F F T

The side effects of propranolol include abdominal cramps, diarrhoea, constipation, fatigue, insomnia, nausea, depression, dreaming, memory loss, fever, impotence, light-headedness, slow heart rate, low blood pressure, cold extremities, sore throat, and shortness of breath or wheezing. Propranolol can aggravate breathing difficulties in patients with asthma, chronic bronchitis, or emphysema. In patients with existing slow heart rates (bradycardias) and heart blocks (defects in the electrical conduction of the heart), propranolol can cause dangerously slow heart rates and even shock. Propranolol reduces the force of heart muscle contraction and can aggravate symptoms of heart failure. In patients with coronary artery disease, abruptly stopping propranolol can suddenly worsen angina and occasionally precipitate heart attacks.

British National Formulary, 61st edn. British Medical Association and Royal Pharmaceutical Society of Great Britain, 2011.

Sasada M, Smith S. *Drugs in Anaesthesia and Intensive Care*. Oxford University Press, 2003.

38. Answers: T T T T T

The aetiology of pericardial diseases is best considered using a modification of the time-honoured pathologic classification of disease into inflammatory, neoplastic, degenerative, vascular, and idiopathic causes. The major causes include:

- viral infection, including HIV
- purulent pericarditis
- tuberculosis
- myocardial infarction
- cardiac surgery
- recent or remote sharp or blunt chest trauma
- cardiac diagnostic or interventional procedure
- drugs and toxins
- metabolic disorders, especially uremia, dialysis, and hypothyroidism
- malignancy, especially lung and breast cancer, Hodgkin lymphoma, and mesothelioma
- mediastinal radiation, recent or remote
- collagen vascular diseases
- idiopathic.

Troughton RW, Asher CR, Klein AL. Pericarditis. *Lancet* 2004; 363: 717.

39. Answers: F F T T F

The Fick principle, based upon the conservation of mass, states that the amount of a substance taken up by an organ (or whole body) per unit time is equal to the arterial minus venous concentration of the substance multiplied by blood flow. Mixed venous samples provided by PAFC allow the arteriovenous oxygen content difference to be calculated. Oxygen consumption is calculated by spirometry.

Allsager CM, Swanevelder J. Measuring cardiac output. *BJA CEPD Rev* 2003; 3(1): 15–19.

40. Answers: T T F F F

Critical temperature is the temperature above which a gas cannot be liquefied, no matter how much pressure is applied. The critical pressure is the pressure needed to liquefy the gas at the critical temperature. A gaseous substance is termed as a gas when it is above its critical temperature and a vapour when it is below it.

As the temperature of a gas approaches its boiling point, the behaviour of the gas deviates from gas laws.

When a mixture of gases is present, there is a specific temperature, the pseudocritical temperature, at which the mixture separates into its constituents.

Davis PD, Kenny GNC. *Temperature. Basic Physics and Measurement in Anaesthesia.* Butterworth Heinemann, 2003.

41. Answers: F F T F F

In laminar flow, the fluid moves in layers called laminas. Laminar flow need not be in a straight line. For laminar flow, the flow follows the curved surface of the airfoil smoothly, in layers. The closer the fluid layers are to the airfoil surface, the slower they move. Moreover, the fluid layers slide over one another without fluid being exchanged between the layers.

In laminar flow, flow is directly proportional to pressure drop, but for turbulent flow, flow is directly proportional to the square root of pressure drop.

The Hagen Poisseulle equation applies to laminar flow:

$$Q = \pi P r^4 / 8 \eta l$$

where Q is the flow in litres/second, η is the viscosity in Pascals/s, P is the pressure in Pascals, r is the radius of the tube in metres, and l is the length of the tube in question in metres.

Davis PD, Kenny GNC. *Temperature. Basic Physics and Measurement in Anaesthesia.* Butterworth Heinemann, 2003.

42. Answers: T F T T F

The thermistor is a metal oxide semiconductor. As thermistors change temperature, there is an exponential decline in resistance. However, in commercial applications where a narrow range is required, the output is often linearized by the device. They are very accurate with 0.1–0.2°C increments possible. Their use is advantageous, in that thermistors can be made very small and are durable, unless subjected to severe changes in temperature.

A thermistor is a type of resistor whose resistance varies significantly with temperature, more so than in standard resistors.

Thermistors are used in Wheatstone bridge circuits, and have the ability to be made in very small sizes. Thermistors used in cardiac output measurement have fast response times. Apart from temperature and cardiac output measurement, thermistors are also used in electronic flowmeters.

However, calibration changes occur during extremes of temperature, e.g. heat sterilization.

Sullivan G, Edmondson, C. Heat and temperature. *Contin Educ Anaesth Crit Care Pain* 2008; 8(3): 104–107.

43. Answers: T T F F T

In 1961, Sellick first described his 'simple manoeuvre' for controlling the regurgitation of gastric or oesophageal contents before intubation with a cuffed endotracheal tube. Since then, cricoid pressure has been utilized to occlude the upper end of the oesophagus by compressing the cricoid cartilage against the bodies of the cervical vertebrae.

Cricoid pressure (at 20–40 N or 2–4 kg) is applied before loss of consciousness. After the jaw has relaxed and succinylcholine-associated fasciculations have ceased, the trachea is intubated.

Pre-oxygenation with oxygen 100% is essential to maximize the oxygen available to the patient from their functional residual capacity during induction. Oxygen is administered for 3–5 min or until the expired oxygen fraction is >85%. A pre-calculated dose of induction agent is administered, followed immediately by a neuromuscular blocking agent. After tube position and adequate seal are confirmed the cricoid pressure may be released.

A nasogastric tube will bypass this artificial obstruction, besides keeping the lower oesophageal sphincter patent. Pre-oxygenation and neck extension, related to prevention of hypoxia during the procedure and aiding ease of intubation, respectively, are not associated with cricoid effectiveness.

Sinclair RCF, Luxton MC. Rapid sequence induction. *Contin Educ Anaesth Crit Care Pain* 2005; 5(2): 45–48.

44. Answers: T T T T T

Complications of supraclavicular brachial plexus blockade include:

- pneumothorax
- phrenic and recurrent laryngeal block
- Horner's syndrome
- subclavian vessel puncture.

Infraclavicular brachial plexus black shares the same complications, but with a reduced risk of pneumothorax.

Interscalene block complications include those of supraclavicular (barring pneumothorax and subclavian puncture) and extradural or intrathecal injections and vertebral artery puncture.

Yentis SM, Hirsch NP, Smith GB. *A–Z of Anaesthesia and Intensive Care*. Butterworth Heinemann, pp 69–71.

45. Answers: F T T F F

The ulnar nerve is a terminal branch of the medial cord of the brachial plexus. It passes behind the medial epicondyle to reach the forearm. The dorsal and palmar cutaneous branches supply:

- ulnar aspect of medial two and a half fingers and the hand and palm
- elbow joint
- flexor carpi ulnaris
- ulnar side of flexor digitorum profundus
- adductor pollicis
- hypothenar muscles
- interossei
- third and fourth lumbricals.

Yentis SM, Hirsch NP, Smith GB. *A–Z of Anaesthesia and Intensive Care*. Butterworth Heinemann, pp 69–71.

46. Answers: T T T T F

The pudendal nerve arises from the sacral plexus. It originates from the ventral rami of S2, S3, and S4. It leaves the pelvis via the greater sciatic foramen after passing between the piriformis and the coccygeus. Then it passes behind the ischial spine and sacrospinal ligament to re-enter the pelvis via the lesser sciatic foramen. The nerve accompanies the internal pudendal artery and the vein.
The pudendal nerve consists of sensory motor and autonomic elements and supplies the innervation to the genitalia, perineum, bladder sphincters, and rectum.

The branches of pudendal nerve are:

- inferior anal nerves
- perineal nerve
- dorsal nerve of the penis/clitoris
- posterior labial nerves.

Pudendal nerve block was first described by Mueller in 1908. The nerve is blocked locally to provide analgesia in obstetrics for forceps and ventouse delivery.

Yentis SM, Hirsch NP, Smith GB. *A–Z of Anaesthesia and Intensive Care*. Butterworth Heinemann, 2004: p. 455.

47. Answers: T F T F T

Compliance describes the elastic properties of various parts of the respiratory system. Compliance represents a volume change per unit change in pressure (200 mL/cm H_2O in the normal lung). The total respiratory compliance consists of combined lung and chest wall compliance and is normally 70–80 mL/cm H_2O.Human lung compliance is approximately 1.5–2 L/kPa (150–200 mL/cmH_2O) and decreases while supine due to a decrease in functional residual capacity. Compliance increases with age and emphysema, and decreases with pulmonary fibrosis, vascular engorgement, and pulmonary oedema. Increased pulmonary venous congestion decreases lung compliance.

Yentis SM, Hirsch NP, Smith GB. *A–Z of Anaesthesia and Intensive Care*. Butterworth Heinemann, 2004: p. 135.

48. Answers: T T T T F

The clinical presentation of pulmonary embolus can be:

- with chest pain
- dyspnea and haemoptysis.

On examination there may be:

- hypotension and tachycardia
- raised jugular venous pressure (JVP)
- bronchospasm
- third and fourth heart sounds present
- ECG changes including:
  - right atrial dilation with peaked P waves in lead II
  - right ventricular strain with right axis deviation, RBBB
  - right precordial T wave inversion.

The classic ECG pattern of an S wave in I, Q, and inverted T in III is rare.

A fall in left atrial pressure due to pulmonary hypertension is common. Hence pulmonary artery occlusion pressure (PAOP) cannot be high.

Simon C, Everitt H, and van Dorp F. *Oxford handbook of general practice*. 3rd ed. Oxford: Oxford University Press, 2010: 823.

Akram A.R., Cowell G.W.. Logan, L.J. et al. (2009) Clinically suspected acute pulmonary embolism: a comparison of presentation, radiological features and outcome in patients with and without PE. *QJM* 102(6), 407–414.

49. Answers: F F T F F

The Valsalva manoeuvre is forced expiration against a closed glottis, after full inspiration. Ideally, 40 mmHg pressure is held for 10 s. The cardiovascular responses are:

- Phase I: increased transthoracic pressure expelling blood from thoracic vessels.
- Phase II: reduced BP due to low venous return, baroreceptor activation, tachycardia and hypertension, BP normalized.
- Phase III: fall in BP as intrathoracic blood pressure drops, pooling blood in pulmonary vessels.
- Phase IV: overshoot; compensatory mechanisms continue operating although BP normalizes.

Pulse-rate changes and overshoot are absent, with persistent low BP in autonomic dysfunction of diabetes.

Square-wave responses: a high BP, which stays high throughout the manoeuvre, returning to normal at the end, is seen in cardiac failure, constrictive pericarditis, cardiac tamponaden, and valvular heart disease.

Yentis SM, Hirsch NP, Smith GB. *A–Z of Anaesthesia and Intensive Care.* Butterworth Heinemann, 2004: p. 551.

50. Answers: T F T F T

Low fixed cardiac outputs indicate inadequate ventricular filling, and common conditions are:

- mitral stenosis
- pulmonary stenosis
- reduced ejection due to fixed obstruction (aortic stenosis).

Ventricular septal defects are associated with increased pulmonary flows and the risk of pulmonary hypertension, rather than ventricular outflow problems.

Myocardial infarction affects muscular contractility and is usually not associated with obstructions to flow.

Kumar P, Clark M. *Clinical Medicine.* Elsevier Saunders, 2005: p. 681.

51. Answers: T F F T F

Hyperthyroidism is most commonly autoimmune in origin. Frequent symptoms in the elderly are atrial fibrillation, tachyarrhthymias, or heart failure. Presentation includes weight loss, irritability, muscle weakness, tremor, breathlessness, palpitation, vomiting, itching, and thirst.

Thyroid-stimulating hormone (TSH) is suppressed in primary disease. Free T4 and T3 are raised. Treatment includes carbimazole and propylthiouracil, which reduce hormone production and are mildly immunosuppressive. Beta blockers (those without intrinsic sympathomimetic activity) are used for rapid control.

Kumar P, Clark M. *Clinical Medicine.* Elsevier Saunders, 2005: p. 963.

52. Answers: T T T T F

Parathyroid hormone is secreted from the chief cells of the four parathyroid hormones. It increases plasma calcium by:

- increasing osteoclastic resorption of bone (rapid)
- increasing intestinal calcium absorption (slow)
- increasing D3 synthesis
- increasing renal tubular absorption of calcium
- increasing renal phosphate excretion.

Hyperparathyroidism may accentuate all these features and cause an increase in serum alkaline phosphatase (from bone).

The biochemical features of primary hyperparathyroidism include:

- high total serum calcium (corrected for albumin) or elevated serum ionized calcium
- hypophosphataemia, phosphaturia
- hyperchloraemia and increased chloride:phosphate ratio
- hypercalciuria (>10 mmol/day) in >75% of hypercalcaemic patients (excess calcium spillage supports a diagnosis of primary hyperparathyroidism but, more importantly, loss of <2 mmol of calcium per day suggests a diagnosis of familial hypercalcaemic hypocalciuria)
- increased concentration of intact parathyroid hormone (PTH); high or non-inhibited PTH concentration in the face of hypercalcaemia is diagnostic of primary hyperparathyroidism
- increased serum alkaline phosphatase and increased urinary excretion of cyclic adenosine monophosphate and hydroxyproline as markers of bone involvement.

System affected symptoms are:

- renal polyuria, back pain, colic, and haematuria
- musculoskeletal aches and pains, bone pain, arthritis, and 'pathological' fractures
- gastrointestinal anorexia, nausea, dyspepsia, constipation, and abdominal pain
- neurological depression, weakness, apathy, lethargy, confusion, and psychosis
- cardiovascular hypertension.

Kumar P, Clark M. *Clinical Medicine*. Elsevier Saunders, 2005: p. 963.

Mihai R, Farndon, JR. Parathyroid disease and calcium metabolism. *Br J Anaesth* 2000; 85(1): 29–43.

53. Answers: F T T T T

Vitamin B12 is synthesized by microorganisms and is hence only available from animal sources, not plants. It is not destroyed by cooking. When ingested as part of food, it is liberated by gastric enzymes, binding to a B12 binding protein (R binder). This complex is released by pancreatic enzymes and becomes bound to an intrinsic factor. This is a glycoprotein secreted by gastric pareital cells along with H^+ ions. The B12 intrinsic factor complex travels to the ileum, where the former is absorbed while the latter stays in the lumen. One per cent of oral B12 is absorbed passively in the duodenum and ileum, without intrinsic factor.

Any condition reducing intrinsic factor production, for example gastrectomy, will impair B12 absorption and lead to anaemia of deficiency. Ileal disorders may impair absorption.

Pregnancy is associated with folate deficiency, usually dietary. Phenytoin inhibits intestinal conjugation of polyglutamate to monoglutamate folate and causes a megaloblastic anaemia. The appropriate treatment for these anaemias is folate, although in the absence of B12 levels both B12 and folate should be given

Kumar P, Clark M. *Clinical Medicine*. Elsevier Saunders, 2005: p. 207.

54. Answers: T F T F F

Normal reticulocyte levels are 0.5–2.5%. An increase indicates RBC production.

Acute leukaemia and aplastic anaemia are associated with reduced production of RBCs and platelets, hence reticulocyte counts are low.

Reticulocytes will be high in chronic, but not acute, haemorrhage, as reticulocytosis does not have time to commence in the latter instance.

Pernicious anaemia is associated with reduced RBC production. Reticulocyte count is thus low, and any increase is a marker of response to therapy.

Kumar P, Clark M. *Clinical Medicine*. Elsevier Saunders, 2005: p. 387.

55. Answers: T T F T T

Dystrophia myotonica is an autonomic dominant condition with triple repeat mutations on chromosome 19. There is a direct correlation between disease severity, age at onset, and the size of mutations. The disease is usually evident between 20 and 50 years of age. Progressive distal muscle weakness ensues. The disease is part of a syndrome comprising cataracts, frontal baldness, mild cognitive impairment, oesophageal dysmotility with aspiration, cardiomyopathy with conduction defects, hypogonadism and a small pituitary, glucose intolerance, and low serum IgG.

Phenytoin or procainamide can help myotonia.

Kumar P, Clark M. *Clinical Medicine*. Elsevier Saunders, pp 19.

56. Answers: T F F T T

Deoxygenated blood in the foetus arrives at the placenta via the umbilical arteries, oxygenated blood returning via the umbilical vein at a PO_2 of 4.7 kPa at 80–90% saturation. Fifty to sixty per cent of this bypasses the hepatic circulation via the ductus venosus to reach the inferior vena cava (IVC). In the IVC, better oxygenated blood streams separately from deoxygenated blood, and is directly preferentially by a flap called the eustacian valve across the foramen ovale into the left atrium. This blood, with 65% oxygen saturation, enters the left ventricle and is ejected in the ascending aorta. The majority of the blood is delivered to the brain coronary circulation. Desaturated blood from the IVC via coronary sinnusis is directed across the tricuspid valve into the right ventricle and ejected into the pulmonary artery. Most (88%) of this enters the descending aorta via the ductus ateriosus due to the high pulmonary arterial pressures.

These high pressures fall at birth, increasing pulmonary venous return to the left atrium. There is a fall in flow in the ductus venosus, hence the IVC. The right atrium pressures fall and equalize with the left atrium pressures, closing the foramen ovale. The shunt in the suctus arteriosus becomes bidirectional. Presumably because of high oxygen partial pressures, the smooth muscles in the wall of the ductus contract, closing it.

Foetal circulation

Foetal lungs do not exchange oxygen. Oxygen is obtained, second hand, via the systemic venous system. Oxygenated blood from the placenta passes through the single umbilical vein and enters IVC.

Deoxygenated blood reaches the placenta via the two umbilical arteries (which arise from the two internal iliac arteries). The placenta receives 60% of the cardiac output.

There are three key anatomical shunts:

- ductus venosus
- foramen ovale
- ductus arteriosus.

Cardiac outputs of the right and left ventricles in the foetus are not equal: left ventricle cardiac output > right ventricle cardiac output.

At birth:

- umbilical cord clamp: ductus venosus closes: ↑SVR
- first breath → lung expansion and ↓HPV, ↓ pulmonary vascular resistance, ↓ venous return to right atrium and↑ venous return to left atrium; atrial pressure gradient reversed—functional closure of foramen ovale
- ↑PaO_2 in ductus arteriosus—closure within 48 h.

Murphy PJ. Fetal circulation. *Contin Educ Anaesth Crit Care Pain* 2005; 5(4): 107–12.

57. **Answers: F T T T F**

Monoamine oxidase inhibitors are non-specific inhibitors of the enzyme, used as antidepressants. Monoamine oxidase catabolizes amines, including catecholamines. Type A enzyme inactivates noradrenaline and 5-hydroxytryptamine (5HT), type B tryptamine and phenylethylamine. Dopamine and tyramine are inactivated by both.

Excessive 5HT activity with pethidine can cause agitation, hyperreflexia, convulsions, hypertension, and tachycardia.

Sympathomimetics can cause exaggerated changes in blood pressure and heart rate. Hypertensive crisis may occur with amphetamines, methyldopa, levodopa, dopamine, epinephrine, norepinephrine, guanethidine, or indirectly acting vasoconstrictors.

The same effect can occur with antidepressants, which can reduce neurotransmitter re-uptake. Benzodiazepines have no interactions with monoamine oxidase inhibitors (MAOIs).

Interaction with opioids may be:

- excitatory: agitation, hypertension, tachycardia, hyperreflexia, hypertonus, pyrexia, convulsions, coma (due to excessive central 5HT and reported with only pethidine, which reduces 5HT uptake from nerve endings)
- depressive: hypoventilation, hypotension, coma (due to impaired hepatic metabolism of opioids, e.g. norpethidine, a metabolite of pethidine metabolism, may accumulate).

Additive hypotension may occur with antihypertensives or spinal anaesthesia.

Additive hypoglycemia may occur with insulins or oral hypoglycemic agents.

Phenelzine may decrease plasma cholinesterase levels.

Patients taking MAOIs may continue taking their medication throughout the perioperative period.

Meperidine, cocaine, and indirect-acting catecholamines should be avoided in these patients.

Yentis SM, Hirsch NP, Smith GB. *A–Z of Anaesthesia and Intensive Care.* Butterworth Heinemann, 2005: p. 362.

58. **Answers: T F T T F**

Long-term use of amiodarone is associated with numerous side effects, most of which resolve when the medication is stopped.

The side effects include:

- respiratory system: interstitial lung disease, pulmonary fibrosis, pneumonitis
- endocrine: hypothyroidism, hyperthyroidism, gynecomastia
- ophthalmic complication: vortex keratopathy (corneal microdeposits), optic neuropathy, optic-disc swelling, visual-field defects
- gastrointestinal and hepatobiliary system: hepatitis, cirrhosis, jaundice, metallic taste
- cardiovascular system: arrythmias, including prolonged QT, AV block, and bradycardia
- neurological: peripheral neuropathy, CNS toxicity
- skin: photosensitivity, discoloration.

Sasada M, Smith S, *Drugs in Anaesthesia and Intensive Care.* Oxford University Press, 2003.

British National Formulary, 61st edn. British Medical Association and Royal Pharmaceutical Society of Great Britain, 2011.

59. Answers: T F F F F

Ritodrine is a β-adrenergic agonist, used as a tocolytic in premature labour. Most complications result from the concurrent activity at the β-1 receptors. The side effects include nausea, vomiting, sweating, and tachycardia. Systolic hypertension and a fall in diastolic pressure, Arrhythmias, and myocardial ischaemia may also be seen. Hepatic impairment and postpartum haemorrhage are also potential complications. Agonists at β-receptors can also cause fluid retention due to decreased water clearance, which can cause tachycardia. This can lead to cardiac failure and pulmonary oedema.

Yentis SM, Hirsch NP, Smith GB. *A–Z of Anaesthesia and Intensive Care.* Butterworth Heinemann, 2004: p. 76.

British National Formulary, 61st edn. British Medical Association and Royal Pharmaceutical Society of Great Britain, 2011.

60. Answers: F T F T F

Pigmentation disorders and birthmarks affect many people. It is important to ascertain the cause of the abnormal pigmention as they can be a sign of underlying systemic disease. Most birthmarks are benign and rarely pose a risk.

Generalized skin pigmentation can occur with liver disease. Examples include haemachromatosis and Cushing's disease.

Melasma presents with brown patches, usually involving forehead, cheeks, lips, and chin. It is more common in women and is seen in pregnancy.

Vitiligo is a skin depigmentation disorder. There is pigment loss due to autoimmune destruction of the melanocytes. Diabetes, pernicious anaemia, and even Addison's may present with pigment loss.

Sheehan's syndrome may give rise to pallor if long standing. Infective endocarditis may give rise to petechiae.

Kumar P, Clark M. *Clinical Medicine.* Elsevier Saunders, 2005.

Single Best Answers

1. Answer: C

The fat emboli may occur by:

- direct entry of depot fat globules from disrupted adipose tissue or bone marrow into the bloodstream in areas of trauma (mechanical)
- production of toxic intermediaries of fat present in the plasma (biochemical).

Tibia fractures of marrow-containing bone have the highest incidence of fat embolism syndrome and cause the largest-volume fat emboli. This may be because the disrupted venules in the marrow remain tethered open by their osseous attachments, therefore the marrow contents may enter the venous circulation with relatively little difficulty. The tibia is a long bone and fracture requires the intramedullary nail. During the process of inserting the intramedullary nail there is increased pressure, which may lead to fat embolism.

Fat embolism syndrome has a classic triad:

- respiratory changes; dyspnoea, tachypnoea, and hypoxaemia are the most frequent early findings
- neurological abnormalities
- petechial rash.

During fat embolism there can be hypoxia, pulmonary odema, coagulation disorder, and loss of carbon dioxide due to sudden increase in the dead space.

Management of fat embolism syndrome involves prevention, early diagnosis, and adequate symptomatic treatment. Supportive care requires maintenance of adequate oxygenation and ventilation, stable haemodynamics, blood products as clinically indicated, hydration, prophylaxis of deep venous thrombosis and stress-related gastrointestinal bleeding, and nutrition.

Mortality is estimated to be 5–15% overall.

Gupta A, Reilly CS. Fat embolism. *Contin Educ Anaesth Crit Care Pain* 2007; 7(5): 148–51.

2. Answer: C

Due to the various changes in lung physiology during one-lung anaesthesia, it is not uncommon to notice a drop in oxygen saturations. All the above steps will have to be performed. However, checking takes time, and interrupting surgery to re-inflate the lungs is a last resort. The first step is ventilation with 100% oxygen, if not doing so already. This will allow time for the necessary equipment checks. Further deterioration may need to be managed by stopping surgery and re-inflating both lungs. Inform the surgeon early before the situation gets out of control. Attention should be paid to maintain perfusion by treating hypotension.

Management of hypoxaemia during one-lung ventilation is as follows:

- increase FiO_2 to 100%
- check the position and patency of the endotracheal tube
- check the rest of the circuit and the anaesthetic machine
- do a fibre-optic bronchoscopy if the airway pressures are high
- treat hypotension and ensure adequate cardiac output
- insufflate oxygen to the non-ventilated lung and apply continuous positive airway pressure (CPAP) if no improvement
- apply positive end-expiratory pressure (PEEP) to the ventilated lung
- if the above measures fail, intermittent inflation of the collapsed lung should be performed
- clamping the pulmonary artery to remove the shunt may be necessary in some thoracic surgeries.

Ng A, Swanevelder J. Hypoxemia during one lung anaesthesia. *Contin Educ Anaesth Crit Care Pain* 2010; 10(4): 9–13.

Gosh S, Latimer RD. *Thoracic Anaesthesia: Principles and Practice.* Butterworth Heinemann, Oxford, 1999.

Gothard J, Kelleher A, Haxby E. *Cardiovascular and Thoracic Anaesthesia in a Nutshell.* Butterworth Heinemann, 2003.

West JB. *Respiratory Physiology—the Essentials,* 7th edn. Lippincott Williams & Wilkins, 2007.

3. Answer: B

Most medications used in psychiatric medicine can be continued until the day of surgery. Lithium is the exception, as it needs to be stopped 24 h pre-operatively. Lithium can prolong neuromuscular blockade by reducing neurotransmitter release. It reduces anaesthetic requirements and can accumulate following NSAID therapy.

The serotonin re-uptake inhibitors (SSRIs) are the most commonly used drugs in the treatment of depression. This is because of their efficacy as antidepressants and preferable side-effect profile. The primary mechanism of action is pre-synaptic serotonin re-uptake inhibition, but they also have an anti-cholinergic effect. SSRIs can be continued up until surgery, but beware the risk of serotonin crisis.

Lithium is used in the treatment of mania and bipolar disorders. The mechanism is poorly understood, but mimics sodium, entering excitable cells during depolarization. This results in a reduction in the release of neurotransmitters in both the central nervous system (CNS) and the peripheral nervous system (PNS). It has a narrow therapeutic ratio and is excreted solely by the kidneys. Prolongation of depolarizing neuromuscular block and a reduction in the anaesthetic agent requirements has been reported. NSAIDs, which reduce the excretion of lithium by the kidneys, can result in toxic plasma levels. Toxic symptoms tend to occur with plasma levels of 1.5 mmol/L. Hence, it is prudent that lithium is stopped at least 24 h before surgery.

Tricyclic antidepressants (TCAs) are used in the treatment of depression, chronic pain, and some forms of acute pain. Their mode of action is by the prevention of presynaptic re-uptake of norepinephrine and serotonin (uptake 1). They also have anti-muscarinic, antihistaminergic and anti-α1-adrenergic effects. Metabolism occurs in the liver, via the cytochrome P450 pathway, with significant interpatient variation. TCAs should be discontinued.

Peck T, Wong A, Norman E. Anaesthetic implication of psychoactive drugs. *Contin Educ Anaesth Crit Care Pain* 2010; 6: 177–81.

4. Answer: D

Central venous pressure (CVP) by itself is an unreliable indicator of fluid status, although trends in CVP may be more accurate. This stems from the fact that CVP readings rely heavily on intact right heart and pulmonary function. Blood pressure may be elevated in hypovolaemia due to sympathetic drive. Heart rate trends, rather than a single reading, are more important. Heart rate itself may be affected by drugs such as sedatives and β-blockers. Septic shock may produce a hypervolaemic circulation with warm peripheries and no lag in capillary refill. Variation of venous return brought about by intrathoracic pressure changes in intermittent positive pressure ventilation (IPPV) is wider in hypovolaemia. A reduced variation of venous return indicates well-filled ventricles.

Gelman S. Venous function and central venous pressure. *Anaesthesiology* 2008; 108: 735–48.

5. Answer: C

Paravertebral block is an advanced regional anaesthesia technique. Thoracic paravertebral block involves injecting local anaesthetic in the vicinity of the thoracic spinal nerves.

Chest deformity may require imaging aids to perform the block but is not a contraindication. There is no evidence that the opiates affect the quality or duration of the regional blocks, but they may do so in central neuraxial blockade. A block above the umbilicus may inhibit the stress response. Generally, ward care of patients following a regional block does not warrant any additional training for the staff looking after these patients, but action on the sympathetic nerve may result in hypotension. This potential complication needs to be monitored for and treated.

Richardshon J, Lonnqvist PA, Naja Z. Bilateral thoracic paravertebral block: potential and practice. *Brit J Anaesth* 2011; 106(2): 164–71.

6. Answer: B

Cerebral palsy is associated with an alteration in neuromuscular sensitivity to muscle relaxation. There is decreased sensitivity to non-depolarizing relaxants. They are less potent and shorter acting, hence larger doses may be required. Depolarizing relaxants do not cause hyperkalemia, and suxamethonium has now been shown to be safe. Anticonvulsant therapy can reduce minimum alveolar concentration (MAC) values by increasing sensitivity to volatile agents, thus risking awareness under anaesthesia. Propofol is preferred both as an induction agent and as an anaesthetic, as it reduces muscle tone. However, there is no risk of malignant hyperthermia.

Prosser DP, Sharma N. Cerebral palsy and anaesthesia. *Contin Educ Anaesth Crit Care Pain* 2010; 10(3): 72–76.

7. Answer: B

Current recommendations on treating malignant hyperthermia recommend simply disconnecting the vaporizer to save time rather than changing the anaesthesia machine and circuit. Hyperventilation with 100% oxygen is recommended. Disconnecting the vaporizer saves time.

Dantrolene needs to be given until cardiac and respiratory systems stabilize, even if the 10 mg/kg dose is exceeded.

Anaesthesia should be maintained with intravenous drugs while surgery is concluded as rapidly as possible. Active cooling measures should be commenced early.

Compartment syndrome might develop later on.

Dantrolene needs to be given till cardiac and respiratory systems stabilize, even if the 10 mg/kg dose is exceeded.

Glahn KPE, Ellis FR, Halsall PJ, *et al*. Recognizing and managing a malignant hyperthermia crisis: guidelines from the European Malignant Hyperthermia Group. *Brit J Anaesth* 2010; 105(4): 417–20.

8. Answer: E

A McCoy laryngoscope, bougie, fibreoptic laryngoscope, and emergency tracheotomy are aids for difficult intubation where a glottis may not be visualized. Retrosternal goitres can compress the trachea, making ventilation impossible. For infra-glottic obstruction and in the circumstances of tracheal collapse, rigid bronchoscopy is the only reliable rescue in an airway emergency.

Nethercott D, Strang T, Krysiak P. Airway stents: anaesthetic implications. *Contin Educ Anaesth Crit Care Pain* 2010; 10(2): 53–58.

9. Answer: C

Although cough, tongue protrusion, hand grip, and generation of inspiratory pressures are good clinical indicators of muscle power, sustained head lift is the only consistent indicator of good recovery.

Clinical assessment:

- sustained head lift for at least 5 s
- generation of a vital capacity of at least 10 mL/kg
- generation of an inspiratory pressure of at least –25 cmH$_2$O.

Tidal volume is not a reliable guide to recovery, since normal volumes can be generated with only 20% functional diaphragm muscle receptors.

Yentis SM, Hirsch NP, Smith GB. *A–Z of Anaesthesia and Intensive Care*. Butterworth Heinemann, 2004: p. 383.

10. Answer: C

The aortic stenosis is a fixed outlet obstruction to left ventricular ejection. Anatomic obstruction to left ventricular ejection leads to concentric hypertrophy of the left ventricular heart muscle. This reduces the compliance of the left ventricular chamber, making it difficult to fill. Contractility and ejection fraction are usually maintained until late stages. Atrial contraction accounts for up to 40% of ventricular filling.

There is a high risk of myocardial ischemia due to increased oxygen demand and wall tension in the hypertrophied left ventricle. Thirty per cent of patients who have aortic stenosis with normal coronary arteries have angina.

Antibiotic prophylaxis is not essential, and needs to be tailored to surgical need. Excessive reduction or increases in peripheral vascular resistance should be avoided. Congenital bicuspid valves present early in life and do not require antibiotic cover.

Yentis SM, Hirsch NP, Smith GB. *A–Z of Anaesthesia and Intensive Care*. Butterworth Heinemann, 2004: p. 39.

11. Answer: C

Autonomic dysreflexia is characterized by massive disordered autonomic responses to stimulation below the level of the spinal lesion. It is rare in lesions lower than T$_7$. Incidence increases with higher lesions. It may occur within 3 weeks of the original injury but is unlikely to be a problem after 9 months. This is due to a loss of descending inhibitory control on regenerating pre-synaptic fibres.

Beta-blockade is only indicated in autonomic hyper-reflexia with tachycardia. Despite a theoretical risk of aspiration, rapid sequence induction of anaesthesia is not indicated for routine surgery. Slight head down or supine position promotes diaphragmatic contractility and improves forced vital capacity (FVC). There is risk of hyperkalaemia after suxamethonium, which usually persists until 9 months post injury. Fertility is not affected in these patients.

Teasdale A. Anaesthesia in spinal cord lesions. In: Allman KG, Wilson IH (eds), *Oxford Handbook of Anaesthesia*. Oxford University Press, 2004: p. 229.

12. Answer: C

Immediate management of airway fire:

- stop laser or diathermy, flood area with 0.9% saline
- disconnect ETT or catheter from the breathing system
- immediately clamp the end to reduce airflow to the burning area
- withhold jet and/or mask ventilation to reduce airflow to the burning area
- monitor pulse oximetry and re-ventilate when the fire is out.

Plastic tapes are more combustible than canvas. The best means of managing the airway in this situation is to avoid intubation and use Venturi devices. Gas mixtures of oxygen and air are better, as nitrous oxide also supports combustion. Matt surfaces do not reflect light and are safer than glossy surfaces.

Sadler J. Laser surgery. In: Allman KG, Wilson IH (eds), *Oxford Handbook of Anaesthesia*. Oxford University Press, 2004: p. 673.

13. Answer: A

Bed rest does not prevent headache, and can promote venous thrombosis instead.

There are a number of theories regarding the cause of post-dural puncture headache (PDPH). The most commonly held belief is that it is due to the CSF leaking through the dural puncture site, leading to intracranial hypotension. This causes settling of the brain and stretching of intracranial nerves, meninges, and blood vessels.

Incidence of PDPH is estimated to be between 30 and 50% following diagnostic or therapeutic lumbar puncture, 0–5% following spinal anaesthesia and up to 81% following accidental dural puncture during epidural insertion in the pregnant woman. It commonly occurs at a rate of about 1% following epidural placement.

The classic features of the headache caused by dural puncture are:

- often frontal-occipital: most headaches do not develop immediately after dural puncture but 24–48 h after the procedure, with 90% of headaches presenting within 3 days; the headache is worse in the upright position and eases when supine
- pressure over the abdomen with the woman in the upright position may give transient relief to the headache by raising intracranial pressure secondary to a rise in intra-abdominal pressure (Gutsche sign).

Other associated symptoms that may be present include nausea, vomiting, neck stiffness, photophobia, tinnitus, visual disturbance, and cranial nerve palsies.

Management of PDPH

Conservative:

- bed rest
- encourage oral fluids and/or intravenous hydration
- reassurance.

A recent Cochrane review concluded that routine bed rest after dural puncture is not beneficial and should be abandoned.

Pharmacological:

- caffeine, either intravenous (e.g. 500 mg caffeine in 1 L of saline) or orally
- synacthen (synthetic adrenocorticotropic hormone (ACTH))
- regular analgesia: paracetamol, diclofenac etc.

Other drugs with insufficient evidence in the literature are 5HT agonists (e.g. sumatriptan), gabapentin, desmopressin (DDAVP), theophyline, and hydrocortisone.

Interventional:

- immediate:
  - insertion of long-term intrathecal catheter placement (15%) and epidural saline bolus (13%)
  - epidural morphine.
- epidural blood patch, which involves injecting approximately 20 mL of the patient's own fresh blood (taken in a strict sterile fashion) into the epidural space near the site of the suspected puncture.

Halker RB et al. Caffeine for the prevention and treatment of postdural puncture headache: debunking the myth. *Neurologist* 2007; 13: 323–27.

Paech MJ. Epidural blood patch—myths and legends. *Can J Anaesth* 2005; 52(Sup 1): R1–5.

Sudlow CLM et al. Posture and fluids for preventing post-dural puncture headache. *Cochrane Database of Systematic Reviews* 2001. http://www2.cochrane.org/reviews/en/ab001790.htm.

14. Answer: B

Ulnar nerve injury is more common in males (3:1) because of reduced fat padding and a smaller carpal tunnel. Fifteen per cent of cases can occur with the patient awake. Additional padding may not make a difference, and although abduction of neutral arm reduces ulnar compression, it can strain the brachial plexus. The injury is more common in older patients, and may be accompanied by reduced nerve conduction in the unaffected arm, indicating pre-operative sub-optimal nerve dysfunction.

Shonfeld A, Harrop-Griffiths W. Regional anaesthesia and nerve injury. In: Allman KG, Wilson IH (eds), *Oxford Handbook of Anaesthesia*. Oxford University Press, Oxford, 2004, p. 1055.

15. Answer: E

Guillain–Barré syndrome is an acute ascending immune-mediated demyelinating polyneuropathy. It is the most common cause of generalized paralysis. Fifty per cent of cases follow a viral illness. Incidence is 1–2 per 100 000 and the male-to-female ratio is 1.5:1. Incidence follows a bimodal distribution, with peaks in age ranges of 15–35 years and 50–75 years.

The major symptom is rapidly progressive paralysis, which, unlike polio, is symmetrical. Paralysis of the lower extremities is followed by paralysis of the upper extremities, and both proximal and distal muscle groups are involved. Deep tendon reflexes are initially reduced and later are absent. One-third of patients require mechanical ventilation.

Management is the ABC approach. The patient requires airway protection (intubation) and respiratory support, such as non-invasive ventilation or tracheostomy, should be considered earlier rather than later because prolonged respiratory support is likely. Patient may need IV fluids, inotropes, and invasive haemodynamic monitoring. After initial management, an attempt should be made to reach a definitive diagnosis (since the initial diagnosis of Guillain–Barré syndrome is clinical). Lumbar puncture and CSF analysis often shows increased CSF protein levels. A neurologist should be consulted if any uncertainty exists as to the diagnosis.

Intravenous immunoglobulins or exchange plasmaphoresis are the disease-modifying treatment. The role of corticosteroids for anti-inflammatory action has no evidence to support it. Other measures are mainly supportive:

- physiotherapy
- prophylaxis against DVT (due to limited mobility for a long time)
- pressure area care
- nutritional support (preferably enteral)
- treatment of infections depending on culture and sensitivity reports.

The best treatment option for Guillain–Barré syndrome is to mange the patient in the critical care unit; providing supportive and immunoglobin therapy has been shown to modify the disease process.

Vucic, S. GBS—an update. *J Clin Neurosci* 2009; 16; 6: 733–41.

16. Answer: C

Carbon monoxide poisoning is treated with oxygen even after clinical improvement beyond 1 day because of the second peak of CO after 24 h. Full-thickness burns can be equally as painful as partial thickness burns, largely due to painful surrounding skin. Lichtenberg flowers appear in lightning strikes. Fluid resuscitation time begins from the initial time of injury.

In carbon monoxide poisoning, when carboxyhaemoglobin (COHb) is >20%, arterial blood gas will appear normal, and SaO_2 will appear normal because both COHb and oxyhaemoglobin absorb at 940 nm. Bench co-oximetry utilizes an additional wavelength of red light, allowing differentiation.

The clinical course of CO poisoning is directly related to the degree and duration of exposure. In the majority of cases those with a COHb level in the blood of less than 10% will have no symptoms, whereas in those with a level of 50% or greater are likely to suffer from coma, cardiac depression, or cardiac arrest. Myocardial injury is common and a predictor of mortality. Some patients may also develop rhabdomyolysis and renal failure.

The classical cherry-pink discolouration of the skin caused by large amounts of COHb is in practice rarely seen. Skin pallor and cyanosis are more usual. Skin blisters may occur as a result of tissue hypoxia.

Table 1.1 shown clinical signs and symptoms seen at different percentage COHb levels.

Table 1.1 Clinical signs and symptoms of carbon monoxide poisoning

COHb level (%)	Clinical signs and symptoms
0–10	In general no symptoms
10–20	Mild headache, slight shortness of breath
20–30	Moderate headache, weakness, difficulty with concentration
30–40	Irritability, nausea/vomiting, dizziness, visual changes
40–50	Tachycardia, tachypnoea, arrhythmias, ataxia, confusion
50–60	Stupor, convulsions, often fatal
60–70	Coma, cardiac depression

Cyanide poisoning (>50 ppm) causes unexplained metabolic acidosis and high venous oxygen saturation. It is common with combustion of plastics and is managed by oxygen therapy.

Nolan J.; The critically ill patient; Early management. In: Allman KG, Wilson IH (eds), *Oxford Handbook of Anaesthesia*. Oxford University Press, Oxford, 2004: Chapter 34, p. 838.

17. Answer: D

Heart and lung transplant patients have altered physiology:

- the heart is denervated, with the resting heart rate usually around 85–95 bpm; some patients will be bradycardic and may have a permanent pacemaker
- the autonomic system responses are obtunded.

Contractility remains the same for the heart, unless rejection is developing.

The heart should be considered as permanently denervated, and hence there will be poor tolerance to acute hypovolaemia.

For pharmacological intervention, direct-acting agents should be used:

- atropine has no effect on the denervated heart
- the effect of ephedrine is reduced and unpredictable

- hydralazine and phenylephrine produce no reflex tachycardia or bradycardia in response to their primary action
- adrenaline, noradrenaline, isoprenaline, and β-blockers act as predicted.

Pulmonary edema can occur due to disrupted pulmonary lymphatics.

Heart–lung transplants should be managed without intubation if possible because of the risk of disruption of the tracheal anastomosis.

Telford R. Cardiovascular disease. In: Allman KG, Wilson IH (eds), *Oxford Handbook of Anaesthesia*. Oxford University Press, 2004: p. 70.

18. Answer: E

The patient is on MAOIs. These work by inhibition of the enzyme monoamine oxidase, which is present on external mitochondrial membranes and inactivates monoamine neurotransmitters in both the central and peripheral nervous systems. MAOIs cause an increase in the level of amine neurotransmitters. Monoamine oxidase exists as two isoenzymes, A and B, which have different properties. MAO-A acts mainly on serotonin, noradrenaline, and adrenaline. It is the main form of MAO found in the human brain. MAO-B preferentially metabolizes non-polar aromatic amines such as phenylethylamine and methylhistamine, and is responsible for 75% of MAO activity, predominating in the gastrointestinal tract, platelets, and most other non-neural cells. Tyramine (a precursor of noradrenaline that is found in cheese and other foods) and dopamine are substrates for both A and B. There are now two generations of MAOIs: the original drugs, which inhibit both forms of MAO non-selectively and irreversibly, and the newer generation, which reversibly inhibit MAO-A. Selegiline, the anti-Parkinsonism drug, is an MAO-B inhibitor.

MAOIs are used as follows:

- non-specific and type A-specific MAOIs (e.g. phenelzine, isocarboxazid, and tranylcypromine) are used for treatment of depression in patients who may not tolerate other modes of therapy (tricyclic antidepressants, SSRIs, or electroconvulsive therapy)
- type B-specific MAOIs (e.g. selegiline) are used as anti-Parkinsonism drugs.

Hypertensive crisis may occur with amphetamines, methyldopa, levodopa, dopamine, epinephrine, norepinephrine, guanethidine, or indirectly acting vasoconstrictors. Hence drugs that have indirect sympathomimetic action are contraindicated in the presence of MAOIs. Direct-acting sympathomimetics (adrenaline, noradrenaline, and phenylephrine) should be titrated to effect in patients on MAOIs, as they may have an enhanced effect due to receptor hypersensitivity.

A bolus of phenylephrine would be the appropriate first line of action with such hypotension.

Luck JF, Wildsmith JAW, Christmas DMB. Monoamine oxidase inhibitors and anaesthesia. *Bull Royal Coll Anaesth* 2003; 21: 1029–34.

19. Answer: B

Down's syndrome is one of the most common chromosomal disorders. Invariably anaesthetists will encounter patients with this syndrome for a variety of procedures.

Screening lateral radiographs in the asymptomatic patients are not indicated. There may be accompanying cardiac defects and leukaemia. Obstructive sleep apnoea and Eisenmenger's syndrome can both increase the chances of pulmonary hypertension and aggravate it.

Down's syndrome is characterized by:

- trisomy of chromosome 21 due to non-dysjunction of chromosomes during germ cell formation; it is the most common congenital anomaly, carrying an incidence of 1.6 per 1000 births

- tonsillar and adenoid hypertrophy due to relative immune deficiency and a degree of upper airway obstruction
- increased tendency (up to 30%) for subluxation/dislocation of the cervical spine due to bony abnormality and laxity of transverse atlantal ligament
- micrognathia, relatively large tongue, short broad neck, and crowding of mid-facial structures, which make intubation more difficult.

Allt JE, Howell CJ. Down's syndrome; *BJA CEPD Rev* 2003; 3(3): 83–86.

Graham H, Uncommon conditions; Down's syndrome. In: Allman KG, Wilson IH (eds), *Oxford Handbook of Anaesthesia*. Oxford University Press, Oxford, 2004: Chapter 13, p. 293.

20. Answer: B

Myasthenia gravis is an autoimmune disease in which IgG auto-antibodies are produced against the nicotinic ACh receptors within the neuromuscular junction. The auto-antibodies lead to destruction of the receptors. Symptoms include a fatigable weakness, which can be localized to specific muscle groups (ocular, bulbar, and respiratory) or become widespread. Treatment may involve cholinesterase inhibitors, plasma exchange, immunosuppressants, and IV immunoglobulins.

Myasthenia gravis patients exhibit a relative resistance to depolarizing neuromuscular blocking agents and the dose used may need to be increased. Conversely, patients show sensitivity to non-depolarizing neuromuscular blocking agents, requiring only 10% of normal dose. Cholinesterase inhibitors should be avoided as they can not only prolong the duration of a depolarizing neuromuscular blocking agents block, but also precipitate a cholinergic crisis. Drugs that interfere with neuromuscular transmission should be avoided. Postoperative ventilation may be necessary.

Marsh S, Ross N, Pittard A. Neuromuscular disorders and anaesthesia. Part 2: specific neuromuscular disorders. *Cont Educ Anaesth Crit Care Pain* 2011; 11(4): 119–23.

21. Answer: D

Geriatric changes increase mortality and morbidity. There is impaired autoregulation, with impaired renal function. There are reduced plasma proteins and body water, affecting drug delivery and metabolism.

There are also respiratory system changes in elderly patients:

- Functional residual capacity (FRC) is unchanged, but closing capacity falls with age, causing lung collapse. Loss of elastic recoil increases pulmonary compliance, but chest wall compliance falls due to degenerative changes in joints. Loss of septa increases alveolar dead space. Closing volume increases to exceed functional residual capacity in the upright posture at 66 years old, resulting in venous admixture. Thus normal PaO_2 falls steadily: $(13.3 - age/30)$ kPa, or $(100 - age/4)$ mmHg and ventilatory reserve declines with age.
- Ventilatory response to hypoxia and hypercapnia declines with risk of postoperative apnoea.
- O_2 consumption and CO_2 production fall by 10–15% by the seventh decade. Patients are able to tolerate a longer period of apnoea following preoxygenation and minute volume requirement is reduced.
- Airway protective reflexes decline, increasing the risk of postoperative pulmonary aspiration.
- In edentulous patients, maintenance of a patent airway and face mask seal may be difficult. Leaving false teeth in situ may help.

Kelly F. Anaesthesia for the elderly. In: Allman KG, Wilson IH (eds), *Oxford Handbook of Anaesthesia*. Oxford University Press, 2004: p. 689.

Jandziol AK, Griffiths R. The anaesthetic management of hip fractures. *BJA CEPD Rev* 2001; 1, 52–55.

22. Answer: A

Compartment syndrome is a painful condition that occurs when pressure within the muscles builds to dangerous levels. This pressure can decrease blood flow, which prevents nourishment and oxygen from reaching nerve and muscle cells.

Muscles are contained in compartments or thick fibrous bands of tissue or fascia. Because of injury, pressure can increase within the compartment, leading to swelling (fluid accumulation) or bleeding. In non-contracting muscle, the compartment pressure is normally about 0–15 mmHg. If the pressure within the compartment increases (usually greater than about 30–45 mmHg; other clinicians use other pressure values that are within 30 mm of the diastolic BP), most individuals develop compartment syndrome. When these high compartment pressures are present, blood cannot circulate to the muscles and nerves to supply them with oxygen and nutrients. Compartment syndrome symptoms such as pain and swelling will then occur.

Muscle compartment measurements via a catheter connected to transducers are important after trauma, particularly in comatose or sedated patients who are otherwise unable to complain of any symptoms.

Mar GJ, Barrington MJ, McGuirk BR. Acute compartment syndrome of the lower limb and the effect of postoperative analgesia on diagnosis. *Brit J Anaesth* 2009; 102: 3–11.

23. Answer: D

The brachial plexus is formed by ventral rami of C5 to C8, with contributions from C4 and T2 in some. It provides nerve supply to the upper limb.

It is composed of:

- roots: C5–C8 and T1 (ventral rami)
- trunks: upper , middle, and lower
- division: anterior and posterior
- cords: medial/lateral/posterior.

At the supra-clavicular region the brachial plexus is in a compact form. The block at this level has the highest probability of blocking all the branches of the plexus. There is increased risk of pneumothorax, but this can be avoided by using ultrasound guidance or avoiding the medial aspect for needle insertion.

Interscalene brachial plexus block could be used, but the area supplied by the C8 and T1 nerve roots may be missed. This may innervate the humeral area.

Yentis SM, Hirsch NP, Smith GB. *A–Z of Anaesthesia and Intensive Care.* Butterworth Heinemann, 2004: pp. 69–71.

24. Answer: D

Severe sepsis, a syndrome characterized by systemic inflammation and acute organ dysfunction in response to infection, is a major healthcare problem affecting all age groups throughout the world. It is crucial to administer appropriate intravenous antimicrobial therapy in the care of patients with severe sepsis who may require surgery to control the source of sepsis. Preoperative resuscitation, aimed at optimizing major organ perfusion, is based on the judicious use of fluids, vasopressors, and inotropes.

Table 1.2 shows parameters for goal directed therapy.

Table 1.2 Goal-directed therapy

Clinical parameter	Goal
Central venous pressure	8–12 mmHg (≥8 mmHg in spontaneously breathing patient, ≥12 mmHg in ventilated patients)
Mean arterial pressure	Between 65 and 90 mmHg
Central venous oxygen saturation	≥70 mmHg
Urine output	≥0.5 mL/kg/h
Haematocrit	≥30%

A haematocrit of ≥30% is a clinical target in goal-directed therapy.

Eissa D, Carton EG, Buggy DJ. Anaesthetic management of patients with severe sepsis. *Brit J Anaesth* 2010; 105(6): 734–43.

25. Answer: E

Complication of neuraxial blockade includes arachnoiditis, meningitis, and abscess, but serious infection following spinal or epidural anaesthesia is rare. Staphylococcus is the most common organism associated with epidural abscess.

The classical triad of fever, backache, and neurological deficit is suggestive of an epidural abscess, but all three features are only present in 13% of cases at the time of diagnosis. It is a time-limited emergency and prognosis in terms of neurological recovery is poor if symptoms are present for longer than 24 h. Delay in diagnosis is associated with increased morbidity and mortality. An urgent MRI to confirm the diagnosis and referral to a neurosurgeon for decompression is indicated.

The catheter tip should be sent for culture and broad-spectrum antibiotics should be instituted, but there should be no delay in decompression once the diagnosis is confirmed.

Grewal S, Hocking G, Wildsmith JAW. Epidural abscesses. *Br J Anaesth* 2006: 96 (3): 292–302.

26. Answer: C

Herpes zoster results from reactivation of the varicella zoster virus. Herpes zoster is a sporadic disease, with an estimated lifetime incidence of 10–20%. The incidence of herpes zoster increases sharply with advancing age, roughly doubling in each decade past the age of 50 years.

Varicella zoster virus is a highly contagious DNA virus. Varicella represents the primary infection in the non-immune or incompletely immune person. During the primary infection, the virus gains entry into the sensory dorsal root ganglia. Reactivation of the virus occurs following a decrease in virus-specific cell-mediated immunity. The reactivated virus travels down the sensory nerve and is the cause for the dermatomal distribution of pain and skin lesions. Patients with disease states that affect cell-mediated immunity, such as HIV infection and certain malignancies, are also at increased risk.

Herpes zoster typically presents with a prodrome consisting of hyperaesthesia, paraesthesias, burning dysaesthesias, or pruritus along the affected dermatome(s). The prodrome generally lasts 1–2 days but may precede the appearance of skin lesions by up to 3 weeks. Some patients may have prodromal symptoms without developing the characteristic rash.

Pain is the most common complaint for which patients with herpes zoster seek medical care. The pain may be described as 'burning' or 'stinging' and is generally unrelenting. Some patients may have insomnia because of the severe pain.

Although post-herpetic neuralgia is generally a self-limiting condition, it can last indefinitely. Treatment is directed at pain control while waiting for the condition to resolve. Pain therapy may include multiple interventions, such as topical medications, simple analgesics, tricyclic antidepressants, anticonvulsants, and a number of non-medical modalities. Occasionally, opioids may be required.

Ryder S, Stannard CF. Treatment of chronic pain: antidepressant, antiepileptic and antiarrhythmic drugs. *Contin Educ Anaesth Crit Care Pain* 2005; 5(1): 18–21.

27. Answer: D

Rheumatoid arthritis is associated with various problems with the airway:

- fixed neck deformity
- narrowing of cricoarytenoid joint
- involvement of the temporomandibular joint
- atlanto-axial subluxation (AAS).

AAS can be anterior (80%), posterior (5%), vertical (10–20%), or lateral. Anterior AAS will produce symptoms on neck flexion while posterior AAS worsens on neck extension with implications for conventional laryngoscopy.

This patient's symptoms are suggestive of posterior AAS and need imaging to diagnose or exclude it. She also has an enlarged thyroid, which may in itself compromise her airway. It would not be appropriate to proceed without further imaging. The patency of the trachea would be important in view of tracheacheal collapse.

Fomban F, Thompson JP. Anaesthesia for adult patients with rheumatoid arthritis. *Contin Educ Anaesth Crit Care Pain* 2006; 6(6): 235–39.

Berry C. Bone, joint, and connective tissue disorders: In: Allman KG, Wilson IH (eds), *Oxford Handbook of Anaesthesia*. Oxford University Press, 2004: p. 185.

28. Answer: B

Compartment syndrome is commonly seen after traumatic fractures in an osseofacial compartment of leg and forearm, but can occur in thigh, upper arm, and foot. Compartment syndrome requires prompt diagnosis and treatment by decompression, otherwise it leads to neurological deficit, muscle necrosis, amputation, and death. Pain is a cardinal feature and regional anaesthesia may mask this and delay diagnosis. The other features are paraesthesia, tense, painful compartment, pain on passive stretch of muscle, and sensory loss. Pulselessness is not common and is a very late feature.

Mar GJ, Barrington MJ, McGuirk BR. Acute compartment syndrome of the lower limb and the effect of postoperative analgesia on diagnosis. *Br J Anaesth* 2009: 102: 3–11.

29. Answer: C

Explanation: fat embolism presents typically 24–72 h after initial trauma, which is usually a long bone fracture. The presentation consists of a classic triad of neurological abnormalities, petechial rash, and respiratory changes. However, these signs are not always reliable and a high index of suspicion is needed. Gurd's criteria (see Table 1.3) are most commonly used to aid diagnosis and have three major and a number of minor criteria described. You need at least one major and four minor criteria for the diagnosis of fat embolism.

Table 1.3 Gurd's criteria

Major criteria

Axillary or subconjunctival petechiae

Hypoxaemia PaO_2 <60 mmHg; FiO_2 = 0.4)

Central nervous system depression disproportionate to hypoxaemia

Pulmonary oedema

Minor criteria

Tachycardia <110 bpm

Pyrexia <38.5°C

Emboli present in the retina on fundoscopy

Fat present in urine

A sudden inexplicable drop in haematocrit or platelet values

Increasing erythrocyte sedimentation rate (ESR)

Fat globules present in the sputum

Reproduced from Amandeep Gupta and Charles S. Reilly, 'Fat embolism', Continuing Education in Anaesthesia Critical Care and Pain, 2007, 7, 5, pp. 148–151 by permission of Oxford University Press and the British Journal of Anaesthesia.

Although the reliability of these criteria has been questioned, they do provide a reasonable basis for the diagnosis of fat embolism.

Gupta A, Reilly CS. Fat embolism. *Contin Educ Anaesth Crit Care Pain* 2007; 7(5): 148–51.

30. Answer: B

Rheumatoid arthritis is a multisystem disorder mainly involving joints. Approximately 25% of patients with severe rheumatoid arthritis have atlanto-axial subluxation, but of these only 25% will have neurological signs or symptoms. It is important to know about tingling of hands or feet, and neck pain, and to assess the range of neck movement. Excessive movement during anaesthesia can lead to cervical cord compression.

Cervical spine radiographs: the role of preoperative cervical spine flexion/extension views is controversial and interpretation is difficult.

Flexion/extension views are mandatory in all patients with neurological symptoms or signs, and also in those with persistent neck pain. Preoperative cervical spine radiographs may help determine management in some patients with severe disease. Specialist radiological advice may be required. All rheumatoid patients should be treated as having an unstable spine. This may involve awake fibreoptic intubation or manual in-line stabilization when undertaking direct laryngoscopy, laryngeal mask airway (LMA) insertion, or moving the patient. MRI and CT may be useful in assessing cord compression.

This patient has suffered a significant trauma to the head, so cervical spinal fracture or further displacement of undiagnosed atlanto-axial subluxation has to be excluded.

Berry C. Bone, joint, and connective tissue disorders. In: Allman KG, Wilson IH (eds), *Oxford Handbook of Anaesthesia*. Oxford University Press, 2004: p. 185.

True/False

1. **Transdermal drug delivery:**
   A. Avoids hepatic first-pass metabolism.
   B. Can often be improved by enzymatic or pH-associated deactivation.
   C. Is unreliable in the vasoconstricted patient.
   D. Is improved if the drug has affinity for both the lipophilic and hydrophilic phases.
   E. Is worse if the drug has high potency.

2. **Regarding beclomethasone dipropionate:**
   A. Dose is 50–100 mcg inhaled 6–12 hourly.
   B. Nebulizer preparation is more effective.
   C. Does not cause HPA suppression in clinical doses.
   D. Has equal glucocorticoid and mineralocorticoid effect.
   E. Works only as prophylactic agent against bronchospasm in asthma.

3. **Carbamazepine:**
   A. Can be used for all types of epilepsy.
   B. Has a narrow therapeutic index compared to phenytoin.
   C. Causes liver enzyme induction.
   D. Should not be given rectally.
   E. Contraindicated in porphyria.

4. **Regarding digoxin:**
   A. Provides no long-term benefit in cardiac failure.
   B. Acts by activating Ca^{++} pump.
   C. Has low volume of distribution.
   D. Slows heart rate by direct effect on the SA node only.
   E. Toxicity more likely with hypercalcemia.

5. **Regarding etomidate:**
   A. Comes with propylene glycol additive.
   B. Is presented as an aqueous solution.
   C. Premixing with lidocaine does not decrease pain on injection.
   D. Steroid synthesis is interfered by single enzyme inhibition of 11 β-hydroxylase.
   E. Reduces cerebral blood flow.

6. **Regarding helium:**
    A. Has more viscosity than oxygen.
    B. Does not support combustion.
    C. Is stored as a gas in cylinders.
    D. Causes voice changes when inhaled.
    E. Decreases the work of breathing in upper airway obstruction.

7. **The following drug causes miosis:**
    A. Cocaine.
    B. Timolol.
    C. Morphine.
    D. Phenylephrine.
    E. Amitryptalline.

8. **Prilocaine hydrochloride:**
    A. Is faster in onset than lignocaine.
    B. Has safer therapeutic index than lignocaine.
    C. Undergoes predominantly hepatic metabolism.
    D. Shorter acting than lidocaine.
    E. Methaemoglobinemia is the most common side effect.

9. **The drug ergometrine maleate:**
    A. Is a partial agonist at serotonin receptors.
    B. Should not be given i.v. because of risk of coronary vasospasm.
    C. Increases the strength and duration but decreases the frequency of uterine contractions.
    D. Contraindicated in asthmatics.
    E. Acts on upper uterine segment more than the lower uterine segment.

10. **With regards to renal function with advancing age in an otherwise healthy individual:**
    A. The functional capacity for glomerular filtration relative to tubular absorption is reduced.
    B. Blood flow is impaired more in the renal cortex than in the medulla.
    C. The capacity to acidify the urine in response to metabolic acidosis is unimpaired.
    D. The ability to concentrate urine is reduced.
    E. Blood creatinine concentration is increased.

11. **NICE and the RCOG recommend magnesium sulphate as the drug of choice for the management of severe pre-eclampsia and eclampsia in the acute clinical setting. What factors should be routinely monitored to ensure that the magnesium levels are not too elevated?**
    A. Urinary magnesium levels.
    B. Therapeutic serum drug level monitoring.
    C. Respiratory rate.
    D. Deep tendon reflexes.
    E. Urine output.

12. Cyanide poisoning:

A. Can occur from prolonged use of sodium nitroprusside.
B. Inhibits cytochrome oxidase system in the mitochondria.
C. Characterized by decrease in arterio-venous oxygen difference.
D. There is no metabolic acidosis.
E. Liver enzyme rhodanese converts cyanide into thiocyanate.

13. About commonly used intravenous fluids:

A. Normal saline (0.9%) has the lowest pH.
B. Colloids are not suited to compensating extracellular fluid losses.
C. 5% dextrose expands intracellular volume more than extracellular volume.
D. Dextrose is mainly metabolized in liver.
E. Hartmann's solution is the ideal fluid for peri-operative fluid replacement.

14. Regarding malignant hyperthermia:

A. Has autosomal dominant inheritance.
B. Always occurs within the first few hours of exposure to triggering agent.
C. Dantrolene 1–2 mg/kg IV up to a maximum of 10 mg/kg is the drug of choice.
D. Mortality is more than 10%, even with the use of dantrolene.
E. Masseter spasm is the first sign.

15. Regarding the distribution of cardiac output (CO) in the resting state:

A. Maximum CO goes to the liver.
B. Heart receives only about 5%.
C. Brain gets about 20%.
D. Autoregulated by organ metabolism.
E. Muscle blood flow is less than kidneys.

16. Regarding pseudocholinesterase enzyme:

A. Present within the RBCs.
B. Normal enzyme has a fluoride number of 80–90.
C. Acquired deficiency can occur in pregnancy.
D. Also present at neuromuscular junction.
E. Acts on mivacurium.

17. Regarding the carotid body:

A. Is a central chemoreceptor.
B. Rate of discharge is increased in cyanide poisoning.
C. Has the highest blood supply per unit weight in the body
D. Is of neuro-ectodermal origin.
E. Has vagal afferents.

18. About an adult cardiac arrest in the community:

A. Compression-only CPR by a lay-person is acceptable.
B. In an unwitnessed arrest, paramedics should do 2 min of chest compression before defibrillation, even for a shockable rhythm.
C. Amiodarone by paramedics should be given after the third shock for a shockable rhythm.
D. Early defibrillation improves mortality outcome.
E. The most common cause is non-shockable rhythm.

19. For the treatment of regular narrow complex tachycardia:

A. Vagal manoeuvres can be tried.
B. Adenosine should be avoided in asthmatics.
C. Verapamil can be given if no response to adenosine.
D. WPW syndrome can cause AV re-entry tachycardia.
E. If pulseless, should be treated with asynchronous shock.

20. About adult cardiac arrest:

A. Certain drugs can be given intra-tracheal if IV access is not available.
B. Atropine is the second-line drug in asystole.
C. There is greater emphasis on early tracheal intubation.
D. Use of capnography can be misleading and is not recommended.
E. Role of precordial thump is de-emphasized.

21. The following are features of acute renal failure:

A. Urine specific gravity > 1.020.
B. Urinary sodium > 40 mmol/L.
C. Urine osmolality > 500 mosmol/L.
D. Urine to plasma creatinine ratio < 20.
E. Renal failure index > 1.

22. Regarding xenon:

A. Has a MAC less than nitrous oxide.
B. Has some respiratory depressant effects.
C. The radioactive isotope Xe-133 is highly dangerous to blood cells.
D. Is environmentally safe and does not have a greenhouse effect.
E. Has the least blood/gas solubility of all known anaesthetic gases.

23. Regarding laudanosine:

A. It is a quarternary amine breakdown product of atracurium by Hofmann degradation.
B. Its half-life is prolonged in renal failure.
C. Blood levels may be clinically significant after several days of infusion, especially in liver failure patients.
D. Is pro-convulsant.
E. Shown to interact with some GABA receptors.

24. Regarding sickle cell anaemia:

A. Is an autosomal recessive genetic disorder.
B. Sickle cell trait (HbAS) may offer survival advantages in certain conditions.
C. HbAS sickles at 5–6 kPa.
D. Oxygen affinity of dissolved HbSS is normal.
E. Pre-operative target of HbS for sickle cell disease patients should be between 20 and 40%.

25. The recurrent laryngeal nerve:

A. Supplies most of the intrinsic muscles of the larynx.
B. Supplies the cricothyroid muscle.
C. Supplies the inferior constrictor muscle.
D. Supplies sensation below the vocal cords.
E. Supplies sensation to the posterior two-thirds of the tongue.

26. The following are characteristic features of myasthenia gravis:

A. Over 90% suffer from diplopia or ptosis at some stage of their illness.
B. Symptoms are usually symmetrical.
C. Muscular weakness is made worse by exercise.
D. Symptoms characteristically remit during pregnancy.
E. Steroids and azathioprine may be effective therapy.

27. Concerning the history of anaesthesia:

A. Thomas Morton gave the first successful public demonstration of ether anaesthesia.
B. August Bier was the first to isolate cocaine and use it for spinal anaesthetic.
C. Thiopentone was discovered by Waters and Lundy in 1934.
D. Humphrey Davey discovered oxygen.
E. John Snow gave ether anaesthesia to Queen Victoria.

28. Signs of fat embolism include:

A. Pyrexia.
B. Bradycardia.
C. Petechial rash.
D. Haemoptysis.
F. Mental changes.

29. Regarding physiology of potassium:

A. Principal intracellular anion.
B. Total daily requirement is 1 mmol/kg/day.
C. Is not easily exchangeable.
D. Is mainly absorbed in the proximal convoluted tubule of the nephron.
E. The amount present within bone and dense connective tissue is more than that present in extracellular fluid.

30. Regarding intra-operative red cell salvage:

A. It is contraindicated in malignancy surgery because of risk of haematogenous metastasis.
B. High suction pressure is needed to effectively suck blood.
C. Blood-soaked swabs can be washed and the fluid used for cell salvage.
D. Use of leucodepletion filters does not decrease contamination from amniotic fluid in obstetric cell salvage.
E. If mother is rhesus negative and foetus is rhesus positive, cell saver can still be used.

31. For severe community-acquired pneumonia:

A. Strep pneumoniae is the most common pathogen.
B. Risk stratification using the pneumonia severity index (PSI) includes for age > 65 years.
C. Patients with a CURB 65 score of 3 or more should be treated aggressively, preferably in ICU.
D. Panton-valentine leukocidin (PVL) producing MRSA is resistant to vancomycin.
E. Tigecycline is a tetracycline antibiotic used to treat MRSA with good tissue penetration.

32. Regarding phaeochromocytomas:

A. Are associated with MEN type 2 and 3 and neurofibromatosis.
B. Approximately 90% occur in the adrenal cortex.
C. May present as polycythaemia.
D. Causes hypoglycaemia.
E. Diagnosed in pregnancy should be treated medically until the patient reaches term.

33. Hyperparathyroidism may present as:

A. Renal stones.
B. Depression.
C. Thirst.
D. Abdominal pain.
E. Tetany.

34. The NICE guidelines on hypertension:

A. Defines hypertension as BP > 160/90 mmHg on two separate visits.
B. Aims to reduce BP < 140/90 mmHg.
C. Patients under 55 years of age should be started on ACE inhibitors or β-blockers.
D. Black patients should be started on calcium channel blockers or ACE inhibitors.
E. β-blockers should be considered first line in women of child-bearing potential.

35. Regarding preconditioning of the myocardium:

A. A short period of ischaemia confers protection against subsequent ischaemia and reperfusion injury.
B. Cardioprotection lasts for several hours after the preconditioning stimulus.
C. The protection only lasts for the first 24 h after the preconditioning stimulus.
D. Preconditioning effects are seen with opioids.
E. Preconditioning effects are not seen with desflurane.

36. Regarding smoking and abstinence from smoking

A. Nicotine increases concentration of circulating catecholamines.
B. Abstinence for more than 3 months decreases overall perioperative cardiovascular risk by 33%.
C. Sustained postoperative abstinence decreases long-term mortality after CABG.
D. Smoking accelerates age-related decrease in FEV1.
E. At least 24 weeks of abstinence is needed to ensure that risk of postoperative respiratory problems requiring intervention is reduced to normal.

37. Regarding postoperative cognitive dysfunction:

A. It is a persistent change in cognitive function as assessed by formal testing.
B. It is particularly common after cardiac surgery.
C. There is now evidence that it persists more than 6 months in elderly patients having major surgery.
D. Is common in elderly patients even after minor surgery.
E. The incidence is significantly higher in patients over 60 years.

38. In obese patients:

A. Platelet activity is reduced.
B. There is decreased concentration of fibrinogen.
C. Obstructive sleep apnoea is seen in 5% of obese patients.
D. Bioavailability of oral drug is affected.
E. There is no increased risk of difficult intubation.

39. Regarding statins, they:

A. Prevent LDL cholesterol production by inhibiting HMG-CoA reductase.
B. Enhance the stability of atherosclerotic plaques.
C. Inhibit vascular smooth muscle proliferation.
D. Inhibit cytokine production.
E. Have anti-oxidant activity.

40. Concerning drug delivery using iontophoresis:

A. The drug diffusion only occurs during current flow.
B. Quantity of drug delivered by iontophoresis is not influenced by the intensity of electric current.
C. Quantity of drug delivered is influenced by duration of electric current.
D. Lidocaine can be successfully administered by iontophoresis.
E. Significant quantity of drug is delivered by passive diffusion during iontophoresis.

41. For a patient for free flap surgery for resection of a tongue cancer, intra-operative management priorities include:

A. Maintenance of haematocrit of 40–50%.
B. Maintenance of a hyperdynamic circulation.
C. Hypothermia to reduce vasodilatation and blood loss.
D. CVP values 3–5 cmH_2O above baseline unless contraindicated.
E. Avoidance of systemic vasodilators.

42. When treating patients of Jehovah's Witness faith:

A. Advanced directives must be respected.
B. They will not accept blood products.
C. 12-year-old boy can be given blood products in an emergency.
D. In an emergency, one is obliged to care for patients in accordance with their wishes.
E. Anaesthetists can refuse to work with the patient.

43. Regarding the physiology of pregnancy:

A. Vital capacity is unchanged in pregnancy.
B. Heart size is markedly increased in the third trimester.
C. In normal pregnancy, blood pressure increases near term.
D. In the latter part of a normal pregnancy. blood urea is elevated above the non-pregnant state.
E. At term the cardiac output can be reduced by up to 40% when the pregnant woman is turned from lateral to the supine position.

44. Regarding the Tuohy needle:

A. Is commonly 16 G or 18 G.
B. Allows passage of a 21 G catheter in paediatric models.
C. Should be held fixed if withdrawing the catheter from beyond the tip during insertion.
D. Available in 5-, 10-, and 15-cm lengths.
E. Tip is called a Huber tip.

45. In the event of accidental injection of thiopentone in an intra-arterial line, the following is appropriate:

A. Stellate ganglion blockade.
B. Intra-arterial injection of lignocaine.
C. Intra-arterial administration of papaverine.
D. Interscalene blockade.
E. Intra-arterial heparin.

46. An elderly patient presents for elective total hip replacement. The following statements are appropriate:

A. The analgesic benefits of epidural over systemic analgesia are limited to the early postoperative period.
B. The hip joint is innervated by the femoral, sciatic, obturator, and ilioinguinal nerves.
C. Lumbar plexus block will reliably block the sciatic nerve.
D. A '3-in-1' technique reliably blocks the lumbar plexus.
E. Complete anaesthesia of the hip joint requires sciatic nerve blockade.

47. The following are changes in the body composition and metabolism seen with advancing old age.

A. Body fat mass declines progressively.
B. Total body water increases.
C. Thyroid hormone production decreases.
D. Glucocorticoid secretion is reduced.
E. Glucose tolerance is reduced.

48. Concerning the decontamination of medical equipment:

A. Semi-critical items are those that are in contact with mucous membranes.

B. Glutaraldehyde is a high-level disinfectant.

C. Re-usable laryngeal mask airways can be sterilized using ethylene oxide.

D. Glutaraldehyde cannot be used to disinfect laryngeal mask airways.

E. High-level disinfection is required for critical items.

49. A brain-stem dead patient is undergoing beating-heart organ retrieval. Which of the following intravenous administrations is appropriate:

A. T3.

B. T4.

C. Insulin.

D. Desmopressin.

E. Growth hormone.

50. A patient is admitted with an Addisonian crisis; the following features are expected:

A. Hypertension.

B. Hypokalaemia.

C. Hypernatraemia.

D. Hyperglycaemia.

E. Pyrexia.

51. The following factors increase the risk of electrocution in the operating theatre:

A. Low-frequency alternating current.

B. Earthed patient contact.

C. Capacitative coupling.

D. Line isolation monitor.

E. High humidity.

52. Injury of the ulnar nerve at the elbow results in:

A. Paralysis of the medial half of the flexor digitorum profundus.

B. Inability to flex the wrist joint.

C. Inability to abduct the thumb.

D. A claw hand deformity worse than ulnar lesions at the wrist.

E. Paralysis of the 3rd and 4th lumbricals, causing hyperextension of the metacarpophalangeal joints.

53. A patient with acute intermittent porphyria:

A. May present with mild abdominal pain.

B. Will have autosomal recessive inheritance.

C. Often has psychosis.

D. Has no skin signs.

E. Has increased urinary porphobilinogens.

54. **The following are 'red flag markers ' for serious spinal pathology in patients with chronic back pain:**
    A. Presentation under the age of 30 years.
    B. Long-term steroid therapy.
    C. Constant progressive sacral pain.
    D. History of trauma.
    E. Non-mechanical pain.

55. **There is good evidence for which of the following in management of musculoskeletal chronic back pain:**
    A. Long-term NSAIDS.
    B. Cognitive behavioural therapy.
    C. Graded exercises.
    D. Tricyclic antidepressants.
    E. Transcutaneous electrical nerve stimulation (TENS).

56. **For spinal nerve root pain:**
    A. It is well localized.
    B. It typically radiates below the knee but rarely goes up to the foot.
    C. Nerve conduction studies are useful in the investigation of this condition.
    D. CT is more useful than MRI in its assessment due to suspected spinal stenosis.
    E. Epidural steroids are useful in its management.

57. **Regarding measurement of data in medical statistics:**
    A. Biological data like weight, height, and blood pressure in humans is normally distributed.
    B. The mean, median, and mode values can be different in Gaussian distribution of data.
    C. Interquartile range is a measure of variability for non-parametric data.
    D. Mode is the only means of measuring central tendency in a dataset containing nominal categorical values.
    E. Skewness is the term describing symmetry and peakedness of the curve.

58. **Regarding trigeminal neuralgia:**
    A. Incidence peaks in the fourth decade.
    B. Bilateral pain is not uncommon.
    C. Vascular compression of the nerve is a quite commonly proposed cause.
    D. Carbamazepine is the drug of choice.
    E. Results of surgical interventions are poor in the long term.

59. **Regarding development of chronic post surgical pain (CPSP):**
    A. Presence of acute pre-operative pain before mastectomy is a strong predictor.
    B. Incidence increases with increasing age.
    C. Risk is lower with use of laparoscope than open surgery.
    D. Regional analgesia techniques are effective in prevention of development of CPSP only when continued in the postoperative period.
    E. Pre-operative gabapentin is very effective in its prevention.

60. Regarding the condition fibromyalgia:

    A. It is more common in females.

    B. Incidence increases with age.

    C. Widespread pain should be present for at least 6 months.

    D. At least nine tender points out of 18 need to be elicited for diagnosis.

    E. There is a common association with Sjogren's syndrome and rheumatoid arthritis.

Single Best Answers

1. **A 70-year-old patient is complaining of feeling heaviness in the chest, lightheadedness and breathlessness. She has a blood pressure of 100/60 mmHg, pulse of 35/min and is getting oxygen by mask. What is the most appropriate next management of this patient?**
    A. Call the intensive care team for review.
    B. Give 500 mcg of IV atropine.
    C. Arrange for transcutaneous pacing.
    D. IV isoprenaline 5 mcg/min.
    E. IV adrenaline 2–10 mcg/min.

2. **A 72-year-old male patient is in recovery after an aorto-femoral bypass surgery under general anaesthesia, which was fairly uneventful. His past medical history includes COPD, ischaemic heart disease, hypertension, and extensive atherosclerosis. A few hours in, the recovery nurse calls you to tell that the patient's heart rate has gone up to 140. The 12-lead ECG shows a narrow complex regular tachycardia with minimal new ST segment depression. The patient is talking to you, is feeling fine and does not seem to be in any pain or discomfort. Which of the following is not appropriate for subsequent management of the patient?**
    A. Vagal manoeuvres such as carotid sinus massage.
    B. IV adenosine.
    C. IV β-blockers.
    D. Preparation for synchronized cardioversion.
    E. High flow oxygen.

3. **While doing a routine urology list on the day surgery unit, one of the patients develops pulseless ventricular tachycardia. Which of the following steps is recommended?**
    A. First priority is defibrillation before chest compression.
    B. Initial 2 min of chest compression is recommended before first shock.
    C. The first shock is delivered at 150–360 J biphasic, with escalating energy for subsequent shocks.
    D. The interval between stopping compression and delivering shock should be less than 10 s.
    E. Give both adrenaline and amiodarone after the third shock.

4. **You have just transferred a 10-year-old boy to recovery after tonsillectomy. Within how many hour(s) of the surgery is the highest risk of post-tonsillectomy haemorrhage?**
    A. 1 h.
    B. 6 h.
    C. 12 h.
    D. 24 h.
    E. 48 h.

5. **Which of the following statements is true regarding children with upper respiratory tract infection (URTI):**
    A. Incidence of laryngospasm and bronchospasm is same in children with concurrent URTI compared to children who had URTI 4 weeks ago.
    B. Children of parents who smoke do not have increased risk of adverse airway events.
    C. Children with recent URTI should be postponed for elective surgery.
    D. There is same incidence of adverse airway events if LMA is used instead of endotracheal tube.
    E. The risk is the same if children have non-productive cough compared to those having productive cough.

6. **You have just given a spinal anaesthetic for an elective caesarean section. Which of the following would you find most useful to decrease the incidence of hypotension for caesarean section under regional anaesthesia?**
    A. Preloading with IV fluids.
    B. Metaraminol bolus.
    C. Prophylactic phenylephrine infusion.
    D. Prophylactic ephedrine bolus.
    E. Low-dose spinal.

7. **The recent RCOA audit on central neuraxial blocks (CNBs) has shown that the incidence of major complications after CNBs is rare. However, in which one of the following is the risk of neurological complications highest when doing a CNB?**
    A. Labour combine spinal epidural.
    B. Paediatric patients under general anaesthesia.
    C. General surgical patients.
    D. Chronic pain patients.
    E. Spinal for orthopaedic procedures.

8. **Which one of the following is an absolute contraindication for doing a central neuraxial block during pregnancy?**
    A. Platelet count of 80 000.
    B. Severe PET with BP 160/100.
    C. HELLP syndrome.
    D. Grade 4 anterior placenta praevia.
    E. Type-3 von Willebrand's disease.

9. **All of the following are proven benefits of epidural analgesia except:**
    A. Early hospital discharge.
    B. Decreased incidence of ileus.
    C. Improved quality of analgesia.
    D. Decreased mortality.
    E. Decreased post-operative pulmonary complications.

10. **A 26-year-old primipara in labour had epidural for labour analgesia. Two hours later she was fine but there was sudden foetal bradycardia on the CTG monitor. With regards to foetal resuscitation, which of the following is the least effective measure?**
    A. Stopping the epidural infusion.
    B. Subcutaneous terbutaline.
    C. Intravenous fluids.
    D. Oxygen by mask.
    E. Lateral position.

11. **An 83-year-old man who slipped and had fracture neck of femur. Based on the NCEPOD recommendations regarding the management of fracture neck of femur in the elderly, the following will improve the outcome except:**
    A. Spinal anaesthesia over GA.
    B. Pre-operative regional analgesia.
    C. Regular input from the geriatric medicine specialists.
    D. Careful fluid management.
    E. Adequate nutritional support.

12. **You have given an interscalene block for a patient undergoing shoulder surgery. However, about 30 min after the block, the patient finds that his voice is getting hoarse and he is finding it difficult to speak. Which of the following is the most likely cause?**
    A. Cervical sympathetic block.
    B. Phrenic nerve block.
    C. LA toxicity.
    D. Horner's syndrome.
    E. Recurrent laryngeal nerve block.

13. **A 35-year-old patient with idiopathic cardiomyopathy is pregnant. When is the highest risk of her developing congestive cardiac failure?**
    A. Between 30 and 32 weeks' gestation.
    B. During first stage of labour.
    C. At term, near 40 weeks' gestation.
    D. Immediately after third stage of labour.
    E. At the peak of uterine contractions in the second stage of labour.

14. **A 25-year-old primipara has an accidental dural tap (ADT) with a 16-G tuohy needle while the anaesthetist was attempting labour epidural analgesia. A day after the ADT, the patient is complaining of severe positional frontal and occipital headache. Which of the following is not appropriate for management?**
    A. Prophylactic bed rest.
    B. Simple analgesics.
    C. Caffeine.
    D. Liberal fluid intake.
    E. Epidural blood patch.

15. **A 75-year-old patient is to undergo an emergency laparotomy for sub-acute bowel obstruction. He suffers from chronic atrial fibrillation and is on warfarin. The patient's INR is 2.0 on admission. What would be the best course of his management?**
    A. Wait for the INR to correct on its own.
    B. Carry on with the surgery with FFP transfused intra-operatively.
    C. Correct INR pre-operatively with FFP.
    D. Correct INR pre-operatively with vitamin K.
    E. Correct INR pre-operatively with vitamin K and prothrombin concentrate.

16. **A 35-year-old young man is sedated and ventilated in critical care following a polytrauma. The plan is to facilitate weaning, and it requires tracheostomy. He is currently on haemofiltration on heparin for renal replacement. However, his platelet count is 70 000 and he is not bleeding. What would be the safest way to manage this situation?**
    A. Give platelet transfusion prior to tracheostomy while continuing haemofiltration.
    B. Do the tracheostomy anyway while continuing haemofiltration with prostacyclin.
    C. Stop the haemofilter and then do the tracheostomy after 3–4 h.
    D. Wait for the haemofilter to clot and then do the tracheostomy without any platelet transfusion, but having it available if needed.
    E. Bedside percutaneous tracheostomy by experienced intensivist.

17. **You are called to the A&E department to assist in the resuscitation of a patient involved in a high-impact traffic accident. The patient is quite hypotensive and bleeding. Which of the following is not appropriate regarding the management?**
    A. Warming the IV fluids.
    B. Pro-active maintenance of normal blood pressure.
    C. Direct haemorrhage control.
    D. Early use of clotting factors and platelets.
    E. Use of near-patient testing for coagulopathy.

18. **An immuno-compromised patient is undergoing revision hip surgery and is worried about the risk of infection from blood products. Which of the following blood components carries the highest risk of bacterial contamination?**
    A. Platelets.
    B. Red cells.
    C. FFP.
    D. Cryoprecipitate.
    E. Fibrinogen concentrate.

19. **A 55-year-old woman is scheduled for total knee replacement. Her only medical condition is hypertension for which she takes atenolol 50 mg. She is consented for awake femoral-nerve block, followed by general anaesthesia. Once the nerve was located 0.5% levo-bupivacaine 20 mL was administered. Suddenly she developed seizures and subsequent cardiorespiratory arrest. Which of the following is not appropriate initial management?**
    A. Call for help and initiate chest compression.
    B. Secure the airway and ventilate with 100% oxygen.
    C. Give 20% intralipid 1.5 mg/mL stat.
    D. Avoid lidocaine as anti-arrhythmic.
    E. Drawing blood for analysis.

20. **Intrathecal diamorphine in a dose of 0.3–0.4 mg is useful for post-operative analgesia after caesarean section, but which of the following is the most common side effect of using it?**
    A. Itching.
    B. Nausea.
    C. Respiratory depression.
    D. Sedation.
    E. Urinary retention.

21. **Which of the following drugs is present in breast milk in such a significant amount that it is recommended to stop it in breastfeeding mothers?**
    A. β-blockers.
    B. Chloramphenicol.
    C. Amiodarone.
    D. Carbamezepine.
    E. Cephalosporins.

22. **A 28-year-old parturient has severe pre-eclamptic toxemia (PET) and is on the PET protocol. Which one of the following is least likely to predict the severity of her condition?**
    A. Raised blood pressure (>160/110 mmHg).
    B. Raised uric acid (>0.5 mmol/L).
    C. Epigastric pain.
    D. Oliguria (<500 mL/24 h).
    E. Low platelets(<100 × 10^9 /L).

23. **Laryngeal mask airway (LMA) is now used more commonly then endotracheal tube while providing general anaesthesia worldwide. Which of the following statements regarding its use is not correct?**
    A. There is high incidence of aspiration when LMA is used in full-stomach patients.
    B. The LMA tip fits the oesophageal inlet but does not seal it completely.
    C. LMA can be used in prone patients for minor surgery.
    D. Aspiration is more common with LMA when positive pressure ventilation is used than in spontaneously breathing patients.
    E. It can be safely used in cardiopulmonary resuscitation as an alternative to endotracheal tube.

24. **A young patient is ventilated in intensive care for 2 weeks with a nasal endotracheal tube. He now develops high fever and raised white cell count of 20 000/mm³. He also indicates a constant headache. The most likely cause is:**
    A. Rhinovirus infection.
    B. Meningitis.
    C. Retropharyngeal abscess.
    D. Maxillary bacterial sinusitis.
    E. Nasal septum fracture.

25. **There is a global epidemic of obesity, which means that more and more patients coming for surgery will be obese. Which of the following statements regarding obesity is incorrect?**
    A. Angina rarely presents in morbidly obese patients.
    B. Moderate obesity (BMI 30–40) is associated with increased risk of complications in the peri-operative period.
    C. The risks are related to the pattern of body fat distribution.
    D. The harmful effects of obesity are mainly on the cardiovascular system.
    E. Male type (android) fat distribution is associated with increased cardiovascular risks.

26. A 5-year-old child who weighs 20 kg presents for elective squint-correction surgery at 08:00 hrs. The child has been fasting from midnight. What is the amount of fluid the child should receive in the first hour of surgery?

    A. 150 mL.
    B. 200 mL.
    C. 300 mL.
    D. 400 mL.
    E. 500 mL.

27. A 30-year-old woman at 28 weeks of gestation is referred to the anaesthetic clinic due to her severe asthma. She is planning to have normal vaginal delivery with the help of labour epidural. With regards to the effect of labour epidural on the respiratory function, which of the following statements is true?

    A. There is increase in peak expiratory flow rate and a decrease in FVC.
    B. There is increase in peak expiratory flow rate and FVC.
    C. There is a decrease in peak expiratory flow rate and an increase in FVC.
    D. There is no change in peak expiratory flow rate and FVC.
    E. There is increase in peak expiratory flow rate and a decrease in FVC.

28. A 49-year-old woman with a history of brittle asthma has come to A&E with severe respiratory distress. Which of the following features would worry you the most?

    A. Respiratory rate of 36 breaths/min.
    B. Widespread wheeze, audible without stethoscope.
    C. PaO_2 of 8.0 kPa.
    D. $PaCO_2$ of 6.8 kPa.
    E. SVT on ECG.

29. A 75-year-old patient is on your list for elective total hip replacement. She is on aspirin, started by her GP, but otherwise very fit with no co-morbidities. She has no particular preference for regional or general anaesthesia and leaves the decision to you. Based on the current literature evidence, which is the most appropriate anaesthetic technique for her?

    A. Spinal anaesthesia with intrathecal opioid.
    B. GA with lumbar plexus block.
    C. GA with fascia iliaca block.
    D. Spinal with lumbar plexus block.
    E. GA with lumbar plexus and sacral plexus block.

30. **You have been called to A&E to assess a patient who has been buried under a collapsed building for over 24 h. The patient is conscious and haemodynamically stable. However, his urine looks dark and you suspect rhabdomyolysis. Which of the following statements about rhabdomyolysis is incorrect?**

    A. Rhabdomyolysis describes the destruction or disintegration of striated muscle and it is an important cause of acute renal failure.

    B. Creatinine kinase concentration is the most sensitive and useful indicator of muscle injury in rhabdomyolysis.

    C. The most important intervention is early aggressive crystalloid fluid resuscitation.

    D. Life-threatening hyperkalaemia is a common cause of death and must be treated promptly.

    E. Myoglobin-induced renal failure has a poor prognosis.

1. Answers: T F T T F

Transdermal drug delivery is defined as the non-invasive delivery of medications through the skin surface. The advantages are more controlled absorption, more uniform plasma drug concentrations, improved drug bioavailability and by avoidance of hepatic first pass metabolism, enzymatic deactivation, and pH-associated deactivation. The disadvantages are local irritation, skin sensitization, unreliability in shocked patients, and the cost of the route of administration.

Absorption rate is proportional to the diffusion coefficient, the constant concentration of drug in the patch, the partition coefficient between the skin and the bathing medium, and the skin thickness. Transdermal drug delivery is improved with molecular weight <500 Da, affinity for both the lipophilic and hydrophilic phases, low melting point and non-ionic ratio of drug, high potency, and short half-life of the drug.

Transdermal preparations are common use among the general public, especially in the chronic pain syndromes population, and anaesthetists should be aware of the limitations and conversions for safe management of these patients within the acute setting.

Bajaj S, Whiteman A, Brandner B. Transdermal drug delivery in pain management. *Contin Educ Anaesth Crit Care Pain* 2011; 11(2): 39–43.

2. Answers: F F T F T

Beclomethasone dipropionate is a steroid used in the prophylaxis of bronchial asthma to prevent bronchospasm by reducing airway inflammation. It does not have any role in an acute attack of bronchospasm. Its dose is 100–800 mcg inhaled 6–12-hourly.

As the drug is poorly soluble, the nebulized preparation is very inefficient for drug delivery and therefore not used. It has only glucorticoid effects and is devoid of any mineralocorticoid effects. Systemic absorption is very low with inhaled dose. so it does not cause HPA suppression. Hoarse voice and oral candidiasis can occur with high doses.

British National Formulary, 61st edn. British Medical Association and Royal Pharmaceutical Society of Great Britain, 2011: Section 3.2.

Yentis SM, Hirsch NP, Smith GB. *A–Z of Anaesthesia and Intensive Care*, Butterworth Heinemann, 2004: p. 58.

3. Answers: F F T F T

Carbamazepine is an anti-convulsant drug used in the treatment of all types of epilepsy except petit mal. It has fewer side effects than phenytoin and has a wider therapeutic index. It is also used in pain management, e.g. in trigeminal neuralgia.

Dosage is 100–200 mg in divided doses of up to 2.0 g per day. It can be given rectally as well. It causes induction of the cytochrome p-450 hepatic enzyme system and can reduce the effects of other drugs such as warfarin. It is contraindicated in atrio-ventricular conduction defects and porphyria.

British National Formulary, 61st edn. British Medical Association and Royal Pharmaceutical Society of Great Britain, 2011: Section 4.8.1.

Yentis SM, Hirsch NP, Smith GB. *A–Z of Anaesthesia and Intensive Care*, Butterworth Heinemann, 2004: p. 85.

4. Answers: T F F F T

Digoxin is a cardiac glycoside used in the treatment of supraventricular arrhythmias, especially in atrial fibrillation for rate control. It can be used both IV and orally. It acts by inhibiting Na^+/K^+ pump and indirectly increasing the intracellular Ca^{2+} concentration. It has a large volume of distribution (700 L). Although it improves short-term cardiac contractility, there are no long-term mortality benefits. It slows the heart rate by an indirect effect via the vagus nerve, as well as a direct effect on AV node conduction.

Side effects are more likely in the presence of hypokalaemia, hypomagnesaemia, and hypercalcaemia.

British National Formulary, 61st edn. British Medical Association and Royal Pharmaceutical Society of Great Britain, 2011: Section 2.1.1.

Yentis SM, Hirsch NP, Smith GB. *A–Z of Anaesthesia and Intensive Care*, Butterworth Heinemann, 2004: p. 91.

5. Answers: T F F F T

Etomidate is a carboxylated imidazole compound presented in 35% propylene glycol. It is used as an IV induction agent for haemodynamically compromised patients as it causes less hypotension and less respiratory depression. It reduces cerebral blood flow and intra-ocular pressure. There is increased incidence of nausea and vomiting. Premixing with 1–2 mL of 1% lidocaine can reduce pain on injection. Intravenous induction dose is 0.2–0.3 mg/kg.

It interferes with adrenal corticosteroid synthesis by inhibiting the enzymes 11β-hydroxylase and 17α-hydroxylase, even after a single dose use.

British National Formulary, 61st edn. British Medical Association and Royal Pharmaceutical Society of Great Britain, 2011: Section 15.1.1.

Yentis SM, Hirsch NP, Smith GB. *A–Z of Anaesthesia and Intensive Care*, Butterworth Heinemann, 2004: p. 190.

6. Answers: F T T T T

Helium is an inert gas, which has the same viscosity as oxygen. It is stored as a gas in brown cylinders at pressure of 137 bar. Helium–oxygen mixture (Heliox) is stored in white cylinders with white/brown shoulders. The ratio of helium:oxygen is 79:21. FiO_2 is a limiting factor when using Heliox mixtures for patients with upper-airway obstruction. Increasing FiO_2 to more than 28% negates the improvement in flow by because of the decreased density of Heliox.

Heliox's density is less than that of nitrogen. It converts turbulent flow into laminar flow by reducing the Reynolds number (which is dependent on density), so it decreases the work of breathing in patients with upper airway obstruction when the flow is turbulent. However, in lower airway obstruction, for example bronchospasm, the benefit of its use is debatable as the airflow is already laminar.

The voice is changed when helium is inhaled because of its lower density compared to nitrogen in air. This results in a laminar flow through the vocal cords instead of the usual turbulent flow, producing a high-pitched squeaky voice.

Yentis SM, Hirsch NP, Smith GB. *A–Z of Anaesthesia and Intensive Care*, Butterworth Heinemann, 2004: p. 243.

7. Answers: F T T F F

Morphine causes miosis by a central effect. Timolol is a ⊠-blocker and miotic used in the treatment of glaucoma. Cocaine, phenylephrine, and amitryptalline are sympathomimetics and therefore cause mydriasis.

Aitkenhead AR, Smith G. *Textbook of Anaesthesia*, 5th edn. Churchill Livingstone, 2006: p. 581.

8. Answers: F T F F T

Prilocaine is an amide local anaesthetic, which is slower in onset than lidocaine but lasts 1.5 times longer and is less toxic. It undergoes both hepatic and renal metabolism. It is used for infiltration, nerve blocks, and IV RA. It is also used for topical anaesthesia of skin in the form of EMLA cream in combination with lidocaine. Maximum safe dose is 5 mg/kg alone and 8 mg/kg with adrenaline. It causes methaemoglobinaemia if the maximum dose is exceeded because of its metabolite, ortho-toulidine.

British National Formulary, 61st edn. British Medical Association and Royal Pharmaceutical Society of Great Britain, 2011: Section 15.2.

Yentis SM, Hirsch NP, Smith GB. *A–Z of Anaesthesia and Intensive Care*, Butterworth Heinemann, 2004: p. 429.

9. Answers: T F F F F

Ergometrine is an ergot alkaloid used as an uterotonic. It possibly acts on serotonin, dopamine, and α-adrenergic receptors. Although the exact mechanism of ergometrine on uterine contractions is not known, it acts as a partial agonist on serotonin receptors, which are present on the myometrium. It acts on both upper and lower uterine segments to cause a sustained uterine contraction. It increases the strength, duration, and frequency of uterine contractions. Normally, used i.m. in a dose of 500 mcg, it can be used IV very cautiously during massive PPH. Care should be taken while using it in coronary disease patients and mild hypertensives. It should be avoided in severe cardiac diseases and eclampsia/PET patients. An aggravating role of ergometrine-induced vasoconstriction has been suggested in aspiration pneumonia in the foetus.

British National Formulary, 61st edn. British Medical Association and Royal Pharmaceutical Society of Great Britain, 2011: Section 9.8.2.

Yentis SM, Hirsch NP, Smith GB. *A–Z of Anaesthesia and Intensive Care*, Butterworth Heinemann, 2004: p. 188.

10. Answers: F T F T F

As people age, there are significant changes in their renal physiology. Essentially, this manifests as globally reduced physiological reserve and subsequent more rapid deterioration in the event of physiological derangement.

The glomerulo-tubular functional balance is well preserved. The excretion of an ammonium chloride load requires almost three times as long as in the young adult. Declining muscle mass reduces creatinine load, and tubular secretion of creatinine is increased. Functional reserve is limited.

Muravchick S. Anesthesia for the elderly. In: Miller RD, (ed) *Anesthesia*, 5th edn. Churchill Livingstone, 2000: 2143–44.

11. Answers: F F T T T

The MAGPIE study has demonstrated that administration of magnesium sulphate to women with pre-eclampsia reduces the risk of an eclamptic seizure. Women allocated magnesium sulphate had a 58% lower risk of an eclamptic seizure (95% CI: 40–71%). The relative risk reduction was similar regardless of the severity of pre-eclampsia. More women need to be treated when pre-eclampsia is not severe (109) to prevent one seizure when compared with severe pre-eclampsia (63). If magnesium sulphate is given, it should be continued for 24 h following delivery or 24 h after the last seizure, whichever is the later, unless there is a clinical reason to continue. When magnesium sulphate is given, regular assessment of the urine output, maternal reflexes, respiratory rate, and oxygen saturation is important. Somnolence, slurred speech, and blurred vision are also features of magnesium toxicity.

Magnesium toxicity is unlikely with these regimens and levels do not need to be routinely measured. Magnesium sulphate is mostly excreted in the urine. Urine output should be closely observed and if it becomes reduced to below 20 mL/h the magnesium infusion should be halted. Magnesium toxicity can be assessed by clinical assessment as it causes a loss of deep tendon reflexes and respiratory depression. If there is a loss of deep tendon reflexes, the magnesium sulphate infusion should be halted. Calcium gluconate 1 g (10 mL) over 10 min can be given if there is concern over respiratory depression.

Hypertension in Pregnancy. NICE guideline (CG107), 2010; http://publications.nice.org.uk/hypertension-in-pregnancy-cg107.

12. Answers: T T T F T

Cyanide poisoning results from industrial accidents, smoke inhalation, prolonged use of sodium nitroprusside, etc. It causes inhibition of the mitochondrial enzyme, cytochrome oxidase, interrupting cellular respiration. Tissues are unable to utilize the delivered oxygen and therefore the arterio-venous oxygen difference is reduced. Metabolic acidosis and increased lactate results from tissue hypoxia. The symptoms are non-specific, and include dizziness, headache, confusion, etc. Cyanide is slowly converted to thiocyanate by the liver enzyme, rhodanase.

Treatment consists of supportive measures and the specific antidote, dicobalt edentate, which combines with cyanide to form inert compounds. Sodium thiosulfate, sodium nitrite, and hydroxycobalamine are also used.

Yentis SM, Hirsch NP, Smith GB. *A–Z of Anaesthesia and Intensive Care*, Butterworth Heinemann, 2004: p. 147.

13. Answers: F T T F T

The choice of IV fluids in resuscitation is contentious, as no single study has yet been assessed for mortality outcome. In rapid major blood loss either crystalloid or colloid is suitable to maintain organ perfusion in the short term. For ongoing losses, colloids offer faster, longer-lasting resuscitation with less volume of infusate. No single colloid solution has been proven to be safer than others. The aim is to restore adequate organ perfusion, avoiding haemodilution, coagulopathy, and hypothermia.

5% dextrose and 4% dextrose with 0.18% saline has the lowest pH (4) amongst commonly used IV fluids. Giving 5% dextrose is like giving free water, as the dextrose is quickly metabolized in the RBCs and the free water then redistributes in the ratio of two-thirds intracellularly and one third extracellularly.

Normal saline (pH 5) can cause hyperchloremic metabolic acidosis if used in large amount.

Hartmanns solution is a balanced salt solution and is the first line for peri-operative fluid replacement.

Self R, Walker D, Mythen M. Blood products and fluid therapy. In: Allman KG, Wilson IH (eds), *Oxford Handbook of Anaesthesia*, 2nd edn. Oxford University Press, 2004: p. 1018–23.

Yentis SM, Hirsch NP, Smith GB. *A–Z of Anaesthesia and Intensive Care*, Butterworth Heinemann, 2004: p. 286.

14. Answers: T F T F F

Malignant hyperthermia (MH) is a pharmacogenetic disease of skeletal muscle induced by exposure to certain anaesthetic agents, such as suxamethonium and all of the halogenated volatile anaesthetic agents. It is inherited as an autosomal dominant condition and caused by loss of normal Ca^{2+} homeostasis at some point along the excitation–contraction coupling process on exposure to triggering agents.

The most likely site is the triadic junction between the T tubule, involving the voltage sensor of the dihydropyridine receptor (DHPR), and the sarcoplasmic reticulum (SR), involving the Ca^{2+} efflux channel of the ryanodine receptor (RYR1).

Clinical diagnosis can be difficult, as the presentation of MH varies. Masseter spasm can be the first sign. Other signs are those of increased metabolism, like tachycardia, dysrhythmias, increased CO_2 production, metabolic acidosis, pyrexia, and DIC. It can be a florid dramatic life-threatening event or have an insidious onset. It rarely develops 2–3 days postoperatively, with massive myoglobinuria and/or renal failure due to severe rhabdomyolysis.

Treatment consists of supportive management and IV Dantrolene 1–2 mg/kg up to 10 mg/kg. Mortality was 60–70% before Dantrolene was available but with the use of Dantrolene, mortality is less than 5%.

Halsall J. Neurological and muscular disorders. In: Allman KG, Wilson IH (eds), *Oxford Handbook of Anaesthesia*, 2nd edn. Oxford University Press, 2004: Chapter 11: p. 260.

Yentis SM, Hirsch NP, Smith GB. *A–Z of Anaesthesia and Intensive Care*, Butterworth Heinemann, 2004: p. 329.

15. Answers: T T F T T

Cardiac output is the volume of blood pumped in a minute (about 5 L/min in a normal adult). Distribution of normal CO in the resting state is as follows (figures are approximate):

- heart: 5%
- brain: 14%
- muscle: 20%
- kidneys: 22%
- liver: 25%
- rest of the body: 14%.

A number of vital organs, such as the brain, heart, liver, and kidneys, auto-regulate their blood flow by various mechanisms, one of which is postulated to be the effects of end products of metabolism, which alter the vessel diameter.

Yentis SM, Hirsch NP, Smith GB. *A–Z of Anaesthesia and Intensive Care*, Butterworth Heinemann, 2004: p. 92.

16. Answers: F F T F T

There are two types of cholinesterase enzymes: acetylcholinesterase and pseudocholinesterase (also called plasma cholinesterase), both of which hydrolyse acetylcholine. Pseudocholinesterase is a circulating enzyme that is synthesized in the liver and released in the plasma.

Actylcholinesterase is present in the brain, liver, kidneys, RBCs, and in the nerve endings and neuromuscular (NM) junction. Almost 70% of suxamethonium given IV is hydrolysed by pseudocholinesterase in the plasma within 1 min, and less than 1% actually reaches the NM junctions. The normal enzyme is present in 94% of the general population and the genotype is homozygote. The enzyme has a dibucaine number (DN) of 75–85 and a fluoride number (FN) of 60.

Abnormal enzyme causes prolonged paralysis after suxamethonium administration, which is caused by abnormal autosomal recessive genes. These genes are mainly of three types:

- Atypical gene: heterozygotes will not be sensitive to suxamethonium unless other contributing factors (e.g. concurrent illness, anticholinesterase administration) are present. Homozygotes (DN 15–25) have a prevalence of 1:3000 and may remain paralysed for 2–3 h after administration of a clinical dose of suxamethonium.
- The fluoride-resistant gene: homozygotes are much rarer (1:150 000) and are moderately sensitive to suxamethonium.
- The silent gene: heterozygotes exhibit a prolongation of the action of suxamethonium, but homozgotes (1:10 000) are very sensitive and develop prolonged apnoea. Usually 3–4 h but may last as long as 24 h.

Pseudocholinesterase metabolizes mivacurium and cocaine, and partially metabolizes esmolol, remifentanil, and diamorphine.

Saddler J. Neuromuscular blockers: reversal and monitoring. In: *Oxford Handbook of Anaesthesia*, 2nd edn. Oxford University Press, 2004: p. 994.

Yentis SM, Hirsch NP, Smith GB. *A–Z of Anaesthesia and Intensive Care*, Butterworth Heinemann, 2004: p. 117.

17. Answers: F T T T F

Carotid bodies are small (2–3 mg) structures, which act as peripheral chemoreceptors involved in chemical control of breathing. They are situated above the carotid bifurcation on each side. They contain glomus cells of neuro-ectodermal origin and glial cells. Afferents pass through the glossopharyngeal nerve to the brain stem.

The rate of discharge from carotid bodies is increased by a decrease in oxygen delivery (reduced arterial PO_2 or reduced cardiac output). It also responds to impaired utilization of oxygen as in cyanide poisoning, rise in PCO_2, or acidosis. They do not respond to decreased oxygen delivery resulting from anaemia and carbon monoxide poisoning. Carotid bodies receive the highest blood flow per 100 g tissue in the body and in fact all its oxygen requirement is met by dissolved oxygen.

Yentis SM, Hirsch NP, Smith GB. *A–Z of Anaesthesia and Intensive Care*, Butterworth Heinemann, 2004: p. 101.

18. Answers: T F T T F

For a lay person, compression-only CPR is better than doing nothing at all, but anyone with a duty to respond should peform CPR with a 30:2 compression-to-ventilation ratio.

In an unwitnessed arrest in the community, the paramedics should start chest compression while defibrillator is being connected and charged but, in the new 2010 guidelines, a specific duration of chest compression is no longer recommended, therefore the shock should be given as soon as the defibrillator is ready.

In the new 2010 guidelines, Amiodarone is given along with the adrenaline after the third shock for a shockable rhythm arrest.

Good quality chest compression and early defibrillation are the only two interventions that have strong evidence in improving mortality outcomes.

The most common cause of arrest in the community is shockable rhythm (VF/pulseless VT). In hospitals, the most common cause is pulseless electrical activity (PEA).

Jewkes F, Nolan J. *Resuscitation Guidelines 2010*. Resuscitation Council (UK), 2010. http://www.resus.org.uk/pages/guide.htm.

19. Answers: T T T T F

The most common cause of regular narrow complex tachycardia is sinus tachycardia, for which the underlying cause should be treated. Narrow complex tachycardia in the absence of adverse features should be initially treated with vagal manoeuvres. If persisting, IV adenosine should be given as a fast bolus up to three times (6 mg + 12 mg + 12 mg). Adenosine is contraindicated in asthmatics. Verapmil 2.5–5 mg over 2 min can be considered if there is no response to adenosine.

Narrow complex tachycardia should be treated with synchronized shock if there is evidence of haemodynamic compromise. However, if pulseless, it should be treated as if it were PEA: CPR should be started and 1 mg IV adrenaline should be given.

Pitcher D, Perkins G. Peri-arrest arrhythmias. In: *Resuscitation Guidelines 2010*. Resuscitation Council (UK), 2010: p. 81. http://www.resus.org.uk/pages/guide.htm.

20. Answers: F F F F T

Tracheal drugs are no longer recommended. Give drugs by intra-osseous route if IV access is not available. Atropine is no longer recommended for asystole. Adrenaline 1 mg along with CPR is the treatment of asystole. Reversible factors should also be ruled out and treated at the same time. In the 2010 guidelines, there is less emphasis on early tracheal intubation unless someone with the relevant skills is present. Supraglottic airway like LMA, I Gel, or bag and mask ventilation are acceptable until such a skilled person arrives. Capnography is recommended to confirm and monitor tracheal tube placement, quality of CPR, and to check for reliable return of spontaneous circulation. Precordial thump has been de-emphasized because of lack of evidence of its efficacy.

Soar J, Nolan J. Summary of changes In: *Resuscitation Council (UK) 2010 Guidelines*, p. 10. http://www. resus.org.uk/pages/guide.htm.

21. Answers: F T F T T

Table 2.1 Investigations used to differentiate between pre-renal azotaemia and acute renal failure

Investigation	Pre-renal azotaemia	Renal failure
Specific gravity	>1.020	<1.010
Urine osmolality (mosmol/kg)	>500	<350
Urine sodium (mmol/L)	<20	>40
Urine/plasma osmolality ratio	>2	<1.1
Urine/plasma urea ratio	>20	<10
Urine/plasma creatinine ratio	>40	<20
Fractional sodium excretion (%)	<1	>1
Renal failure index	<1	>1

Renal failure index is ratio of urine sodium to urine/plasma creatinine ratio (see Table 2.1).

Yentis SM, Hirsch NP, Smith GB. *A–Z of Anaesthesia and Intensive Care*, Butterworth Heinemann, 2004: p. 45.

22. Answers: T T F T T

Xenon is an inert gas making up less than 0.00001% of air. It has anaesthetic properties, with a MAC of 63% and blood–gas partition coefficient of 0.14 (which is the least amongst anaesthetic agents), resulting in an extremely rapid uptake and washout. It has a respiratory depressant effect but no cardiovascular effects. Its lack of any adverse environmental effects, unlike nitrous oxide, has led to extensive investigations into xenon despite its high cost. Its radioactive isotope Xe^{133} is used in estimations of organ blood flow and in ventilation perfusion scans.

Yentis SM, Hirsch NP, Smith GB. *A–Z of Anaesthesia and Intensive Care*, Butterworth Heinemann, 2004: p. 549.

Jordan BD, Wright E. Xenon as an anesthetic agent. *AANA J* 2010; 78(5): 387–92.

23. Answers: F T F T T

Laudanosine is a tertiary amine breakdown product of atracurium by Hofmann degradation. Being a tertiary amine, it can cross the blood/brain barrier more easily. The compound is epileptogenic, with increased EEG activity in animals. The clinical significance of laudanosine in humans is debatable.

Its half-life of 2–3 h is doubled in renal failure. Blood levels in humans, even after several days' infusion of atracurium in patients with renal and liver failure, rarely rises to clinically significant levels. Recently, laudanosine has been found to have some analgesic effects in animals and to interact with central GABA, acetylcholine, and opioid receptors.

Yentis SM, Hirsch NP, Smith GB. *A–Z of Anaesthesia and Intensive Care*, Butterworth Heinemann, 2004: p. 315.

24. Answers: T T F T T

Sickle cell disease (SCD) is an autosomal recessive condition caused by substitution of glutamic acid by valine on the sixth position of the β chain of haemoglobin. It presents in the homozygous state (HbSS: sickle cell anaemia), the heterozygous state (HbAS: sickle cell trait), or in combination with another haemoglobin β chain abnormality such as haemoglobin C (HbSC disease) or haemoglobin D (HbSD) disease. It is thought to have originated as a spontaneous genetic mutation in Africa, with subsequent selection owing to the relative resistance of sickle cell trait (HbAS) against malaria.

Deoxygenated HbSS polymerizes and precipitates within RBCs at PaO_2 5–6 kPa, causing sickling of the RBCs, which are then haemolysed in the spleen as well as causing infarcts in various organs because of increased blood viscosity and impaired flow.

Sickle cell trait (HbAS) polymerizes at a much lower PaO_2 of 2.5–4 kPa, and therefore has less of a sickling tendency. Exposure to cold, dehydration, and acidosis also increases sickling.

The O_2 affinity of dissolved HbSS is normal.

Exchange transfusions have a role in some vaso-occlusive crises (acute chest syndrome, stroke). Always discuss with a haematologist. For patients with high perioperative risk, transfusing to achieve an HbS level of <30% may decrease complications but is controversial.

Other peri-operative precautions include avoiding hypoxia, dehydration, hypothermia, acidosis, and hypercarbia.

Purday J. Haematological disorders. In: Allman KG, Wilson IH (eds), *Oxford Handbook of Anaesthesia*, 2nd edn. Oxford University Press, 2004: pp. 200–2.

Yentis SM, Hirsch NP, Smith GB. *A–Z of Anaesthesia and Intensive Care*, Butterworth Heinemann, 2004: p. 471.

25. Answers: **T F F T F**

The recurrent laryngeal nerve, which is a branch of the vagus, supplies all the muscles of the larynx except the cricothyroid. It carries sensory afferent fibres from below the vocal cords. It also supplies the inferior constrictor muscle via the pharyngeal plexus and gives branches to the cardiac plexus as well.

Damage to the recurrent laryngeal nerve can occur during thyroid surgery or due to invasive neck tumour or neck trauma. If unilateral it causes hoarseness but if bilateral can cause respiratory distress.

The posterior two-thirds of the tongue is supplied by glossopharyngeal nerve.

Yentis SM, Hirsch NP, Smith GB. *A–Z of Anaesthesia and Intensive Care*, Butterworth Heinemann, 2004: p. 314.

26. Answers: **T T T F T**

Myasthenia gravis is characterized by muscle weakness, which is typically worse on exertion and improves with rest. It is caused by autoimmune disruption of postsynaptic acetylcholine receptors at the neuromuscular junction, with up to 80% of functional receptors lost. Auto-antibodies are detectable in up to 90% of patients. The disease may occur at any age but is most common in young adult females. It may be associated with thymus hyperplasia, with 15% of affected patients having thymomas. Symptoms are usually symmetrical and range from mild ptosis to life-threatening bulbar palsy and respiratory insufficiency. Management is usually with oral anticholinesterase medication, with or without steroid therapy. Severe disease may require immunosuppressant therapy, plasmapheresis, or immunoglobulin infusion with positive-pressure ventilation.

Myasthenic crisis can be precipitated by drug omission, infection, stress, pregnancy, and drugs such as aminoglycosides.

Anaesthetic considerations

All patients with myasthenia are sensitive to the effects of non-depolarizing muscle relaxants. Plasmapheresis depletes plasma esterase levels, prolonging the effect of suxamethonium, mivacurium, ester-linked local anaesthetics, etc.

Suxamethonium may have an altered effect—patients may be resistant to depolarization due to reduced receptor activity, requiring increased dose. This, in conjunction with treatment-induced plasma esterase deficiency, leads to an increased risk of non-depolarizing (Phase II) block.

Teasdale A. Neurological and muscular disorders. In: Allman KG, Wilson IH (eds), *Oxford Handbook of Anaesthesia*, 2nd edn. Oxford University Press, 2004: pp. 246–51.

Yentis SM, Hirsch NP, Smith GB. *A–Z of Anaesthesia and Intensive Care*, Butterworth Heinemann, 2004: p. 351.

27. Answers: **T F F F F**

William Thomas Morton was the first person to give public demonstration of successful anaesthesia using ether, at Massachusetts General Hospital, Boston on 16 October 1846.

Albert Niemann, a German chemist, first isolated cocaine in 1859 but it was used for the first spinal anaesthetic by August Bier in 1889.

Volwiler and Tabern from Abbott Laboratories first discovered thiopentone in the early 1930s. However, Ralph Waters, and later John Lundy, first used thiopentone in humans in 1934. Thiopentone fell in to disrepute after being attributed to causing many deaths when used in the patients in shock after the Pearl Harbour attacks in 1941.

Joseph Priestley discovered oxygen, while Humphrey Davy discovered nitrous oxide.

John Snow used chloroform for the labours of Queen Victoria in 1853 and 1857.

Wilkinson DJ. *History of Anaesthesia*. RCOA website. http://www.rcoa.ac.uk/index.asp?PageID=200.

28. Answers: T F T T T

Fat embolism syndrome is associated with trauma or surgery and has an extremely variable presentation; diagnosis is often made by exclusion. Although embolization of fat occurs frequently, the syndrome is comparatively rare (1–3% of single long-bone fractures).

Its features (as defined by Gurd) are:

- major
  - ◆ respiratory symptoms: tachypnoea, dyspnoea, bilateral crepitations, haemoptysis, diffuse shadowing on CXR
  - ◆ neurological signs: confusion, drowsiness
  - ◆ petechial rash.
- minor
  - ◆ tachycardia
  - ◆ retinal change: fat or petechiae
  - ◆ pyrexia
  - ◆ renal: oliguria or anuria.

Laboratory test findings show thrombocytopenia, raised ESR, and fat macroglobulaemia.

Treatments are:

- early resuscitation and stabilization are vital
- early O_2 therapy may prevent onset of syndrome
- may require mechanical ventilation (10–40% of patients)
- steroid use is controversial
- FES usually resolves within 7 days.

Worms R, Griffiths R. Orthopaedic surgery. In: Allman KG, Wilson IH (eds), *Oxford Handbook of Anaesthesia*, 2nd edn. Oxford University Press, 2004: p. 447.

Yentis SM, Hirsch NP, Smith GB. *A–Z of Anaesthesia and Intensive Care*, Butterworth Heinemann, 2004: p. 203.

29. Answers: F T F T T

Potassium is the principal intracellular cation, present in a concentration of 135–150 mmol/L. Plasma concentration is 3.5–5 mmol/L. Daily requirement is about 1 mmol/kg/day. Total body content is 3200 mmol, of which 90% is intracellular, 7.5% is within bone and dense connective tissue, and 2.5% in extracellular fluids. 90% of it is easily exchangeable. It is important in the maintenance of cell membrane potential and the generation of action potential.

Potassium filtered in the nephrons is mostly reabsorbed in the proximal convoluted tubule. It is secreted in the distal tubule under the effect of aldosterone hormone, in exchange for sodium and hydrogen ions.

Yentis SM, Hirsch NP, Smith GB. *A–Z of Anaesthesia and Intensive Care*, Butterworth Heinemann, 2004: p. 424.

30. Answers: F F T F T

Indications of intra-operative cell salvage in surgery are:

* anticipated blood loss of >1000 mL or >20% estimated blood volume
* patients with a low Hb or increased risk factors for bleeding
* patients with multiple antibodies or rare blood types
* patients with objections to receiving allogeneic (donor) blood.

During surgery, blood loss can be removed from the operative site by a combination of suction and swabs. Depending on the type of surgery, blood loss to swabs during surgery has been estimated at between 30% and 50% of the total surgical blood loss. By washing swabs, the blood that is normally discarded can be collected and the overall efficiency of red cell recovery improved. To reduce haemolysis the vacuum pressure should always be set as low as practicable.

NICE has approved the use of ICS in urological malignancies. Aspiration of blood from around the tumour site should be avoided to minimise contamination of salvaged blood with malignant cells. There is in-vitro evidence that blood filtration through leucodepletion filters significantly reduces malignant cell numbers.

NICE has also approved ICS use in obstetrics, in conjunction with use of leucodepletion filters. This decreases amniotic fluid contamination. Rhesus incompatibility between mother and foetus is also not a contraindication, as the mother will receive anti-D antibodies anyway, which should prevent immunization against foetal rhesus positive cells.

Wee MYK, Thomas D, Verma R, *et al. Intra-operative Cell Salvage Guidelines.* AAGBI, September 2009. http://www.aagbi.org/sites/default/files/cell%20_salvage_2009_amended.pdf.

31. Answers: T F T F F

Streptococcus pneumoniae is the most common pathogen causing community-acquired pneumonia. The risk stratification using the pneumonia severity index (PSI) includes age over 50 years. Patients with a CURB 65 score of three or more should be treated aggressively, preferably in critical care. The panton-valentine leukocidin (PVL) producing community-acquired MRSA, which causes necrotizing pneumonia, is not resistant to vancomycin. Tigecycline is a glycylcycline antibiotic used to treat MRSA and *Acinetobacter* with good tissue penetration.

Sadashivaiah JB, Carr B. Severe community-acquired pneumonia. *Contin Educ Anaesth Crit Care Pain* 2009; 9(3): 87–91.

32. Answers: T F T F F

Phaeochromocytomas are associated with von Hippel Lindau disease as well as with MEN type 2 and 3 and neurofibromatosis. Approximately 90% occur in the adrenal medulla. They may present as polycythaemia and can cause hyperglycaemia.

If diagnosed in a pregnant patient, they should be removed before 24/40 weeks and should not be left untreated till term, due to the risk of spontaneous labour precipitating hypertensive crisis.

Pace N, Buttigieg M. Phaeochromocytoma. *Contin Educ Anaesth Crit Care Pain* 2003; 3(1): 20–23.

33. Answers: T T T T F

The four parathyroid glands are responsible for maintaining calcium homeostasis via secretion of parathyroid hormone. Parathyroid hormone acts on the bones and kidneys to increase serum calcium and decrease serum phosphate. It stimulates osteoclasts to release calcium and phosphate into the extracellular fluid, and simultaneously increases phosphate excretion and calcium re-absorption in the kidney.

The most common indication for surgery is primary hyperparathyroidism (PHP) from a parathyroid adenoma. The incidence of PHP is thought to be 25 per 100 000 of the UK population, and as high as 1 in 500 of women over the age of 45 years.

An increased circulating parathyroid hormone concentration causes hypercalcaemia, which leads to fatigue and bone, abdominal, urological, and mental symptoms. Thus PHP has been described historically as a disease of 'stones, bones, abdominal groans, and psychic moans'.

PHP is also associated with a higher incidence of cardiovascular deaths related to hypercalcaemia, impaired glucose tolerance, increased fracture risk, and poorer quality-of-life scores than the normal population. Traditionally, parathyroidectomy involved a collar incision, bilateral exploration of the neck, identification of all four glands, and removal of the diseased gland or glands. This requires a general anaesthetic technique similar to that for thyroid surgery, although airway encroachment is rare.

Aguilera M, Vaughan RS. Calcium and the anaesthetist. *Anaesthesia* 2000; 55: 779–90.

Malhotra S, Sodhi V. Anaesthesia for thyroid and parathyroid surgery. *Contin Educ Anaesth Crit Care Pain* 2007; 7(2): 55–58.

34. Answers: F T F F T

NICE guidelines on hypertension define hypertension as SBP >140/90 mmHg on two separate visits. The aim is to reduce the BP to less than 140/90 mmHg.

β-blockers are no longer the first-line treatment. Black patients should be started on calcium channel blockers and not ACE inhibitors. β-blockers should be considered first-line treatment in women of child-bearing potential.

Sever P. New hypertension guidelines from the National Institute for Health and Clinical Excellence and the British Hypertension Society. *J Renin Angiotensin Aldosterone Syst* 2006; 7(2): 61–3.

Hypertension. NICE guideline, February 2011. http://www.nice.org.uk/CG034.

35. Answers: T T F T F

Preconditioning was originally described following short periods of ischaemia, which conferred protection against subsequent ischaemia-reperfusion injury. The cardioprotection lasts for several hours after the preconditioning stimulus. A second window of protection appears after 24 h, and this lasts for 2 days. This is called late ischaemic preconditioning. Preconditioning effects are seen with sevoflurane, desflurane, isoflurane, and opioids. The effects are mediated by simulation of mitochondrial K^+ ATP-channel opening, which preserves mitochondrial function during reperfusion and reduces cytosolic calcium overload.

Preconditioning refers to changes at the biomolecular level that enable specialized tissues to better tolerate a major adverse event (e.g. ischaemia) if those tissues have already been exposed to minor adverse events.

Ischaemic preconditioning is an evolutionary conserved response that can protect the myocardium from hypoperfusion and ischaemia.

Ischaemic preconditioning can be mimicked pharmacologically by a variety of substances, including the volatile anaesthetic agents. This is termed anaesthetic preconditioning.

There is evidence of improvements in biochemical markers, echocardiographic findings, and clinical data after anaesthetic preconditioning.

Anaesthetic preconditioning may reduce perioperative myocardial injury during cardiac surgery and possibly non-cardiac surgery.

Loveridge R, Schroeder F. Anaesthetic preconditioning. *Contin Educ Anaesth Crit Care Pain* 2010; 10(2): 38–42.

36. Answers: T T T T F

Nicotine increases sympathetic activity as there is rise in circulating catecholamines. It has a half-life of about 1 h. Carboxyhemoglobin has a half-life about 4 h, which impedes release of O_2 to tissues, leading to increased frequency of cardiac arrhythmias. Abstinence from smoking for more than 3 months decreases overall perioperative cardiovascular risk by 33%. Preoperative abstinence for even 12 h should theoretically decrease perioperative ischaemia risk. Sustained postoperative abstinence decreases long-term mortality after CABG. Cough and wheezing takes several months to resolve and at least 12 weeks of abstinence is needed to ensure that risk of postoperative respiratory problems requiring intervention is reduced to normal.

Incidence of wound complications is normalized after 4 weeks of preoperative abstinence.

Werner DO. Perioperative abstinence from smoking. *Anaesthesiology* 2006; 104: 356–67.

Tønnesen H. Smoking and alcohol intervention before surgery: evidence for best practice. *Br J Anaesth* 2009; 102(3): 297–306.

37. Answers: T T F F T

Deficits in cognition in the postoperative period can cause severe problems, and are linked to significant increases in morbidity and mortality. Postoperative cognitive delirium and postoperative cognitive dysfunction are the two main entities of this cognitive decline. Persistent changes in cognitive function, as assessed by formal testing, are particularly common after cardiac surgery. The incidence varies depending on when and which tests are performed and the criteria used to determine the deficits. The cause is usually multifactorial. Postoperative cognitive dysfunction is only evident after major surgery and the incidence is significantly higher in patients aged over 60 years. There is little evidence for postoperative cognitive dysfunction persisting after 6 months, even in elderly patients having major surgery.

Rudolph JL, Schreber KA, Culley DJ, *et al*. Measurement of post-operative cognitive dysfunction after cardiac surgery: a systematic review. *Acta Anaesthesiol Scand* 2010; 54(6): 663–77.

Warltier DC. Postoperative cognitive dysfunction. *Anaesthesiology* 2007; 106: 572–90.

38. Answers: F F T F F

Obesity is defined as having BMI of greater than 30. The incidence is greater in females. Patients with high BMI have impaired cell-mediated immune function and increased plasma leptin concentration, which stimulates pro-inflammatory responses.

There is also platelet hyperactivity and increased concentration of fibrinogen. There is increased risk of ischaemic heart disease and diabetes mellitus. Obstructive sleep apnoea is seen in about 5% of obese patients. Difficult intubation is encountered in 16% of obese patients and in 33% of morbidly obese patients. The bioavailability of oral drugs is unaffected in obese patients. The volume of distribution is increased for propofol and midazolam.

Peri-operative Management of the Morbidly Obese Patient. The Association of Anaesthetists of Great Britain and Ireland, 2007. http://www.aagbi.org/publications/guidelines/peri-operative-management-morbidly-obese-patient.

Lotia S, Bellamy MC. Anaesthesia and morbid obesity. *Br J Anaesth* 2008; 8: 151–6.

Blanshard H. Endocrine and metabolic disease. In: Allman KG, Wilson IH (eds), *Oxford Handbook of Anaesthesia*, 2nd edn. Oxford University Press, 2004: pp. 182–184.

39. Answers: T T T T T

Cholesterol is a component of cell membranes and precursor of steroid hormones and bile acids. High serum cholesterol concentration is an important risk factor for cardiovascular disease. The contribution of dietary cholesterol exerts relatively small effects on serum cholesterol. Seventy per cent of cholesterol is synthesized in the liver. HMG-CoA reductase is a rate-limiting enzyme in cholesterol synthesis. Statins act by inhibiting the HMG-CoA reductase and preventing (LDL) cholesterol production. Statins have antioxidant activity. Atorvastin metabolite inhibits LDL oxidation and upregulates catalase, which is a free radical scavenger. Statins enhance stability of atherosclerotic plaques and inhibit vascular smooth muscle cell proliferation.

The use of statins is widespread and many patients presenting for surgery are regularly taking them. There is evidence that statins have beneficial effects beyond those of lipid lowering, including reducing the perioperative risk of cardiac complications and sepsis. Statins appear to have actions on vascular nitric oxide through the balance of inducible and endothelial nitric oxide synthase. There is reasonably strong evidence that patients already taking statins should continue on them perioperatively.

Brookes ZLS, McGown CC, Reilly CS. Statins for all: the new premed? *Br. J. Anaesth* 2009; 103(1): 99–107.

40. Answers: T F T T F

Drug delivery by iontophoresis involves use of electric current to transport ionized drug molecules actively across the skin and into the systemic circulation. Current drives ionized drug molecules from the reservoir into the sub-dermal tissue via electro-repulsion of similarly charged molecules and bulk fluid flow resulting from electro-osmosis. Drug diffusion into skin only occurs during current flow and passive diffusion plays a insignificant role when iontophoresis is active. There is a fixed dose of drug delivered per activation. This mode of drug delivery is well tolerated. However, erythema is seen in 10% of the subjects.

The quantity of drug delivered is influenced by the surface area of skin in contact with the electrode compartment. It also depends on the duration and intensity of electric current. Drugs that can be successfully administered using iontophoresis include lidocaine, fentanyl, and dexamethasone.

Grond S, Hall J, Spacek A, *et al*. Iontophoretic transdermal system using fentanyl compared with patient-controlled intravenous analgesia using morphine for postoperative pain management. *Br J Anaesth* 2007; 98(6): 806–15.

Margetts L, Sawyer R. Transdermal drug delivery: principles and opioid therapy. *Contin Educ Anaesth Crit Care Pain* 2007; 7(5): 171–177.

41. Answers: F T F T T

Principles of anaesthesia and perioperative management for free tissue transfer surgery are aimed at providing optimal physiological conditions for perfusion and flow. Perfusion pressure must be maintained and excessive vasoconstriction must be avoided, as this will compromise blood flow and increase blood viscosity resulting in flap failure. For these reasons hypothermia must be avoided.

A non-linear relationship exists between blood viscosity and haematocrit and, while haemodilution improves flow dynamics, it also reduces the oxygen-carrying capacity of the blood; a haematocrit of 30% is thought to be optimal. Systemic vasodilators should also be avoided as this may cause a steal phenomenon and divert blood away from the flap, as the vessels will already be maximally dilated. A hyperdynamic circulation maintains cardiac output with a low systemic vascular resistance, providing optimal conditions for microcirculatory flap perfusion.

Adams J, Charlton P. Anaesthesia for microvascular free tissue transfer. *Contin Educ Anaesth Crit Care Pain* 2003; 3: 33–7.

42. Answers: **T F T T T**

Patients should be individually consulted to ascertain which treatments are acceptable. Advanced directives state the desire of a competent individual and must be respected. In a life-threatening emergency for a child unable to give competent consent, all life-saving treatment should be given, irrespective of the parents' wishes. Departments should keep a regularly updated list of those senior members prepared to care for followers of the Jehovah's Witness faith.

Management of Anaesthesia for Jehovah's Witnesses, 2nd edn. Association of Anaesthetists of Great Britain and Ireland, 2005.

43. Answers: **T F F F T**

FRC is reduced but vital capacity is unchanged.

Heart size is apparently increased and apex beat displaced to the left by diaphragm elevation caused by the enlarged uterus.

Blood pressure is unchanged due to a fall in systemic vascular resistance in the latter part of pregnancy.

As there is an increase in cardiac output, renal plasma flow, and glomerular filtration rate during pregnancy, urea, creatinine, urate clearance and excretion of bicarbonate are increased, causing plasma concentrations to be less than in the non-pregnant population.

This is caused by aortocaval compression. Miller notes that 10% of pregnant patients develop shock symptoms when placed supine near term.

Heidemann BH, McClure JH. Changes in maternal physiology during pregnancy. *BJA CEPD Rev* 2003; 3(3): 65–68.

Kuczkowski KM. Anesthetic implications of drug abuse in pregnancy. *J Clin Anesthes* 2003; 15(5): 382–94.

Glosten B. Anesthesia for obstetrics. In: Miller RD, (ed.). *Anesthesia,* 5th edn. Churchill Livingstone, 2000: pp. 2025–30.

44. Answers: **T T F T T**

An epidural needle is simply a needle that is placed into the epidural space. To provide continuous epidural analgesia or anaesthesia, a small hollow catheter may be threaded through the epidural needle into the epidural space, and left there while the needle is removed. There are many types of epidural needles as well as catheters, but in modern practice in UK, disposable materials are used to ensure sterility.

Types of epidural needles include:

- Crawford
- Tuohy
- Husted
- Weiss
- Eldor

Epidural needles are designed with a curved tip to help prevent puncture of the dural membrane. The bevel on the needle is slightly curved superiorly (to direct the catheter cephalad), and the leading edge is curved, not pointed as in a typical needle. This tip, the Huber tip, is considerably blunter than another needle of equivalent size with a standard cutting tip (a Quincke tip). The bluntness adds to the force required to advance the needle through the tough ligaments of the spine, but this contributes to its safety, as the 'feel' of the needle is improved, and it is less likely to puncture the dura accidentally.

In order to apply force to advance the needle, it has wings attached to the hub, which make it easier to push on. These are called Mackintosh wings.

During insertion the needle should be removed with the catheter, to avoid risk of catheter shearing by the oblique bevel (named the Huber point). The 10-cm model is most commonly used, but 5- and 15-cm models exist.

Frolich MA, Caton D. Pioneers in epidural needle design. *Anesth Analg* 2001; 93: 215–20.

45. Answers: T T T T F

The morbidity associated with intra-arterial injection of thiopentone relates to the change in pH, which results in precipitation of microcrystals within the artery, causing arterial spasm, endarterial obstruction, and release of vasoactive mediators, which results in thrombosis and necrosis.

Priorities of management are stopping the injection, immediate dilution, followed by methods to establish maximal arterial vasodilatation of the affected limb, including sympathetic blockade of the stellate ganglion or brachial plexus blocks. Saline washout is an effective treatment after accidental extravasation. Papaverine is a smooth-muscle relaxant, structurally related to atracurium. Local anaesthetics such as lignocaine are appropriate options. Intravenous anticoagulation with heparin is also indicated as a priority. Early anticoagulation is an important intervention in accidental IA injection with tissue ischaemia. Prompt management improves outcome and early referral to a plastic surgeon should be considered.

Lake C, Beecroft CL. Extravasation injuries and accidental intra-arterial injection. *Contin Educ Anaesth Crit Care Pain* 2010; 10(4): 109–13.

46. Answers: T F F F T

A Cochrane systematic review concluded that epidural analgesia may be useful for postoperative pain relief following major lower-limb joint replacements. However, the benefits may be limited to the early (4–6 h) postoperative period. The hip joint is innervated by the femoral, sciatic, and obturator nerves, with cutaneous innervation supplied by the lateral cutaneous nerve of the thigh (LCNT). Thus the sciatic nerve must be blocked for complete anaesthesia. A lumbar plexus block will reliably block the femoral and obturator nerves and the LCNT. The sciatic nerve (L4,5 and S1,2,3) is derived from the sacral plexus and is thus not reliably blocked. A Winnie or '3-in-1' block attempts to block the femoral, obturator, and LCNT with one injection; complete lumbar plexus block occurs in only 35% of patients.

Choi P, Bhandari M, Scott J, Douketis J. Epidural analgesia for pain relief following hip or knee replacement. *Cochrane Database Syst Rev* 2003; 3: CD003071.

47. Answers: F F T F T

Body fat increases in the middle years but declines in extreme old age. There are gender differences. Total body water decreases and, significantly, intracellular fluid decreases. Glucocorticoid secretion remains similar to young people. The response to stress differs slightly but the clinical significance is questioned.

The basal metabolic rate falls by 1% per year after the age of 30. Fall in metabolic activity and reduced muscle mass may cause impaired thermoregulatory control.

Murray D, Dodds C. Perioperative care of the elderly *Contin Educ Anaesth Crit Care Pain* 2004; 4(6): 193–96.

Hornick T. Effects of advanced age on body composition and metabolism. In: Fleisher LA, Prough DS, (eds), *Management of the Elderly Surgical Patient*. Lippincott-Raven, 1997: pp. 461–70.

48. Answers: T T F T F

The Spaulding classification categorized medical devices according to the risk of infection associated with their use as critical, semi-critical, and non-critical; critical items must be sterile as they enter sterile tissue or the vascular system, while semi-critical items describe those in contact with mucous membrane or intact skin. Decontamination processes can be divided into cleaning, and low- and high-level disinfection and sterilization; high-level disinfection kills vegetative bacteria, fungi, and viruses (but not all endospores), but with sufficient contact time will produce sterilization, provided thorough cleaning has been carried out. Laryngeal mask airways should not be cleaned with glutaraldehyde, iodine, or phenols and should only be sterilized using a steam autoclave.

Sterilization, Disinfection and Cleaning Medical Devices and Equipment: Guidance on Decontamination from the Microbiology Advisory Committee to Department of Health Medical Devices Agency, Part 1–3. Medical Devices Agency, Department of Health, London, 1996–2000.

Sabir N, Ramachandra V. Decontamination of anaesthetic equipment. *Contin Educ Anaesth Crit Care Pain* 2004; 4(4): 103–106.

49. Answers: T F T T F

There is a severe shortage of organs for donation from brainstem-dead heart-beating donors. Diagnosing brainstem death is good intensive care practice and should be performed irrespective of any possibility of organ donation. All potential organ donors should be discussed with transplant services; the organ donor register should always be checked.

Pathophysiological changes during and after brainstem death lead to organ damage. Optimal medical management of the organ donor increases the number of potential organs suitable for transplantation and may also improve outcome.

In a brainstem-dead patient undergoing a beating-heart organ donation, endocrine failure dictates a requirement for hormone supplementation. Hypothalamo–pituitary axis dysfunction causes a significant fall in ADH, causing diabetes insipidus necessitating replacement with DDAVP (desmopressin). TSH levels decrease, leading to a fall in T3. Although debated, the supplementation of T3 to the donor has been shown to improve donor heart function in the recipient. T4 does not appear to undergo peripheral conversion to its active form of T3 in a brain-dead patient. Hyperglycaemia is common and thus insulin is required. The United Network for Organ Sharing recommends a three-drug 'hormone-resuscitation', which has led to a 22% increase in the number of organs recovered. It comprises:

- vasopressin: 1 unit bolus, infusion at 0.5–2.5 U/h
- T3: 4 mg bolus, infusion at 3 mg/h
- insulin: 1 IU/h minimum, titrated to blood glucose
- in addition, high-dose methylprednisolone 15 mg/kg is also recommended

Edgar P. Management of the potential heart-beating organ donor *Contin Educ Anaesth Crit Care Pain* 2004; 4(3): 86–90.

50. Answers: F F F F T

Addison's disease is characterized by reduced or absent secretion of glucocorticoids, usually associated with deficient mineralocorticoid activity. Destruction of the adrenal cortex by autoantibodies is the cause of primary hypoadrenalism in 80% of cases; other causes include tuberculosis, metastatic carcinoma, bilateral adrenalectomy, and haemorrhage (e.g. meningococcal sepsis). Secondary hypoadrenalism results from prolonged corticosteroid therapy and hypopituitarism. Aldosterone secretion is maintained and the fluid and electrolyte disturbances are less marked.

An Addisonian crisis is a potentially life-threatening condition caused by acute glucocorticoid (and to a lesser extent mineralocorticoid) deficiency. In chronic insufficiency states, a crisis can be precipitated by an acute stress or intercurrent illness, whereby the ability to secrete glucocorticoids is exceeded by demand. Most commonly the cause is abrupt cessation of steroid therapy coupled with hypothalamo–pituitary and adrenal suppression; other causes include adrenal destruction due to haemorrhage, infection (tuberculosis), or autoimmune disease. Features include the sequelae of glucocorticoid and mineralocorticoid deficiency: hypotension unresponsive to catecholamines, hyperkalaemia, hyponatraemia (may be normal), and hypoglycaemia. Pyrexia is common and may be due to an underlying infection.

Davies M, Hardman J. Anaesthesia and adrenocortical disease. *Contin Educ Anaesth Crit Care Pain* 2005; 5(4): 122–26.

51. Answers: T T T F F

Electrocution or macroshock can result from completion of an electrical circuit through bodily contact with two conducting parts at different voltage potentials. The effect of the current on the body depends on the current density, duration of contact, current frequency (higher frequencies present less hazard), and also on location of contact. An earthed patient represents a path for current completion, and isolation transformers are therefore used to isolate the operating theatre power supply from the patient. Two live unearthed lines exist for use with operating equipment, and line isolation monitors are therefore used to measure the potential for current flow from the isolated wire to earth. An alarm is actuated if the current detected is high (2–5 mA); a circuit-breaker interrupts flow in such circumstances, but these are not usually incorporated in operating theatre power supplies. Conductive flooring increases the risk of electrical hazard; capacitative coupling occurs when electrosurgical equipment induces stray currents in nearby conductors. High levels of humidity (>50%) significantly reduce the risk of sparking.

Boumphrey S, Langton JA. Electrical safety in the operating theatre. *BJA CEPD Rev* 2003; 3(1): 10–14.

52. Answers: T T F F T

All perioperative nerve injuries involve the ulnar nerve. The classic site of injury is the exposed ulnar groove behind the medial epicondyle of the humerus. At this point, the nerve is exposed to both direct trauma from the sides of the operating table and indirect trauma from stretch.

The ulnar nerve arises from the medial cord of the brachial plexus and enters the forearm, passing behind the medial epicondyle.

Complete injuries at the elbow result in paralysis of the medial flexor digitorum profundus (FDP) and flexor carpi ulnaris, which leads to a claw deformity; injuries at the wrist are worse as the FDP is not affected and therefore causes marked flexion of the phalanges. In addition, the small muscles of the hand will be paralysed except for the thenar muscles and the first and second lumbricals, supplied by the median nerve; inability to adduct the thumb will also result but abduction and opposition is provided by the median nerve. On flexion of the wrist, a degree of abduction will result, due to flexor carpi radialis paralysis.

McCahon RA, Bedforth NM. Peripheral nerve block at the elbow and wrist. *Contin Educ Anaesth Crit Care Pain* 2007; 7(2): 42–44.

53. Answers: T F T F T

The acute porphyrias include acute intermittent porphyria (AIP), variegate porphyria (VP), hereditary coproporphyria (HCP), and the very rare plumboporphyria (PP). With the exception of PP, which is recessive, these porphyrias are inherited as non-sex-linked, autosomal dominant conditions with variable expression.

Acute attacks of porphyria are most commonly precipitated by events that decrease haem concentrations, thus increasing the activity of ALA synthetase and stimulating the production of porphyrinogens.

Acute exacerbations may be precipitated by a number of factors, including physiological hormonal fluctuations (such as those occurring with menstruation), fasting, dehydration, stress, and infection. The enzyme-inducing drugs are by far the most important trigger factors, particularly in relation to anaesthesia.

Acute attacks are characterized by severe abdominal pain, autonomic instability, electrolyte disturbances, and neuropsychiatric manifestations.

Neuromuscular weakness, which may progress to quadriparesis and respiratory failure, is the most prominent and potentially lethal neurological manifestation, but sensory losses also occur.

Central nervous system involvement with upper motor neuron lesions, cranial nerve palsies, and involvement of the cerebellum and basal ganglia are less commonly seen.

Permanent neurological lesions, especially parasympathetic dysfunction, can occur, particularly in AIP, although this is rarely seen unless the attacks have been multiple or of long duration.

James MFM, Hift RJ. Porphyrias. *Br J Anaesth* 2000; 85(1): 143–53.

54. Answers: F T F T T

Chronic back pain can be triaged into three categories: simple musculoskeletal back pain (95%), spinal nerve root pain (4–5%), and serious spinal pathology (1%).

Table 2.2 shows 'red flag markers for serious spinal pathology.

Table 2.2 Red-flag markers for serious spinal pathology

Presentation <20 or >55 years
History of significant trauma
Constant progressive thoracic pain
Past history of cancer, steroid therapy, IV drug abuse or HIV infection
Unexplained weight loss
Systemically unwell
Cauda equina syndrome (saddle anaesthesia, gait/sphincter disturbance)
Structural deformity
Marked restriction of lumbar flexion (<5 cm)
Non-mechanical pain

Reproduced from Mark A Jackson and Karen H Simpson, 'Chronic back pain', Continuing Education in Anaesthesia Critical Care and Pain, 2006, 6, 4, pp. 152–155 by permission of Oxford University Press and the British Journal of Anaesthesia.

Patients with one or more of these markers should be referred to specialists for advanced radiological investigations at the earliest opportunity.

Jackson M, Simpson K. Chronic back pain. *Contin Educ Anaesth Crit Care Pain* 2006; 6(4): 152–55.

55. Answers: T T T T F

Evidence supports the use of non-steroidal anti-inflammatory drugs (NSAIDs) and opioids in the management of back pain, although the long-term use of NSAIDs requires careful assessment of benefits and risks. Initial management is often regular acetaminophen and NSAID, with or without a weak opioid. A strong opioid may be appropriate; opioid prescribing in this context should follow agreed recommendations, such as those produced by the British Pain Society. The use of immediate-release opioids should usually be avoided. There is evidence supporting the use of tricyclic antidepressants and anticonvulsants for neuropathic pain. There is strong evidence to support the use of graded exercise therapy and some psychological approaches (e.g. cognitive behaviour therapy) to manage chronic pain in adults, either as an individual therapy or in a group setting. There is no evidence to support the use of caudal and lumbar epidural injections in the treatment of simple musculoskeletal back pain. These treatments may have a role in the early treatment of nerve root pain in some patients. Transcutaneous electrical nerve stimulation may be more effective than placebo in reducing pain in the short term, but there is little evidence to support its long-term use.

Jackson M, Simpson K. Chronic back pain. *Contin Educ Anaesth Crit Care Pain* 2006; 6(4): 152–55.

56. Answers: T F F T T

Spinal nerve root pain can be caused by disc herniation, spinal stenosis, and epidural adhesions. Spinal nerve root pain is often well localized, radiating down the leg in a dermatomal pattern. The radicular element is characteristically much worse than the associated back pain because it is neuropathic. The pain typically radiates below the knee into the foot. It is described as a sharp, electric-shock-like pain and is well localized. Nerve root pain should not be confused with referred back pain; the latter rarely extends below the knee and is poorly localized. Plain radiographs are of no benefit in the assessment of nerve root pain. CT scan will show bone architecture better, while MRI scan shows the soft tissue better. Hence MRI scan is the investigation of choice for assessing soft tissues. MRI is more useful than CT as an investigation for nerve root pain, unless the history is suggestive of spinal stenosis, when CT may be more appropriate. Nerve-conduction studies are not recommended for investigating nerve root pain; they have a high false-positive rate and often lack the sensitivity to make a specific diagnosis. However, they can be useful for distinguishing between a radicular and peripheral neuropathic pain.

Nerve root pain and simple back pain can be managed within a pain management clinic using a multidisciplinary approach. There is no evidence to support the use of caudal and lumbar epidural injections in the treatment of simple musculoskeletal back pain. These treatments may have a role in the early treatment of nerve root pain in some patients. Transforaminal nerve root injections have been shown to be effective in reducing the need for disc surgery.

Surgical procedures for spinal stenosis and surgical discectomy can provide pain relief for nerve root pain.

Jackson M, Simpson K. Chronic back pain. *Contin Educ Anaesth Crit Care Pain* 2006; 6(4): 152–55.

57. Answers: T F T T F

The most important and useful distribution of data in statistical analysis is the normal or Gaussian distribution. It is also often referred to as a parametric distribution because two key parameters that fully describe its shape can be defined: the mean and standard deviation (SD). A normal distribution is characterized by a unimodal, symmetrical, bell-shaped curve when interval data are represented by a histogram or line graph. All three measures of central tendency, i.e. mean, median, and mode, are equal. Much biological data such as height and mean arterial blood pressure in healthy adults are normally distributed.

Mode is strictly a measure of the most popular (frequent) value in a dataset and is often not a particularly good indicator of central tendency. Despite its limitations, the mode is the only means of measuring central tendency in a dataset containing nominal categorical values.

The interquartile range (IQR) is often quoted as a measure of variability when referring to interval data that is not normally distributed.

Kurtosis describes the peakedness of the curve, whereas skewness describes the symmetry of the curve.

McCluckey A, Lalkhen AG. Statistics II: Central tendency and spread of data. *Contin Educ Anaesth Crit Care Pain* 2007: 7(4): 127–30.

58. Answers: F F T T F

Trigeminal neuralgia (TGN) has an incidence of 3–5/100 000, with a peak onset in the fifth and sixth decades. The hallmark is agonizing, paroxysmal, lancinations confined strictly to one or more branches of the trigeminal nerve. The pain is nearly always unilateral. About 80% of cases are associated with vascular compression of the trigeminal nerve. TGN is diagnosed in up to 5% of patients with multiple sclerosis. Other causes include schwannoma, meningioma, epidermoid cyst, pontine infarction, and Chiari malformation. About 70% of patients with TGN can initially be controlled non-surgically. The drug of choice is carbamazepine. Those that fail medical treatment may respond to one of the surgical options available. Percutaneous neuroablative techniques, aimed at denervating the gasserian ganglion, include glycerol gangliolysis, radiofrequency thermocoagulation, microcompression, and stereotactic radiosurgery. All are safe and well-tolerated procedures. Microvascular decompression surgery through the posterior fossa is directly aimed at the proposed cause, the target area being the nerve–pons junction. It provides prolonged analgesia with pain relief in 90% of patients short-term, and 55–70% long-term.

Farooq K, Williams P. Headache and chronic facial pain. *Contin Educ Anaesth Crit Care Pain* 2008: 8(4): 138–42.

59. Answers: F F T T F

The existence and intensity of preoperative pain is a risk factor for the development of CPSP after hernia repair, thoracotomy, amputation, and mastectomy; for the latter two procedures continuous preoperative pain for more than 1 month predicts CPSP. Laparoscopic surgical approaches result in less chronic pain after hernia repair and cholecystectomy.

Increasing age is inversely related to the development of CPSP.

Epidural analgesia, when commenced before surgery and continued into the postoperative period, reduces the incidence of CPSP in patients undergoing thoracotomy and laparotomy. Similarly, paravertebral block initiated before incision and continued into the postoperative period reduces the incidence of CPSP in thoracic and breast cancer surgery patients. It may be that establishing sufficient afferent block before the surgical incision and continuing this well into the postoperative period reduces the nociceptive barrage that results in central sensitization.

The preventative effects of perioperative gabapentin have been studied, but with inconclusive results. Perioperative IV ketamine infusion has been used to prevent development of CPSP in patients undergoing mastectomy, thoracotomy, and rectal cancer surgery. Clonidine, when used in conjunction with local anaesthetics as a regional anaesthetic technique, may reduce the incidence of CPSP. There are limited data to suggest that multimodal analgesic techniques (such as a combination of local anaesthesia and gabapentin or intra-articular bupivacaine, morphine, and clonidine) may help reduce CPSP.

Gabapentin failed to reduce the incidence of chronic pain after amputation when given during the perioperative period and for 30 days afterwards.

Searle RD, Simpson KH. Chronic post-surgical pain. *Contin Educ Anaesth Crit Care Pain* 2010; 10(1): 12–14.

60. Answers: T T F F T

Regarding fibromylgia, there is no difference in gender incidence in childhood, but in adults the ratio of women to men with fibromyalgia varies between 9:1 and 20:1. The condition is mostly diagnosed between the ages of 20 and 50. The incidence increases with age, so that by the age of 80, 8% of adults meet the diagnostic criteria.

Fibromyalgia is defined on the basis of criteria laid down by the ACR. The first criterion is a history of spontaneous chronic widespread pain for a continuous period of 3 months. The second criterion requires the patient to elicit tenderness in at least 11 of the 18 defined tender points when palpated digitally.

Fibromyalgia has been reported to co-exist in 25% of patients with rheumatoid arthritis, in 30% of those with systemic lupus erythematosus, and 50% of those with Sjogren's syndrome.

Dedhia J, Bone M. Pain and fibromyalgia. *Contin Educ Anaesth Crit Care Pain* 2009; 9(5): 162–66.

Single Best Answers

1. Answer: B

The 2010 ALS Bradycardia algorithm suggests 500 mcg IV atropine as the first line of management in patients with symptomatic bradycardia with adverse features. The other options mentioned form part of the subsequent management of this patient.

Adult Bradycardia Algorithm. Resuscitation Council UK, 2010. http://www.resus.org.uk/pages/medimain.htm.

2. Answer: A

All the above mentioned steps are part of the adult algorithm for management of narrow complex tachycardia, so will be appropriate in any other situation. Cardioversion is not recommended in stable narrow complex tachycardia unless the patient has adverse signs or symptoms but, given this patient's medical history and the onset of ST depression on ECG, it would be sensible to be ready for cardioversion if pharmacological treatment does not work.

However, this particular patient has significant atherosclerosis and carotid sinus massage might therefore not be very safe because of the risk of embolization from an undiagnosed atheromatous plaque present in the carotid artery. High-flow oxygen should be given even in a COPD patient who is unwell post-operatively and in an acute situation.

Adult Tachycardia Algorithm. Resuscitation Council UK, 2010. http://www.resus.org.uk/pages/medimain.htm.

3. Answer: E

Even for a shockable rhythm, chest compression should be started while waiting for the defibrillator to be attached and/or charged, but once ready, the first shock should delivered without delay. The first shock is delivered at 150–200 J biphasic, with subsequent shocks at 200–360 J biphasic. The time between stopping chest compressions and shock delivery should ideally be less than 5 s. The new guidelines suggest both adrenaline and amiodarone should be given after the third shock.

Adult Tachycardia Algorithm. Resuscitation Council UK, 2010. http://www.resus.org.uk/pages/medimain.htm.

4. Answer: B

Seventy-five per cent of post-tonsillectomy haemorrhage occurs within the first 6 h, and the rest occurs within the first 24 h. The most common cause of early haemorrhage is the pain, which causes hypertension and re-bleeding.

Haemorrhage occurring after a few days is secondary to infection.

Ravi R, Howell T. Anaesthesia for paediatric ear, nose, and throat surgery. *Contin Educ Anaesth Crit Care Pain* 2007; 7(2): 33–37.

Deakin C, Nolan J, Perkins G, *et al*; Adult advanced life support. In: *Resuscitation Guidelines 2010.* Resuscitation Council (UK), 2010. http://www.resus.org.uk/pages/als.pdf.

Roberts F. Ear, nose, and throat surgery. In: Allman KG, Wilson IH (eds), *Oxford Handbook of Anaesthesia*, 2nd edn. Oxford University Press, 2004: pp. 612–614.

5. Answer: A

There is no difference in laryngospasm or bronchospasm during elective surgery when children had active URTI or URTI in the last few weeks. Independent risk factors for adverse respiratory events in children with URTI include history of reactive airway disease, history of prematurity, parental smoking, airway surgery, use of endotracheal tube, productive cough, and nasal congestion. If a patient has normal appetite and activities, no fever, and does not look systemically unwell, it is probably safe to proceed with the surgery.

Larson CP. Laryngospasm—the best treatment. *Anesthesiology* 1998; 89: 1293–94.

Tait AR, Malviya S. Anesthesia for the child with an upper respiratory tract infection: still a dilemma? *Anesth Analg* 2005; 100: 59–65.

6. Answer: C

Historically the recommended first-line drug treatment for hypotension associated with regional anaesthesia in obstetrics is ephedrine. This is because early animal studies suggested that ephedrine, which is a predominantly β-adrenergic agonist, was better at increasing maternal arterial pressure while preserving uterine blood flow than other vasopressors. However, the use of ephedrine to prevent or treat hypotension associated with regional anaesthesia might even worsen foetal acidosis.

Metaraminol is a mixed α- and β-adrenergic agonist that has predominant α effects at doses used clinically. When used by infusion to maintain arterial pressure during spinal anaesthesia for caesarean section, metaraminol was associated with less neonatal acidosis and more closely controlled titration of arterial pressure than ephedrine.

There is evidence that the metaraminol and phenylephrine are safe and are associated with better foetal acid–base status. If infusions of phenylephrine or metaraminol are used, umbilical cord blood gases are significantly better than with ephedrine, but decreases in maternal heart rate are more common with metaraminol. The bradycardia is usually a baroreceptor-mediated event and resolves on stopping the infusion.

Prophylactic infusion of phenylephrine 100 mcg/min decreased the incidence, frequency, and magnitude of hypotension, with equivalent neonatal outcome, compared with a control group receiving IV bolus phenylephrine.

Ngan Kee WD, Shaw KS, Ng FF, Lee BB. Prophylactic phenylephrine infusion for preventing hypotension during spinal anesthesia for cesarean delivery. *Anesth Analg* 2004; 98(3): 815–21.

Emmett RS, Cyna AM, Andrew M, Simmons SW. Techniques for preventing hypotension during spinal anaesthesia for caesarean section. *Cochrane Database Syst Rev* 2002; 4: CD002251.

7. Answer: C

National Audit Project 3 showed the highest incidence of complications in epidurals performed in adult patients undergoing general surgical procedures, which reflects the co-morbidities that these patients have as well as the fact that they usually have thoracic epidurals, which are technically more difficult and challenging.

Third National Audit Project of the Royal College of Anaesthetists. *Major Complications of Central Neuraxial Block in the United Kingdom*. http://www.rcoa.ac.uk/docs/NAP3_web-large.pdf.

8. Answer: E

Von Willebrand's disease Type 3 results in a complete absence of von Willebrand's factor, platelet dysfunction, and severe coagulopathy, so regional techniques are contraindicated.

All others situations mentioned are amenable to regional techniques. You can still give a single-shot spinal in pre-eclampsia with platelet count of 80 000, or in a patient with severe PET or HELLP syndrome if the coagulation is normal and the risk of giving GA is considered to be high when assessed by an experienced anaesthetist.

Von Willebrand's disease (vWD) is characterized by either a shortage or defect (or both) in a protein in the blood called von Willebrand factor (vWF), which helps to make blood clot. It thus takes longer with vWD for the blood to clot and for bleeding episodes to stop. vWD is the most common of bleeding disorders, affecting 1% to 2% of the population nationwide, and is named after the Finnish haematologist who first reported it. It varies in severity, and in its milder form often goes undetected, unless unusual bleeding occurs during tooth extraction, surgery, or an accident. Most people with vWD live completely normal lives.

Symptoms can also change over time and include:

- prolonged bleeding from minor skin cuts
- easy bruising
- frequent epitasis nose bleeds
- unusual bleeding from mouth or gums
- bleeding in the gastrointestinal tract
- bleeding into muscles and joints
- excessive haemorrhage after injury, dental work, or surgery

The different types of vWD are:

- Type 1 A
- Type 2: 2A, 2B, 2M and 2N
- Type 3

Von Willebrand's disease. The Haemophilia Society website. http://www.haemophilia.org.uk/information/Bleeding+Disorders/von+Willebrands+Disease.

Francis S, May A, Pregnant women with significant medical conditions: anaesthetic implications *Contin Educ Anaesth Crit Care Pain* 2004; 4(3): 95–97.

9. Answer: D

Epidural analgesia as a part of enhanced recovery programme has been shown to shorten hospital stay. It also has been shown to decrease ileus, provide better analgesia, and improve pulmonary function. However, none of the epidural studies or systematic reviews has shown long-term survival benefits.

Nimmo SM. Benefit and outcome after epidural analgesia. Contin Educ Anaesth Crit Care Pain 2004; 4(2): 44–47.

10. Answer: A

In-utero resuscitation consists of steps taken to improve the placental perfusion in a compromised foetus. Lateral position removes aorto-caval compression. Terbutaline causes tocolysis. Oxytocin should be stopped as well if being used. IV fluids and oxygen also improve placental perfusion. Epidural infusion is generally stopped during the resuscitation but it does not help in immediate in-utero resuscitation.

Maharaj D. Intrapartum fetal resuscitation: a review. *Internet J Gynecol Obst* 2008; 9(2).

11. Answer: A

There is no evidence that using spinal or GA in management of fracture of neck of femur makes a difference to the overall outcome of the patients. The other points are recommended in the NCEPOD report.

Pre-operative regional anaesthesia by doing fascia–iliaca block is recommended to relieve the pain of the fracture and operation within 24 h. A systematic review found no robust evidence that spinal/epidural anaesthesia confers any benefit over general anaesthesia with regards to overall mortality at 3, 6 and 12 months following surgical repair of hip fracture in older people (6.9% versus 10%; relative risk, 0.69; confidence interval, 0.5–0.95).

An Age Old Problem: Review of Care Received by Older Patients Undergoing surgery. NCEPOD 2010. http://www.ncepod.org.uk/2010pn.htm.

Parker MJ, et al. *Anaesthesia for hip fracture surgery in adults.* Cochrane Database of Systematic Reviews 2004, 4: CD000521 (Guideline Ref ID: 8 PARKER2004B).

Regional (spinal or epidural) versus general anaesthesia. In: *The Management of Hip Fracture in Adults.* NICE guideline, 2011: pp. 82–90. http://www.nice.org.uk/nicemedia/live/13489/54918/54918.pdf.

12. Answer: E

Recurrent laryngeal nerve block is a well-known complication after interscalene block, which can cause hoarseness of voice due to ipsilateral paralysis of vocal cord. The other mentioned complications are possible but are unlikely to be responsible for change in voice.

Miller RD, Eriksson LI, Fleisher LA, et al. *Miller's Anesthesia*, 7th edn, Churchill Livingstone, 2009: pp. 409, 1640–3.

13. Answer: D

The maximum increase in cardiac output occurs at the end of the third stage of labour, when the placenta separates and there is autotransfusion of blood from placental circulation back into maternal circulation. This is the time when the risk of congestive cardiac failure is highest.

Boyle RK. Anaesthesia in parturients with heart disease: a five year review in an Australian tertiary hospital. *Int J Obstet Anesth* 2003; 12: 173–77.

Tamhane P, O'Sullivan G, Reynolds F. Oxytocin in parturients with cardiac disease. *Int J Obstet Anesth* 2006; 15: 332–33.

14. Answer: A

There is no evidence for prophylactic bed rest in post-dural puncture headache. All the other mentioned treatments have some benefit, with the blood patch having the best results.

Management of PDPH

Conservative management approaches include:

- bed rest
- encouraging intake of oral fluids and/or intravenous hydration
- reassurance.

A recent Cochrane review concluded that routine bed rest after dural puncture is not beneficial and should be abandoned.

Pharmacological approaches include:

- caffeine—either intravenous (e.g. 500 mg caffeine in 1 L saline) or orally
- synacthen (synthetic ACTH)
- regular analgesia: paracetamol, diclofenac etc.
- other drugs with insufficient evidence in the literature are:
  - 5HT agonists (e.g.sumatriptan)
  - gabapentin, DDAVP
  - theophyline
  - hydrocortisone.

Interventional approaches include:

- immediate:
  - insertion of long-term intrathecal catheter placement (15%) and epidural saline bolus (13%)
  - epidural morphine

- epidural blood patch, which involves injecting approximately 20 mL of the patient's own fresh blood (taken in a strict sterile fashion) into the epidural space near the site of the suspected puncture. It is successful in the majority of cases, and the onset of relief from headache may be immediate (but occasionally takes up to 24 h). In patients in whom a blood patch is not successful, or where relief is temporary, it may be repeated, although the likelihood of improvement is reduced.

Sudlow CLM, Warlow CP. Posture and fluids for preventing post-dural puncture headache. *Cochrane Database Syst Rev,* 2001. http://www2.cochrane.org/reviews/en/ab001790.html.

Apfel CC. Prevention of postdural puncture headache after accidental dural puncture: a quantitative systematic review. *Br J Anaesth* 2010; 105(3): 255–63.

15. Answer: E

Warfarin is a coumarin derivative, which inhibits synthesis of the vitamin-K-dependent clotting factors (factors II, VII, IX and X) in the liver, by preventing the reduction of oxidized vitamin K required for carboxylation of clotting factor precursors. The management of patients on warfarin for emergency surgery requires administration of prothrombin complex concentrate (PCC), which contains the necessary factors, although fresh frozen plasma at 15 mL/kg can be administered, but this presents a risk of anaphylaxis and transmission of blood-borne pathogens, and is the most common cause of transfusion-related acute lung injury (TRALI). The best course of management for this patient would be to correct INR with vitamin K and PCC if the surgery is not very urgent. FFP is to be given only if there is significant ongoing bleeding or PCC is not available.

Red cell transfusion. In: *Blood Transfusion and the Anaesthetist.* AAGBI guidelines, 2005. http://www.aagbi.org/sites/default/files/red_cell_08.pdf.

16. Answer: D

Tracheostomy in ICU is usually not an emergency procedure and can wait for some time. There is no need to give platelets for invasive procedures unless the platelet count is less than 50 000 or the patient is bleeding with platelet count between 50 000 and 80 000. Severe thrombocytopenia has been described as a contraindication for percutaneous tracheostomy, but here the platelet count is 70 000 and when performed by experienced personnel is relatively safe. Stopping the haemofilter for this non-emergency procedure is also not recommended.

Red cell transfusion. In: *Blood Transfusion and the Anaesthetist.* AAGBI guidelines, 2005. http://www.aagbi.org/sites/default/files/red_cell_08.pdf.

Kluge, S, Meyer A, Kühnelt P, *et al.* Percutaneous tracheostomy is safe in patients with severe thrombocytopenia. *Chest* 2004; 126(2): 547–51.

17. Answer: D

The aim for resuscitation for a polytrauma patient should be to maintain a low normal blood pressure rather than aggressive management of hypotension. All the other steps are recommended in the management of major haemorrhage.

Management of massive haemorrhage. In: *Blood Transfusion and the Anaesthetist.* AAGBI guidelines, 2005. http://www.aagbi.org/sites/default/files/massive_haemorrhage_2010_0.pdf.

18. Answer: A

Platelets are stored in an oxygen-permeable bag at 22°C, which increases the risk of bacterial growth. The risk of bacteraemia is therefore highest with platelets and they should be used at the earliest opportunity.

Blood component therapy: In: *Blood Transfusion and the Anaesthetist*. AAGBI guidelines, 2005. http://www.aagbi.org/sites/default/files/bloodtransfusion06.pdf.

19. Answer: E

Cardiac arrest following LA toxicity should be initially managed with standard ALS guidelines: 20% intralipid in a dose of 1.5 mL/kg over 1 min followed by an infusion of 15 mL/kg/h. In a case of poor response, two more boluses of same dose can be given 5 min apart, and the infusion rate doubled. Total cumulative dose should not exceed 12 mL/kg. Recovery in LA-toxicity cardiac arrest may take more than 1 h, so resuscitation should continue well beyond 1 h.

Management of Severe Local Anaesthetic Toxicity. AAGBI guidelines, 2010. http://www.aagbi.org/sites/default/files/la_toxicity_2010_0.pdf.

20. Answer: A

The incidence of itching after intrathecal diamorphine is 60–80%, although only a minority actually need treatment. Nausea occurs in about 30%. Respiratory depression is quite rare as pregnancy increases the sensitivity of respiratory centre. Sedation is also rare. Urinary retention is uncommon and does not matter as the patients are catheterized anyway.

Dashfield A. Acute pain epidural analgesia. In: Allman KG, Wilson IH (eds), *Oxford Handbook of Anaesthesia*, 2nd edn. Oxford University Press, 2004: p. 725.

21. Answer: C

Amiodarone is excreted in significant amounts in breast milk, so should be stopped while breastfeeding. Other drugs are excreted in breast milk in insignificant amounts.

Eldridge J. Obstetric anaesthesia and analgesia; breast feeding and drug transfer. In: Allman KG, Wilson IH (eds), *Oxford Handbook of Anaesthesia*, 2nd edn. Oxford University Press, 2004: p. 729.

22. Answer: B

Currently, there is no single, reliable, and cost-effective laboratory test for the diagnosis of pre-eclampsia. Uric acid levels are not sensitive or specific for diagnosis or prognosis of the severity of PET. All other factors are indicative of severe PET.

The Management of Hypertensive Disorders during Pregnancy. NICE clinical guideline, CG107, August 2010. http://www.nice.org.uk/cg107.

Lim KH, Friedman SA, Ecker JL, et al. The clinical utility of serum uric acid measurements in hypertensive diseases of pregnancy. *Am J Obstet Gynecol* 1998; 178: 1067–71.

23. Answer: A

There have been number of prospective trials and case series where LMA was used in full stomach patients but even then the incidence of aspiration was surprisingly quite low. However, it does not provide a reliable seal of the oesophagus or airway. LMA has been used in prone patients but not very routinely. The risk of aspiration with LMA is more when positive-pressure ventilation is used. LMA has been included as an alternative to endotracheal tube during CPR when the arrest team does not have intubation skills.

Barash PG, Cullen BF, Stoelting RK. *Clinical Anesthesia*, 5th edn. Lippincot Williams and Wilkins, 2005: p. 604.

24. Answer: D

Although nasal intubation is considered to be more comfortable and secure for the patient, it has some complications associated with it. Prolonged nasal intubation can cause bacteraemia, epistaxis, sinusitis, otitis media, and retropharyngeal abscess. However, the presence of a constant headache with other signs of infection indicates it is most likely bacterial maxillary sinusitis. Meningitis is relatively rare after nasal intubation unless there is a breach in the base of skull with CSF leak.

Miller RD, Eriksson LI, Fleisher LA, et al. Miller's Anesthesia, 7th edn. Churchill Livingstone, 2009: p. 1445–1446.

25. Answer: D

Angina is uncommon in the morbidly obese because of their limited mobility. Even moderate obesity increases risk of peri-operative complications. Pattern of fat distribution, such as the truncal fat seen in men, predisposes to cardiovascular risks. Obesity affects not only the cardiovascular system but also the respiratory, endocrine, musculoskeletal, metabolic, and gastrointestinal systems.

Barash PG, Cullen BF, Stoelting RK. Clinical Anesthesia, 5th edn. Lippincot Williams and Wilkins, 2005: p. 1040.

26. Answer: C

According to the '4–2–1' fasting fluid requirement formula, the child needs 60 mL/h ($10 \times 4 + 10 \times 2$).

The total fasting deficit is 480 mL (60×8). Half of this, i.e. 240 mL, plus the hourly maintenance of 60 mL, should be given in the first hour, a total of 300 mL.

Berg S. Paediatric and neonatal anaesthesia. In: Allman KG, Wilson IH (eds), Oxford Handbook of Anaesthesia, 2nd edn. Oxford University Press, 2004: p. 763.

Consensus Guideline on Perioperative Fluid Management in Children, v1.1. Association of Paediatric Anaesthetists, 2007. www.apagbi.org.uk/docs/perioperative_fluid_management_2007.pdf.

27. Answer: B

Lumbar epidural analgesia during labour is widely accepted. The impact of epidural analgesia is based on mixtures of low-dose local anaesthetic solutions, and lipophilic opioid on most clinically relevant obstetric outcomes is minimal. Although epidural analgesia can cause some degree of motor block, in patients with long-term asthma it would be important to know the effects on the respiratory system as there is potential for the compromise of the respiratory function. In the study, parturients underwent spirometry ante partum and after receiving epidural analgesia and it was found there is minimal increase of a 7% in forced vital capacity (FVC) and a 2% increase in peak expiratory flow rates (PEFR).

Von Ungern-Sternberg BS, Regli A, Bucher E, et al. The effect of epidural analgesia in labour on maternal respiratory function. Anaesthesia. 2004; 59(4): 350–53.

28. Answer: A

Acute severe asthma:

- PEF: 33–50%
- respiratory rate: >25/min
- heart rate: >110/min
- inability to complete a sentence in one breath

Although there is a rise in $PaCO_2$, an isolated rise $PaCO_2$ in comparison to high respiratory rate is a life-threatening sign of asthma, which is also sign of exhaustion and carries a higher mortality rate.

Asthma Guidelines. BTS/SIGN, 2011. http://www.brit-thoracic.org.uk/guidelines/asthma-guidelines.aspx.

29. Answer: A

Total hip replacement (THR) is not as painful as total knee replacement. The hip joint has complex innervation and therefore there is no single nerve block that reliably provides analgesia for THR. There is evidence that central neuraxial block decreases the blood loss, decreases risk of thromboembolism, and provides better immediate post-operative analgesia. The addition of long-acting opioids will prolong the analgesia. The evidence therefore favours a spinal with a long-acting opioid for THR.

Grant CRK, Checketts MR. Analgesia for primary hip and knee arthroplasty: the role of regional anaesthesia. *Contin Educ Anaesth Crit Care Pain* 2008; 8(2): 56–61.

30. Answer: E

Myoglobin induced acute renal failure (ARF) has a good prognosis. The renal failure occurs because of blockage of the renal tubules with myoglobin, which precipitates in acidic urine. It also causes renal vasoconstriction and oxidative injury to the tubules, but all this is reversible. Patients with creatinine kinase >5000 Units/L develop renal failure in more than 50% of cases. Aggressive fluid resuscitation and urinary alkalization has been shown to prevent ARF. The hyperkalemia results from the release of intracellular K+ from the injured muscle fibres.

Hunter JD, et al. Rhabdomyolysis. *Contin Educ Anaesth Crit Care Pain* 2006; 6(4): 141–43.

True/False

1. **Regarding potassium:**
   A. It is the most important determinant of intracellular osmotic pressure.
   B. It is not as important as sodium as a determinant of extracellular osmotic pressure.
   C. Infusion of potassium should not normally exceed 40 mmol/h.
   D. Changes in extracellular hydrogen ion concentration do not directly affect extracellular $[K^+]$.
   E. Changes in circulating insulin levels can directly alter plasma $[K^+]$ independent of glucose transport.

2. **Regarding intra-aortic balloon pumps:**
   A. It is inserted in a retrograde fashion.
   B. The balloon lies just distal to the left subclavian artery.
   C. It may be inserted via the subclavian artery.
   D. They inflate during the diastole, beginning with closure of aortic valve.
   E. Can be inflated with CO_2.

3. **In a patients with head injury:**
   A. GCS after the initial resuscitation is the most important prognostic indicator.
   B. The motor score of GCS is the most useful component.
   C. Marshall grading system correlates with mortality.
   D. Involvement of abducens nerve reflects injury in middle fossa.
   E. Involvement of 7th cranial nerve reflects injury in middle fossa.

4. **Regarding myasthenia gravis, the following statements are true:**
   A. May present with autonomic disturbances.
   B. More common in women.
   C. Muscarinic symptoms usually suggest over-treatment with acetylcholinesterase inhibitors.
   D. Commonly associated with other autoimmune diseases.
   E. Auto-antibodies are detected in less than 50% of patients with generalized myasthenia gravis.

5. **In renal failure:**

    A. It is not safe to use suxamethonium in the presence of renal failure, even if the serum potassium concentration is below 5 mEq/L.
    B. Intermittent haemodialysis (IHD) is efficient at removing urea.
    C. More than 500 mL/h fluid volume can safely be removed with IHD.
    D. Usually fluid overload causing pulmonary oedema is easier to treat than patients with acute kidney injury due to excessive fluid administration.
    E. Significant accumulation of atropine can occur in patients with renal impairment.

6. **Regarding N- acetylcysteine (NAC) and paracetamol overdose:**

    A. Provides complete protection against hepatotoxicity if given early in non-staggered overdose of paracetamol.
    B. Can be continued indefinitely in cases of acute liver failure.
    C. Prothrombin time is the most sensitive prognostic marker in paracetamol overdose.
    D. Patients with PT more than 36 s at 36 h are very likely to develop acute liver failure.
    E. Initial treatment dose in paracetamol poisoning is 0.5 g/kg over 15 min.

7. **In a patient with cocaine poisoning which of the following can happen:**

    A. Gastrointestinal perforation.
    B. Haemorrhagic stroke.
    C. Ischaemic stroke.
    D. Impairment of haemostasis.
    E. Non-cardiogenic pulmonary oedema.

8. **Regarding magnesium:**

    A. Absorption occurs in jejunum.
    B. Excretion is via the kidney.
    C. Prevalence of hypomagnesaemia is about 50% in intensive care patients.
    D. Ataxia may be a sign of hypomagnesaemia.
    E. Should not be used as a tocolytic drug.

9. **In a case of rib fracture:**

    A. More than three fractured ribs is an indication for hospitalization.
    B. Reported mortality with seven or more rib fractures is about 30%.
    C. Only the first seven ribs are called true ribs.
    D. Epidural analgesia tends to reduce mortality in patients with multiple rib fracture.
    E. 11th rib is a vertebral rib.

10. **Regarding intracranial pressure:**

    A. It reflects cerebral metabolism and blood flow.
    B. It does not correlate with survival in severe head injury.
    C. ICP greater than 60 mmHg is associated with 100 % mortality.
    D. It is normally 1–2 kPa.
    E. In lateral recumbent position, lumbar CSF pressure is normally equal to the supratentorial CSF pressure.

11. The drug clonidine:

    A. Is an imidazole, with $\alpha2$-adrenergic antagonist activity.

    B. Has an antisialogogue effect.

    C. Decreases intraocular pressure.

    D. Increases thyroid function.

    E. Increases gastric motility.

12. Regarding the condition β-thalassaemia major:

    A. It is due to a single gene defect.

    B. It is usually present with severe anaemia immediately after birth.

    C. It causes hypochromic macrocytic anaemia.

    D. Patients may have a normal concentration of HbA2.

    E. Patients synthesize normal amount of α chains.

13. Concerning central venous pressure (CVP):

    A. 'y' descent in CVP waveform is produced by closing of tricuspid valve in diastole and blood flowing into right ventricle.

    B. Massive 'v' wave indicates significant tricuspid regurgitation.

    C. 'x' descent is caused by downward movement of ventricle during diastole.

    D. 'c' wave is caused by elevation of tricuspid valve into right atrium during early ventricular contraction.

    E. Inspiratory fall in CVP indicates fall in CO likely on application of PEEP.

14. Acute kidney injury is defined as:

    A. An abrupt reduction in kidney function, usually within 48 h.

    B. An absolute increase in serum creatinine of more than or equal to 26.4 µmol/L (0.3 mg/dL).

    C. A percentage increase in serum creatinine of more than 25%.

    D. A reduction in urine output of less then or equal 0.5 mL/kg/h for more than 4 h.

    E. 1.5-fold increase in serum creatinine from baseline.

15. Regarding ketamine:

    A. The racemic mixture of ketamine contains both S(+) and R(−) isomers in equal concentrations.

    B. Ketamine has a pKa of 7.5.

    C. R(−) ketamine enantiomers have a greater affinity for the NMDA receptor.

    D. Ketamine has no effect on opiate tolerance and hyperalgesia.

    E. The R(−) isomer of ketamine is more potent.

16. Concerning etomidate:

    A. It has analgesic properties.

    B. Hypnosis occurs through action on the NMDA receptor.

    C. Etomidate can lead to pain during injection.

    D. Etomidate has high lipid solubility.

    E. Adrenocortical suppression is usually temporary.

17. Regarding the determinants of speed of recovery when using an inhalation anaesthetic agents:

A. Using high fresh gas flow to prevent rebreathing increases elimination rate of inhaled anaesthetics.

B. The higher the blood solubility of a volatile, the shorter the recovery time.

C. Blood and tissue solubilities of a volatile are bigger determinants of recovery time than duration or depth (mean inspired concentration) of anaesthesia.

D. Halothane recovery time is same as that of isoflurane, despite having a higher blood gas partition coefficient.

E. In obese patients, prolonged procedures may result in prolonged recovery; this is due to high oil–gas partition coefficient.

18. Regarding the second gas effect when using inhalation anaesthetic agents:

A. The second gas effect persists during the anaesthesia maintenance phase.

B. The ventilation perfusion (V/Q) heterogeneity in the lung further increases the second gas effect.

C. The second gas effect applies to existing alveolar gases, e.g. oxygen. PaO_2 increases after starting to inspire 70% N_2O.

D. High concentration of newly introduced gas in alveolus results in rapid uptake of the gas into pulmonary capillary blood, up its concentration gradient.

E. Rapid uptake of new gas from alveolus results in active concentration of all other gases within alveolus.

19. Regarding physiologic factors affecting induction:

A. Hyperventilation speeds up induction with volatile anaesthetic.

B. Obese patients achieve equilibrium between inspired and alveolar concentration of the volatile agents relatively quickly.

C. Induction time is shorter in patients with atelectasis.

D. Decreased cardiac output prolongs induction time.

E. Increase in cardiac output accelerates anaesthetic uptake and transport to the brain.

20. Regarding blood supply of the spinal cord:

A. The anterior spinal artery is formed by the joining of branches of the vertebral artery.

B. The posterior spinal arteries can arise directly from the vertebral artery.

C. Aortic dissection or aortic atherosclerotic disease can send emboli to the anterior spinal artery, mainly affecting the sensory tracts.

D. The aorta provides segmental blood vessels in the midthoracic region.

E. The artery of Adamkiewicz is on the left side of the vertebral column in 78% of patients and is variably located between segments T8 and L4, usually T9–T11.

21. **Regarding the condition central post-stroke pain:**
    A. It is a form of neuropathic pain associated with lesion of the CNS.
    B. It can be associated with injury to the spinal cord.
    C. It is often associated with ischemic lesion within thalamus.
    D. Allodydia is an uncommon feature in central post-stroke pain.
    E. It develops in 8% of stroke patients.

22. **Regarding transthoracic echocardiography (TTE):**
    A. Ejection fraction (EF) is a relatively poor index of myocardial contractility on resting TTE.
    B. In patients in ICU on IPPV, the interposition of air-filled lung between body surface and heart limits access while performing TTE.
    C. Diastolic function is difficult to quantify using TTE.
    D. Qualitative assessment of chamber size and function can be done with TTE.
    E. A simplified Bernoulli equation is used for quantitative assessment of gradient across valves.

23. **Regarding early goal-directed therapy (EGDT) the therapeutic components and goals include:**
    A. Avoiding antibiotics.
    B. Titration of crystalloid infusion to achieve CVP greater than 12 mmHg.
    C. Administration of inotrope if mean arterial pressure (MAP) is less than 70 mmHg.
    D. Administration of vasodilator if MAP is greater than 90 mm Hg.
    E. Applying PEEP if patient is hypoxic.

24. **Concerning heparin:**
    A. Heparin-induced thrombocytopaenia (HIT) is caused by shortened platelet survival time.
    B. Heparin-induced thrombocytopaenia is associated with bleeding.
    C. Heparin-induced thrombocytopaenia is associated with thrombosis.
    D. Long-term therapy can cause hyperkalaemia.
    E. Long-term therapy can stimulate osteoblasts and result in new bone formation.

25. **Concerning acute hyponatraemic encephalopathy (AHE):**
    A. Hypoxia is the main cause of brain damage in patients with symptomatic hyponatraemia.
    B. Elderly males are resistant to AHE.
    C. Children are generally resistant to AHE.
    D. Brain cannot increase in volume by more than 10% without herniation.
    E. It is more common in men.

26. **Regarding intrathecal administration of drugs**
    A. Normobaric drugs given intrathecally are distributed rapidly within the cerebrospinal fluid and are detectable within the cisterna magna within 20–30 min of injection.
    B. Lipophilic drugs penetrate the spinal cord and traverse the dura to enter the epidural space.
    C. Vascular uptake accounts for the limited duration of action of lipophilic opioids.
    D. Morphine is more hydrophilic than fentanyl and binds less to fat within the epidural space.
    E. Analgesia distribution with intrathecal morphine is relatively unaffected by site of injection.

27. Regarding critical illness myopathy (CIM):

A. It can present as failure to wean in ventilated patients.
B. Muscle biopsy characteristically shows a diffuse non-necrotizing myopathy accompanied by fibre atrophy.
C. CIM usually resolves, with long-term sequelae.
D. Does not occur together with critical illness polyneuropathy.
E. Usually there is evidence of sensory neuropathy.

28. The following applies for antiretroviral drugs:

A. The aim of therapy is to achieve an undetectable viral load.
B. Treatment should be initiated only when CD4 cell counts are <350 cells/mm^3.
C. Zidovudine is a nucleoside reverse transcriptase inhibitor.
D. Indinavir inhibits processing of viral proteins.
E. Triple therapy consists of two protease inhibitors combined with a nucleoside reverse transcriptase inhibitor.

29. Regarding the nerve supply to the lower limb:

A. The terminal branch of the femoral nerve supplies sensation to the majority of the skin of the forefoot.
B. The lateral cutaneous nerve of the thigh is a branch of the femoral nerve.
C. The deep peroneal nerve pierces the anterior intermuscular septum.
D. The deep peroneal nerve lies medial to the dorsalis pedis artery in the foot.
E. The sural nerve accompanies the long saphenous vein.

30. Regarding the breathing systems, the following statements are correct:

A. Coaxial Mapleson A is efficient for mechanical ventilation.
B. Mapleson D requires a fresh gas flow of 70–100 mL/kg/min for mechanical ventilation.
C. Magill requires a fresh gas flow of 70–100 mL/kg/min for spontaneous ventilation.
D. Mapleson C is efficient for spontaneous ventilation.
E. Lack requires a fresh gas flow of 70–100 mL/kg/min for spontaneous ventilation.

31. Regarding the condition with long QT syndrome:

A. The duration of the QT interval depends on the heart rate.
B. There can be association with deafness.
C. Congenital long QT syndrome is autosomal dominant.
D. Hyperkalaemia makes the condition worse.
E. May be caused by dietary irregularities.

32. Congenital heart disease:

A. The most common congenital heart defect is an atrial septal defect.
B. Ostium primum holes are the most common type of atrial septal defect.
C. Eisenmenger's syndrome is a right-to-left shunt associated with pulmonary hypertension and cyanosis.
D. Spontaneous closure of a VSD occurs in <10% of patients.
E. Ebstein's anomaly is a congenital defect of the tricuspid valve in which the opening of the tricuspid valve is displaced towards the apex of the right ventricle of the heart.

33. **Chronic regional pain syndrome:**
    A. May be associated with osteoporosis.
    B. May be associated with an increase in skin temperature.
    C. Often presents with pain as the presenting complaint.
    D. Is associated with vasomotor disturbances.
    E. Is more common in athletes.

34. **The following statements are true regarding xenon:**
    A. It is manufactured by fractional distillation of natural gas.
    B. It has a MAC value of 63.
    C. It decreases airway resistance.
    D. It does not produce preconditioning.
    E. It is flammable.

35. **Regarding compartment syndrome:**
    A. No pain when limb is passively flexed.
    B. Occurs only in lower limbs.
    C. May cause acute tubular necrosis due to myoglobinaemia.
    D. Is diagnosed by an absent pulse.
    E. Manifest by paraesthesia in a peripheral nerve distribution.

36. **Regarding propofol infusion syndrome:**
    A. Usually seen in patients who have had propofol infusion for over 96 h.
    B. Usually seen if infusion rates are greater than 4 mg/kg/h.
    C. Presents with metabolic alkalosis.
    D. Presents with enlarged fatty liver.
    E. Presents with hyperlipidaemia.

37. **Indications for temporary pacing after cardiac surgery do not include:**
    A. Prolonged AV delay.
    B. Type II second-degree block.
    C. New bifasicular block.
    D. Prolonged QTc with bradycardia.
    E. Atrial flutter.

38. **The following statement is true regarding tetanus:**
    A. The manifestations of tetanus are caused by the tetanolysin neurotoxin released by the
       C. tetani bacterium.
    B. Can be treated with ciprofloxacin.
    C. Can cause type 1 or type 2 respiratory failure or both.
    D. Is diagnosed from culture of the *C. tetani* bacterium.
    E. Autonomic dysfunction is the major cause of mortality in the developing world.

39. Regarding conventional transdermal drug delivery:

A. The drugs diffuse through the stratum corneum by passive transport.
B. The drugs undergo first-pass metabolism.
C. Can be used for rapid delivery of drugs.
D. The drugs should have high lipophilicity for transdermal diffusion.
E. The drugs should have low melting point for transdermal diffusion.

40. The following are suggestive of croup rather than epiglottitis:

A. Barking cough.
B. Temperature > 39°C.
C. Stridor sounds harsh.
D. Sudden onset.
E. Drooling.

41. The recurrent laryngeal nerve:

A. Is a branch of the vagus nerve.
B. Left is shorter than the right.
C. Supplies the inferior constrictor muscle.
D. Contributes fibres to the cardiac plexus.
E. Supplies sensation to the posterior two-thirds of the tongue.

42. Severe hypercapnia is associated with:

A. Papilloedema.
B. Raised central venous pressure.
C. Rapid thready pulse.
D. Cool periphery.
E. Raised blood pressure.

43. Finger clubbing is seen in the following conditions:

A. Asbestosis.
B. Chronic bronchitis.
C. Fibrosing alveolitis.
D. Thalassemia.
E. Broncheictasis.

44. Regarding physiologic factors affecting induction:

A. Hyperventilation speeds up induction with volatile anaesthetic.
B. Obese patients achieve equilibrium between inspired and alveolar concentration of the volatile agents relatively quickly.
C. Induction time is shorter in patients with atelectasis.
D. Decreased cardiac output prolongs induction time.
E. Increase in cardiac output accelerates anaesthetic uptake and transport to the brain.

45. In a patient with spinal cord infarction the following sensation modalities are usually preserved:

A. Pain.

B. Temperature.

C. Joint proprioception.

D. Two-point discrimination.

E. Vibration.

46. Concerning confidence intervals:

A. Confidence intervals are larger with large sample size.

B. They indicate the presence or absence of a statistical difference between two groups.

C. A 95% confidence interval means that 95% of all observed values fall within that interval.

D. In an odds ratio, the 95% confidence should include unity for there to be any difference between the values compared in the study.

E. Confidence interval gives a range of values within which the true value will lie.

47. Regarding measures of central tendency:

A. Mode is the measurement below which half the observations fall.

B. Median is the most frequently occurring observed value.

C. The arithmetic mean, median, and mode are always identical.

D. The median is shifted to the left in the negatively skewed distribution curve.

E. The shape of the normal distribution curve is completely determined by the mean and standard deviation.

48. Patients using psychoactive drugs frequently present for both elective and emergency surgery with significant implications for anaesthesia such as:

A. Tricyclic antidepressants (TCAs) can cause prolongation of QT interval leading to perioperative arrhythmias.

B. Selective serotonin reuptake inhibitors (SSRIs) can precipitate serotonin syndrome with the use of tramadol or pethidine.

C. Lithium can reduce the duration of depolarizing neuromuscular block.

D. Haloperidol can produce features of Parkinsonism and tardive dyskinesia.

E. Quetiapine can produce postural hypotension and neuroleptic malignant syndrome.

49. Regarding autonomic neuropathy:

A. Autonomic neuropathy can be central or peripheral.

B. Can be sympathetic or parasympathetic.

C. Patients are not at risk of developing severe hypotension with extradural anaesthesia unlike spinal anaesthesia.

D. Patients are at increased risk of aspiration.

E. Autonomic neuropathy seen in Shy–Drager syndrome is generally progressive.

50. Presence of bias in a study implies that:

   A. The results of study are not precise and accurate.
   B. The results of the study are not precise.
   C. There is a systematic difference between the obtained results and the expected results.
   D. The results of the study may be accurate but not precise.
   E. The results of the study are not accurate.

51. The following conditions are associated with central pontine myelinosis:

   A. Hyponatraemia.
   B. Alcoholism.
   C. Malnutrition.
   D. Diuretic therapy.
   E. Liver transplantation.

52. Regarding cricothyroidotomy:

   A. Incision is performed above the thyroid cartilage.
   B. The cricoid cartilage is at the level of C6 vertebrae.
   C. May be performed for trans-tracheal injection of local anaesthetic to facilitate awake intubation.
   D. Incision is performed below the cricoid cartilage.
   E. Barotraumas may result when passive expiration is not allowed.

53. Regarding diaphragm:

   A. The central tendon is attached to the pericardium.
   B. Both the crura attach to the upper lumbar vertebrae.
   C. It is pierced by the splanchnic nerves and the left phrenic nerve.
   D. The right phrenic nerve is transmitted through the opening for inferior vena cava.
   E. Lower intercostal nerves provide sensory supply to the diaphragm.

54. Concerning spinal vertebrae:

   A. Axis lacks a body.
   B. All 12 thoracic vertebrae articulate with the corresponding ribs.
   C. Pedicle extends between the transverse processes and the spinous processes.
   D. The laminae extends between the vertebral body and the transverse processes.
   E. In children the spinal cord ends at L3.

55. Concerning advance directive:

   A. Advance directive can only be made by a competent adult over 18 years of age.
   B. Individual can be coerced into making an advanced directive if there is a foreseeable condition that will incapacitate them in the near future.
   C. It is not necessary for the individual to have sufficient information about the medical prognosis when they make an advance refusal.
   D. Advance directive is a way of prolonging the autonomy of the patient.
   E. Advance directive can request treatment that is not in the patient's best interests.

56. Regarding consent:

A. The patient can make a choice that is not sensible.
B. A highly irrational decision may indicate underlying mental illness.
C. In case of incapacity the patient's relatives can consent to medical or surgical treatment.
D. Best interests include personal, social, and financial factors.
E. The anaesthetic room is an acceptable place to consent a patient.

57. Concerning analysis of arterial blood gas:

A. Excess heparin in the sample increases the pH reading.
B. Air bubble in the sample will increase the partial pressure of oxygen.
C. If the sample is stored at room temperature before analysis, the partial pressure of carbon dioxide increases.
D. The normal hydrogen ion concentration is 40 nmol/mL.
E. It is possible to measure the partial pressure of carbon dioxide by measuring pH.

58. When a face mask is used during anaesthesia:

A. There is no significant effect on the apparatus dead space.
B. It is essential for the rubber mask to be covered by carbon particles, as an antistatic measure.
C. It is essential to check and inflate the cuff of the mask.
D. The face masks have a 15-mm end to connect to the catheter mount.
E. Goldman nasal inhaler is a nasal mask that can be used for dental procedures.

59. Regarding epidural catheters:

A. It has a length of 90 cm.
B. The side ports are the points of weakness where the catheter may break.
C. At least 5 cm of the catheter should be advanced into the epidural space.
D. Catheters with side port have a reduced incidence of dural puncture compared to those with single port.
E. The filter should be changed every 24 h.

60. The concentration of the following clotting factors increase during pregnancy:

A. IX.
B. X.
C. XI.
D. XII.
E. XIII.

Single Best Answers

1. **After a difficult intubation on a 65-year-old with cervical spondylosis, the patient presents with paralysis of upper limbs but only weakness of the lower limbs. Cervical spine X-ray shows only degenerative changes. What is the diagnosis?**
    A. Central cord syndrome.
    B. Brown–Sequard syndrome.
    C. Posterior cord syndrome.
    D. Anterior cord syndrome.
    E. Transverse myelitis.

2. **An adult male who was an unrestrained driver in an accident is rushed to the hospital. He has multiple bruises over anterior chest and abdominal wall. His blood pressure is 70/30 mmHg and his pulse rate is 100/min. Trachea is midline. Pulmonary capillary wedge pressure (PCWP) is 12 mmHg. After rapid administration of 1 L crystalloid, the PCWP is 22 and BP is 75/30 mmHg with pulse rate 123/min. The likely diagnosis is:**
    A. Myocardial contusion.
    B. Pulmonary embolism.
    C. Pneumothorax.
    D. Hypovolaemic shock.
    E. Neurogenic shock.

3. **A 46-year-old heavy smoker has decreased breath sounds at the right lung base on the second day following upper abdominal surgery. He is afebrile and his vital signs are stable, but he is hypoxaemic. Chest X-ray shows a triangular opacity in the right lower chest. The most effective strategy to prevent this condition is:**
    A. Broad-spectrum antibiotics given preoperatively.
    B. Broad-spectrum antibiotics given postoperatively.
    C. Smoking cessation 1 week before surgery.
    D. Preoperative use of glucocorticoids.
    E. Active breathing exercises.

4. **A 45-year-old patient on warfarin for atrial fibrillation presents with acute abdomen. X-ray shows gas under the diaphragm. His blood results show haemoglobin of 9.2, platelet count of 90 000/mm³, and INR of 2.1. Which of the following is the best initial treatment preoperatively?**
    A. Fresh frozen plasma.
    B. Vitamin K.
    C. Packed RBC transfusion.
    D. Desmopressin.
    E. Platelet transfusion.

5. On day 3 following severe traumatic brain injury, an adult patient still
    has raised intracranial pressure (ICP), despite adequate sedation,
    elevation of head end, and removal of CSF. How can hyperventilation
    decrease ICP in this patient?

    A. By decreasing capillary leak.
    B. By increasing PO_2.
    C. By causing cerebral vasoconstriction.
    D. Increased venous outflow from head.
    E. By causing cerebral vasodilatation.

6. A 1-day-old term neonate is transferred to your regional paediatric
    ICU. A congenital diaphragmatic hernia has been diagnosed. The baby
    is already intubated and receiving artificial ventilation. Which of the
    following is incorrect about this condition?

    A. Stomach should be deflated using oro-gastric tube to reduce lung compression.
    B. Early enteral nutrition should be commenced.
    C. Adequate sedation usually obviates need for paralysis.
    D. Allow (permissive) hypercapnia, as aggressive ventilatory support may damage the
        vulnerable lungs.
    E. Surgery will improve lung function and oxygenation.

7. A previously fit 24-year-old patient has been admitted to your intensive
    care unit with an isolated severe head injury. Eighteen hours after
    admission he develops polyuria. Which of the following is not a feature
    of central diabetes insipidus?

    A. Urine osmolality less than 200 mOsmol/kg.
    B. Urinary sodium concentration 20–60 mmol/L.
    C. Plasma osmolality less than 280 mOsmol/kg.
    D. Serum sodium concentration greater than 145 mmol/L.
    E. Urinary specific gravity less than 1.005.

8. One day after admission for traumatic fracture of femur a young man
    is found to have petechial rash, and he is confused and tachypneic. ABG
    shows pH 7.49, PO_2 6.7, and PCO_2 3.7. The most probable diagnosis is:

    A. Haematoma of the thorax.
    B. Pulmonary embolism.
    C. Fat embolism.
    D. Staphylococcus aureus pneumonia.
    E. Pulmonary oedema.

9. **A COPD patient presents with aching in both wrists, clubbing, and weight loss. The skin is warm and red. X-ray of wrists shows periosteal thickening and possible infection. Which of the following is the most appropriate treatment?**
    A. Perform chest radiograph.
    B. Aspirate wrist joint.
    C. Treat the patient with methotrexate.
    D. Obtain ESR.
    E. Treat with antibiotics.

10. **A 68-year-old patient with congestive heart failure is to receive total hip replacement. Which of the following is the best prophylaxis to prevent pulmonary embolism, if the patient has no other significant medical history?**
    A. Early mobilization.
    B. Clopidogrel 75 mg/day.
    C. Aspirin 325 mg/day.
    D. Warfarin (to maintain INR between 2 and 3) or low molecular weight heparin (LMWH).
    E. Subcutaneous heparin 5000 units every 12 h.

11. **A 54-year-old patient admitted to the intensive care unit has low-grade fever. On examination of chest, he has decreased excursion on right side and reduced fremitus. The percussion note is dull and breath sounds are decreased on right side. The trachea is deviated to left. The most likely diagnosis is:**
    A. Pneumonic consolidation.
    B. Atelectasis.
    C. Chronic obstructive pulmonary disease.
    D. Pleural effusion.
    E. Pneumothorax.

12. **An alcoholic patient with poor oral hygiene presents with cough and fever. Chest X-ray reveals air-fluid level in the superior segment of right lower lobe. The most likely causative organism is:**
    A. *Mycoplasma pneumoniae.*
    B. Anaerobic agents.
    C. Legionella.
    D. *Haemophillus influenza.*
    E. Streptococcus pneumoniae.

13. **A 65-year-old patient with pulmonary oedema is intubated and ventilated. Echocardiogram shows ejection fraction of 44%, with severe mitral regurgitation (MR). There is no improvement even after aggressive treatment with furosemide. What is the next best step in treating this patient?**
   A. Start the patient cautiously on a second-loop diuretic.
   B. Start the patient on enalapril.
   C. Start the patient on β-blocker.
   D. Patient will need placement of intra-aortic balloon pump (IABP).
   E. Arrange for mitral valve replacement surgery.

14. **A 19-year-old primiparous at 32 weeks presents with BP of 158/98 mmHg, 1+ proteinuria, and tonic clonic seizure. Which of the following is indicated in immediate treatment for this patient?**
   A. Antihypertensive therapy.
   B. Emergency caesarean section.
   C. Magnesium sulphate.
   D. Load the patient with phenytoin.
   E. Aspirin.

15. **A 30-year-old with placenta praevia has a caesarean section under general anaesthesia. Which of the following is contraindicated in this patient with uterine atony?**
   A. Intramuscular methylergometrine.
   B. Hemabate suppository.
   C. Misoprostol suppository.
   D. Intravenous terbutaline.
   E. Prostaglandin E2 suppository.

16. **Following an emergency caesarean section under general anaesthesia, the patient presents with respiratory distress and tachycardia in recovery. Auscultation reveals coarse crepitations in right lower lobe. Her condition is most likely due to:**
   A. Endotracheal intubation.
   B. Positive pressure ventilation.
   C. Extubation of patient in semi-erect position.
   D. Extubation of the patient in lateral recumbent position with lowered head.
   E. Administration of antacid prior to induction.

17 **A 5-year-old boy presents to A&E having sustained a cerebrovascular accident. On examination there is increased muscle tone. Lesion of which structure is unlikely in this patient?**
   A. Spinal chord.
   B. Basal ganglia.
   C. Internal capsule.
   D. Cerebellum.
   E. Pyramidal tract.

18. **A 38-year-old presents with ulnar nerve injury following ulnar nerve block just above the wrist. The patient will be unable to:**
    A. Extend his wrist.
    B. Flex his wrist.
    C. Spread his fingers.
    D. Oppose the thumb and index finger.
    E. Flex the distal phalages of fourth and fifth digits.

19. **After receiving deep intramuscular steroid injection for neck pain a 45-year-old patient presents with wrist drop. The site of injury could be:**
    A. Brachial plexus: posterior cord.
    B. Brachial plexus: medial cord.
    C. Brachial plexus: lateral cord.
    D. Spinal root: T1.
    E. Spinal root: C5.

20. **A 34-year-old female patient presents with pain on the right side of the face. Trigeminal neuralgia is diagnosed. Which of the following is not true about this condition?**
    A. It is almost exclusively unilateral pain in the distribution of trigeminal nerve.
    B. Episodes of severe pain can occur spontaneously without any triggering factor.
    C. It can occur due to tumour or disease such as multiple sclerosis.
    D. It is easier to treat in comparison with trigeminal neuropathy.
    E. Microvascular decompression (MVD) in the treatment of this condition involves mobilizing the veins and dividing the arterial branch of the superior cerebellar artery compressing the trigeminal nerve.

21. **The MRI scan of a 20-year-old man following a head injury shows multiple foci of punctuate haemorrhage. This is suggestive of:**
    A. Ischemic infarction of brain.
    B. Diffuse axonal injury.
    C. Malignant hypertension.
    D. Amyloid angiopathy.
    E. Coagulopathy.

22. **A 66-year-old patient in intensive care is intubated and ventilated for a neurological condition requiring prolonged ventilatory support. The patient is started on systemic cephalosporins for the first four days in the unit. Which of the following is true about selective digestive tract decontamination?**
    A. Aims to prevent incidence of ventilator associated pneumonia (VAP).
    B. Rate of pneumonia in intensive care patients doubles if they are ventilated.
    C. Aims to eliminate anaerobic intestinal flora through selective use of antibiotics.
    D. Has not been shown to reduce mortality in intensive care unit.
    E. Comprises use of intravenous ciprofloxacin.

23. **A 45-year-old patient with neuropathic pain in right leg is implanted with spinal cord stimulator implant. Which of the following is not true about patients with spinal chord stimulators?**
    A. Can have 1.5-T MRI head scan.
    B. Can have simultaneous cardiovascular implantable electronic device.
    C. Can have artefacts on ECG.
    D. Pre-existing permanent pacemaker (PPM) should be considered as a general contraindication for neurostimulation therapy, due to the electromagnetic interference between the two devices.
    E. Patients with failed back surgery syndrome and treated with spinal cord stimulator implants do better than re-operation.

24. **A 28-year old multiparous woman at 35 weeks gestation presents with vaginal bleeding. On examination her blood pressure is 90/60, her pulse is 116/min, and she has a respiratory rate of 16. Which of the following is the most appropriate next step in management?**
    A. Emergency referral to the obstetrician.
    B. Obtain venous access with two large-bore cannula.
    C. Immediate caesarean section.
    D. Check full blood count, PT/INR, and PTT.
    E. Internal vaginal examination.

25. **Eight hours after receiving labour epidural anaesthesia, examination shows that cervix is soft, 50% effaced, and still 2 cm dilated, which is unchanged. The patient had a normal vaginal delivery for her first pregnancy, for which she required an episiotomy. The estimated foetal weight is 7.5 lb. The most likely cause of the prolonged labour is:**
    A. Early epidural anaesthesia.
    B. Perineal scarring.
    C. False labour.
    D. Cephalopelvic disproportion.
    E. Possible cervical dysfunction.

26. **A 56-year-old man is admitted with fracture of the right sixth and seventh ribs after a fall. His blood pressure is 140/88 mmHg, heart rate is 92/min, and respiratory rate is 24/min and shallow. Which of the following is the most important goal in management of the fracture in this patient?**
    A. Ensure adequate ventilation after intubation.
    B. Use only colloids for fluid resuscitation.
    C. Provide mechanical stabilization of the chest wall.
    D. Ensure adequate analgesia.
    E. Give prophylactic antibiotics.

27. **After a motor vehicle collision, a 25-year-old is found to have blood pressure of 90/60 mmHg and pulse rate of 126/min. After administering 2 L of Hartman's solution, the BP is 110/70 mmHg and pulse is 90/min. His abdomen is tender in the left upper quadrant and ultrasound shows fluid in spleno-renal angle. What is the most appropriate next step?**
    A. Perform emergency laprotomy.
    B. Perform CT scan.
    C. Transfer the patient to intensive care .
    D. Perform laproscopy.
    E. Administer blood.

28. **A 36-year-old man presents to A&E with massive haemoptysis and bright red foamy sputum. His blood pressure is 100/60 mmHg and his pulse rate is 110/min. Breath sounds are audible on both sides. Chest X-ray shows opacity in right lower lobe. The next best step is to:**
    A. Organize a urgent CT scan.
    B. Perform upper gastrointestinal tract endoscopy.
    C. Rigid bronchoscopy.
    D. Perform pulmonary arteriography with embolism.
    E. Prepare the patient for emergency thoracotomy.

29. **Three days after an elective cholecystectomy, a 63-year-old patient presents with blood pressure of 148/100 mmHg, pulse rate of 92/min, and SpO_2 of 90%. Which of the following will increase her functional residual capacity significantly?**
    A. Decrease the total opioid dose being administered to the patient.
    B. Nebulized salbutamol.
    C. Administer intravenous naloxone.
    D. Elevation of the head of the bed and making the patient sit up.
    E. Pneumatic compression device to her lower limbs.

30. **Twenty-four hours after surgical repair of infra-renal aortic aneurysm, a patient develops progressive abdominal pain and bloody diarrhoea. He was given cefuroxime antibiotic prophylaxis perioperatively. His temperature is 38.6°C, blood pressure 110/65 mmHg, and pulse rate 22/min. He has a distended and tender abdomen.**
    A. Infectious diarrhoea caused by *E. coli*.
    B. Pseudomembranous colitis caused by bacterium *Clostridium difficile*.
    C. Bowel ischaemia or infarction.
    D. Aortoenteric fistula.
    E. Iatrogenic bowel perforation.

True/False

1. Answers: T T T F T

Potassium is the most important determinant of intracellular osmotic pressure, and sodium is the most important determinant extracellular osmotic pressure.

Some factors that influence potassium shift between various compartments include.

- changes in the extracellular pH
- circulating catecholamines
- insulin levels
- osmolality of plasma
- temperature (hypothermia).

Insulin and catecholamines decrease plasma [K^+] by acting on the Na^+–K^+ ATPase activity and changes in circulating insulin levels can alter plasma [K^+] independent of glucose concentration. Generally the treatment of electrolyte disorder is empirical and is based on published literature and expert opinion. The patient's clinical condition and the pathophysiology of the disorder should dictate the speed of correction. The current recommendation for correction of hypokalaemia is infusion of potassium with a rate not exceeding 40 mmol/h.

Morgan GE, Mikhail MS, Murray MS. Management of patients with fluid and electrolyte disturbances. In: *Clinical Anaesthesiology*, 4th edn. McGraw-Hill, 2006.

Paradis OC. *Fluids and Electrolytes*, 2nd edn. Lippincott, 1999.

2. Answers: T T T T T

The intra-aortic balloon pump (IABP) is considered to be the single most effective and widely used device for temporary mechanical assistance of the failing heart.

The IAB catheter consists of a polyurethane balloon mounted on a catheter, which is inserted into the patient's descending thoracic aorta, just distal to the left subclavian artery and above the renal arteries. The IAB catheter is connected to a pneumatic pump that shuttles helium in and out of the balloon to inflate and deflate it in time with the mechanical cardiac cycle. IABP exerts its effect by volume displacement, which augments coronary blood flow by the following methods.

- Increasing aortic pressure during diastole (i.e. increases myocardial oxygen delivery); this is achieved by balloon inflation. Inflation of balloon is timed to occur as soon as the aortic valve closes (dicrotic notch).
- Decreasing aortic pressure during systole to reduce workload of LV (i.e. decreases myocardial oxygen demand); this is achieved by balloon deflation.

Balloon deflation is timed to occur immediately before the aortic valve opens (and the IABP wave upstroke).

Papaioannou TG, Stefanadis C. Basic principles of the intraaortic balloon pump and mechanisms affecting its performance. *ASAIO J* 2005; 51(3): 296–300.

3. Answers: T T T F T

Cranial nerve lesions in head injury may reflect the site of injury:

- anterior fossa (1–6 CN)
- middle fossa (7–8 CN)
- posterior fossa (9–10 CN).

Marshall grading system (Table 3.1) comprises four grades defined by CT brain appearance in head injury patients with diffuse axonal injury. Glasgow Coma Score after initial resuscitation is a good prognostic indicator for patients with head injury.

Table 3.1 Marshall grading system

Grade	CT changes	Mortality %
1	No intracranial injury visible.	10
2	Cisterns present. Midline shift 0–5 mm and small, high or mixed density lesions <25 cc	14
3	Cisterns compressed or absent	34
4	Midline shift >5 mm +1, 2, or 3	56

Marshall LF, Marshall SB, Klauber MR, et al. The diagnosis of head injury requires a classification based on CAT. J Neurotrauma 1992; 9(Suppl 1): S287–92.

4. Answers: F T T T F

Myasthenia gravis (MG) is an autoimmune condition characterized by easy fatigability of skeletal muscles. It is more common in women, and women typically present with this condition in their third decade while men have the highest incidence in their sixth and seventh decades. The post-synaptic acetylcholine receptors at the neuromuscular junction (NMJ) are thought to be destroyed by autoantibodies. IgG autoantibodies against nicotinic acetylcholine receptors in NMJ are found in about 90% of patients with generalized myasthenia gravis and in about 60% of patients with ocular myasthenia gravis. More than half the patients have thymic hyperplasia and about 10% develop thymoma. Patients generally present with asymmetric weakness, which may be confined to one group of muscles, or generalized weakness. Ocular muscles are most commonly affected. Patients with bulbar involvement present with dysarthria and difficulty with swallowing, which may result in aspiration. The autonomic nervous system is not involved in myasthenia.

Treatment of mild disease includes anticholinesterase drugs to improve muscle weakness by increasing the available acetylcholine at NMJ. However, overdose of this drug results in cholinergic crisis.

A combination of anticholinesterases and immunomodulators is used to treat moderate-to-severe conditions. Patients with respiratory failure and bulbar involvement may need plasmapheresis. A majority of patients show improvement after thymectomy.

Thavasothy M, Hirsch N. Myasthenia gravis. BJA CEPD Rev 2002; 2(3): 88–90.

Teasdale, A. Neurological and muscular disorders: myasthenia gravis. In: Allman KG, Wilson IH. Oxford Handbook of Anaesthesia. Oxford University Press, 2006: pp. 246–250.

5. Answers: F T T T T

Intermittent haemodialysis (IHD) is efficient at removing urea. The clearance rate is 198 mL/min, compared to 30 mL/min for continuous veno-venous haemodiafiltration.

IHD requires a shorter time and is less labour-intensive in the ITU. More than 500 mL/h of fluid can be safely removed. Enflurane must be avoided as fluoride ions can accumulate.

Suxamethonium can be safely used if $[K^+]$ is less than 5 mEq/L. Atropine and glycopyrrolate have a potential for significant accumulation in renal failure. In groups that can be compared there is no difference in mortality between intermittent haemodialysis and continuous veno-venous haemodiafiltration. Pulmonary oedema caused by fluid overload can often be effectively treated when diagnosed early.

Pannu N, Klarenbach S, Wiebe N, et al. Renal replacement therapy in patients with acute renal failure a systematic review. JAMA 2008; 299(7): 793–805.

6. Answers: T T T T F

In paracetamol toxicity there is depletion of hepatic glutathione. Toxic metabolic intermediates rely on glutathione accumulate in the body. N-acetyl-p-benzoquinone imine is a toxic minor metabolite, which is normally conjugated by glutathione. It interacts with hepatic enzymes and damages the hepatocytes in patacetamol overdose.

Dosage of intravenous N-acetylcysteine (NAC) in adults (refer to Toxbase):

1. Start with 150 mg/kg in 200 mL of 5% dextrose over 15 min.
2. This is followed by 50 mg/kg 500 mL of 5% dextrose over 4 h.
3. Then 100 mg/kg in 1000 mL of 5% dextrose given over 16 h.

N-acetylcysteine, if given within 12 h, will provide complete protection against hepatotoxicity. In acute liver failure it can be give at 150 mg/kg/day until improvement occurs or transplant is performed. The efficacy is, however, not proven. About 50% of the overdose patients with PT greater than 36 s at 36 h will develop acute liver failure. NAC acts as a sulfhydryl donor to restore the glutathione stores.

Other uses of NAC include:

- mucolytic agent
- for sulphate repletion in autism
- nephroprotective agent in prevention of contrast induced nephropathy
- in decontamination of sputum (Petroff's method)
- in psychiatric disorders.

Dargan PI, Jones A. Acetaminophen poisoning: an update for intensivist. Crit Care 2002; 6: 108–10.

Vale JA, Proudfoot AT. Paracetamol (acetaminophen) poisoning. Lancet 1995; 346: 547–52.

7. Answers: T T T F T

In cocaine poisoning there is increased platelet activation and decreased protein C and antithrombin 3 levels, which results in a hypercoagulable state. This predisposes to arterial thrombosis, stroke, and MI. Hypertensive crisis can cause haemorrhagic stroke. Cerebral vasospasm can also cause ischaemic stroke. Extrapyramidal movement disorder suggests accumulation of dopamine in basal ganglia due to chronic ingestion. Cocaine poisoning can also manifest as pulmonary infarction, haemorrhage, asthma, and pneumonitis.

Shanti CM, Lucas CE. Cocaine and the critical care challenge. Crit Care 2003; 31(6): 1851–9.

Montoya ID, McCann DJ. Drugs of abuse: management of intoxication and antidotes. EXS 2010; 100: 519–41.

Ward C, Sair M. Oral poisoning: an update. Contin Educ Anaesth Crit Care Pain 2010; 10(1): 6–11.

8. Answers: F T T T F

Magnesium is an intracellular cation which acts as a cofactor in several important enzyme pathways. Normal magnesium (Mg) levels in serum are 0.7–1 mmol/L. The prevalence of deficiency of Mg in intensive care patients is 50–60%. Only about 30% of the magnesium is absorbed. It is absorbed in terminal ileum and mainly excreted in the kidneys.

Distribution of the body's magnesium stores is:

1. bone (67%)
2. intracellular compartment (31%)
3. extracellular fluid (1–2%).

Hypomagnesaemia in critically ill patients is a common problem that is often overlooked. This is usually accompanied with hypokalaemia and hypophosphatemia.

Use of β-adrenergic agonists can cause transient hypomagnesaemia due to uptake by adipose tissue. The clinical features include muscle weakness, fasciculations, paraesthesia, ataxia, and convulsions. In critical care settings when hypomagnesaemia cannot be corrected orally, 1–2 mg magnesium sulphate can be administered intravenously over 60 min.

Watson VF, Vaughan RS. Magnesium and the anaesthetist. *BJA CEPD Rev* 2001; 1(1): 16–20.

9. Answers: T T T T

The first to seventh ribs are connected by the costal cartilages, with the vertebral column behind and with the sternum in front. They are hence called true, or vertebrosternal, ribs. Ribs 8–10 have cartilages that are attached to the cartilage of the rib above; these are the vertebrochondral ribs. The last two ribs are free anteriorly. The 11th and 12th ribs are called floating or vertebral ribs. More than six fractured ribs in an elderly patient is a strong indication for admission to the high dependency unit or ICU. Ziegler *et al.* reported that patients with one or two rib fractures had a 5% mortality rate, and patients with seven or more fractures had a 29% mortality rate. The average blood loss per fractured rib is estimated to be 100–150 mL. However, compared to other bones rib fractures heal early. Adequate analgesia and chest physiotherapy are vital in patients with multiple rib fractures.

Sirmali M, Türüt H, Topçu S, et al. A comprehensive analysis of traumatic rib fractures: morbidity, mortality and management. *Eur J Cardiothorac Surg* 2003; 24(1): 133–8.

Ziegler DW, Agarwal NN. The morbidity and mortality of rib fractures. *J Trauma* 1994; 37(6): 975–9.

10. Answers: T F T T T

The cranial vault, which has a fixed volume, consists of the:

- brain (80%)
- blood (12%)
- cerebrospinal fluid (8%).

Intracranial pressure (ICP) usually means supratentorial cerebrospinal fluid (CSF) pressure measured in the lateral ventricles or over the cerebral cortex. In lateral recumbent position, lumbar CSF pressure is normally equal to the supratentorial CSF pressure.

Normal ICP is 7–17 mmHg (1–2 kPa).

ICP is a crude way to estimate blood flow and cerebral metabolism, but correlates with survival in head injury.

Expected mortality in head injury is as follows:

- with ICP less than 20 mmHg the expected mortality is about 18%
- with ICP between 20 and 40 mmHg, it is 45%
- with ICP between 40 and 60 mmHg, the mortality is 74%
- with ICP greater than 60 mmHg, mortality is 100%.

Steiner LA, Andrews PJD. Monitoring the injured brain: ICP and CBF. *Br J Anaesth* 2006; 97: 26–38.

11. Answers: F T T F F

Clonidine is a selective α2-adrenergic receptor agonist, with a wide spectrum of activity. It stimulates the CNS at presynaptic α2-adrenergic receptors, resulting in decreased catecholamine release. It may also have an action on inhibitory postsynaptic α1-receptors. Clonidine has a half-life of 23 h. Conidine stabilizes the circulatory system but is also known to cause hypotension. It has sedative, anxiolytic, analgesic, and diuretic effects. Clonidine has some role during the perioperative period. When used in premedication it has a lot of advantages: it causes sedation, has anxiolytic properties, reduces secretion of saliva, stabilizes the circulatory system, diminishes stress reaction, and augments action of anaesthetic and analgesic drugs. When used during the operation, it regulates the circulatory system, and prolongs and amplifies central and peripheral blocks. Clonidine diminishes patients' requirement for opioids and local anaesthetics during postoperative and long-term pain therapy. Its side effects include bradycardia, hypotension, and respiratory depression.

Sanderson PM, Eltringham R. The role of clonidine in anaesthesia. *Hosp Med* 1998; 59(3): 221–3.

12. Answers: F F F T F

Thalassemia is a haematological disease characterized by a defect in production of subunits of haemoglobin. The incidence of this condition is high in people of African, Mediterranean, and Indian origin. There is reduced production of α or β chains. The patients may have normal concentration of HbA. The degree of impairment in the production of the subunits determines the severity of the disease. The abnormal subunit composition of the haemoglobin can result in altered red cell membranes. There is haemolysis due to the defective haemoglobin and the patients present with microcytic anaemia. The haematopoiesis is also affected, which can present as hypertrophy of the bone marrow and skeletal abnormality. These patients may have difficult airways due to hypertrophy of maxilla.

In β-thalassemia there are mutations in the HBB gene on chromosome 11. The mode of inheritance is autosomal recessive. A variety of diverse mutations can result in β-thalassemia. The nature of the mutation dictates the severity of the disease. In β-thalassemia major, the most severe form of β thalassemia, the mutations prevent the formation of β chains. This results in relative excess of the α chain, which binds to the red cell membrane damaging it. There is also derangement in α chain production in this condition.

Wilson M, Forsyth P, Whiteside J. Haemoglobinopathy and sickle cell disease. *Contin Educ Anaesth Crit Care Pain* 2010; 10(1): 24–28.

13. Answers: F T F T T

Central venous pressure (CVP) is the hydrostatic pressure in large central vein relative to an arbitrary reference level (midpoint of right atrium). The CVP waveform has three waves and two descents:

- 'a' wave: due to contraction of right atrium
- 'c' wave: caused by elevation of tricuspid valve into right atrium during early ventricular contraction
- 'x' descent: caused by downward movement of ventricle during systolic contraction
- 'v' wave: secondary to blood filling right atrium while tricuspid valve closed
- 'y' descent: produced by tricuspid valve opening in diastole and blood flowing into right vetricle.

Massive 'v' wave indicates significant tricuspid regurgitation.

Intermittent large 'v' waves may be associated with short runs of VT.

Intermittent large 'a' wave indicates a–v dissociation or ventricular pacing without atrial sensing.

A large 'y' descent, of more than 4 mmHg, indicates restricted right ventricular filling (stiff ventricle or excessively volume loaded: unlikely to respond to further volume loading).

Loss of 'x' and 'y' descent suggests tamponade.

Inspiratory fall in CVP indicates fall in cardiac output, likely on application of PEEP.

Patients with no inspiratory fall in CVP unlikely to respond to volume loading.

Izakovic M. Central venous pressure evaluation, interpretation, monitoring, clinical implications. *Bratisl Lek Listy* 2008; 109(4): 185–7.

14. Answers: T T F F T

Acute kidney injury (AKI) is an abrupt (within 48 h) reduction in kidney function, defined as one of the following:

- an absolute increase in serum creatinine of more than or equal to 26.4µmol/L (0.3 mg/dL)
- a percentage increase in serum creatinine of ≥50% (1.5-fold from baseline)
- a reduction in urine output of ≤0.5 mL/kg/h for more than 6 h.

AKI confers independent mortality. Early recognition and intervention are essential. Recognition and resuscitation of the acutely ill patient is essential (NICE CG 50). Even a modest increase in serum creatinine of 26.4 µmol/L is associated with a dramatic impact on the risk of mortality, hence 'acute kidney injury'.

Mehta RL, Kellum JA, Shah SV, *et al*; Acute Kidney Injury Network: report of an initiative to improve outcomes in acute kidney injury. *Critical Care Med* 2007; 11: R31.

Chertow GM, Burdick E, Honour M, *et al.* Acute kidney injury, mortality, length of stay, and costs in hospitalized patients. *J Am Soc Nephrol* 2005; 16: 3365–70.

Lassnigg A, Schmidlin D, Mouhieddine M, *et al.* Minimal changes of serum creatinine predict prognosis in patients after cardiothoracic surgery: a prospective cohort study. *J Am Soc Nephrol* 2004; 15: 1597–1605.

15. Answers: T T F F F

Ketamine is a unique induction agent that has potent analgesic effects. It was released for clinical use in 1970 after initially being used on American soldiers during the Vietnam conflict. Ketamine is a phencyclidine derivative.

S-(þ)-ketamine is more potent than its racemic mixture and has a faster recovery time; this has prompted reconsideration of the place of ketamine in anaesthetic practice. Ketamine is a dissociative anaesthetic that also provides profound analgesia. Pharyngeal and laryngeal muscular tone is maintained. Ketamine should be considered for use as an anaesthetic agent in patients suffering haemodynamic compromise, for patients with active bronchospastic disease, and as an adjunct/supplement to regional or local anaesthesia. The use of ketamine in pain relief is growing. Ketamine plays a major role in field hospitals, in emergency retrieval, in developing countries, and in veterinary surgery.

However, it has a number of adverse psychological effects, which limit its routine use. More recently there has been much renewed interest in ketamine due to its effect on opiate tolerance, hyperalgesia, and the availability of S(+)-ketamine. Ketamine has two optical isomers (S(+) and R(−)), weighs approximately 238 Kd, has a high lipid solubility, and has a pKa of 7.5. S(+)-ketamine is more effective at producing analgesia than R(−)-ketamine and can be administered through the epidural route.

The racemic mixture of ketamine contains both S(+) and R(−) isomers in equal concentrations and contains a preservative, benzathonium chloride, which is potentially neurotoxic. S(+)-ketamine is twice as potent as racemic ketamine. S(+)-ketamine enantiomers have a greater affinity for the NMDA receptor.

Ketamine is a highly versatile agent that is used in both adult and paediatric settings as an alternative to other, standard anaesthetic drugs such as propofol and thiopentone.

Pai A, Heining M. Ketamine. *Contin Educ Anaesth Crit Care Pain* 2007; 7(2): 59–63.

16. Answers: F F T F T

Etomidate is an imidazole hypnotic, with a very stable haemodynamic profile and minimal respiratory depression. Etomidate formulations for clinical use contain the purified R− enantiomer. Etomidate has a pKa of 4.2 and is hydrophobic at physiologic pH. To increase solubility, it is formulated as a 0.2% solution either in 35% propylene glycol (Amidate; Hospira Inc, Lake Forest, IL) or lipid emulsion (Etomidate-Lipuro; B. Braun, Melsungen, Germany). Eight formulations in cyclodextrins have also been developed. Early clinical studies determined that intravenous bolus doses of 0.2–0.4 mg/kg provided hypnosis for 5–10 min. After a bolus, maintenance of general anaesthesia can be achieved by continuous infusion of etomidate at 30–100 g/kg/min. Oral transmucosal etomidate has been used to induce sedation, and rectal administration has been used to induce general anaesthesia in paediatric patients.

Etomidate has a very stable haemodynamic profile and minimal respiratory depression but, due to the inhibition of adrenocortical steroid synthesis either after a single dose or with drug infusion, the popularity of etomidate has declined. It can causes hypnosis through its action on the GABA receptor system.

Etomidate reduces CBF and CMRO2 while maintaining the MAP and CPP.

An induction dose of etomidate of 0.3 mg/kg reduces intra-ocular pressure.

Administration of etomidate has been associated with grand mal seizures and it also seems to cause myoclonic movements (which is not associated with seizure-like activity on EEG).

It produces delta wave activity on the EEG prior to burst suppression. Brainstem-evoked potentials are not influenced by administration of etomidate, but on auditory-evoked potentials it leads to a dose-dependant increase in latency and a decrease in amplitude of the cortical component.

Forman SA. Clinical and molecular pharmacology of etomidate. *Anesthesiology* 2011; 114(3): 695–707.

17. Answers: T F T T T

The main determinants of speed of induction and recovery when using an inhalational anaesthetic are:

- during recovery, anaesthetic agent moves back from tissue depots to lungs down concentration gradients
- using high fresh gas flow (FGF) to prevent rebreathing increases elimination rate of inhaled anaesthetics
- blood and tissue solubilities of volatiles are bigger determinants of recovery time than duration or depth (mean inspired concentration) of anaesthesia
- the lower the blood solubility of volatile, the shorter the recovery time
- volatile with low blood gas partition coefficient (BGPC) is undetectable in systemic arterial circulation (after single passage through pulmonary circulation) once its inspired concentration is zero
- volatile with high OGPC prolongs recovery time in obese patients if duration of anaesthesia >4 h
- halothane recovery time is the same as that of isoflurane, despite having higher BGPC, because halothane cleared by both lungs and liver (15–40% is metabolized); ISO metabolism insignificant.

Peyton PJ, Horriat M, Robinson GJ, *et al*. Magnitude of the second gas effect on arterial sevoflurane partial pressure. *Anesthesiology* 2008; 108: 381–7.

18. Answers: T T T F T

Second gas effect

A high concentration of (newly introduced) gas in the alveolus results in rapid uptake of the gas into pulmonary capillary blood, down its concentration gradient. Rapid uptake of gas from the alveolus results in more gas moving in from the airways and breathing circuit, effectively increasing V_A.

Rapid uptake of new gas from the alveolus results in active concentration of all other gases within the alveolus.

Starting to inspire a high concentration of N_2O results in rapid rate of rise of N_2O concentration in FRC, and an equally rapid rate of rise of alveolar concentration for all newly introduced gases given concomitantly. These other gases will be both concentrated and subjected to increased V_A, and so have a faster rate of rise of alveolar concentration than if given alone.

The effect applies to existing alveolar gases, e.g. O_2: PaO_2 increases after starting to inspire 70% N_2O.

Inspiring 70% N_2O results in peak N_2O uptake rate of 500 mL/min and the 'second gas effect' increases (by >20%) the rate of rise of the (arterial SEVO partial pressure)/(inspired SEVO partial pressure) ratio.

V/Q heterogeneity in lung further increases the second gas effect: uptake of N_2O occurs mainly in lung compartments with moderately low V/Q ratio. Compartments that receive most BF predominantly determine the composition of gases in the arterial blood. The rate of N_2O uptake in these compartments is large relative to their alveolar ventilation.

This second gas effect persists during anaesthesia maintenance phase.

Peyton PJ, Horriat M, Robinson GJ, *et al*. Magnitude of the second gas effect on arterial sevoflurane partial pressure. *Anesthesiology* 2008; 108: 381–7.

19. Answers: T T F F T

Physiological factors affecting induction are:

- hyperventilation increases speed of equilibration between inspired gas and alveoli, so speeds up induction (clinically insignificant for SEVO)
- reduced FRC (e.g. obese patients) associated with smaller intrapulmonary distribution space, which accelerates equilibrium between inspired and alveolar concentrations
- V/Q mismatch (e.g. atelectasis) decreases rate of increase of arterial concentration; induction time prolonged
- increase in cardiac output accelerates anaesthetic uptake and transport to brain, but alveolar-inspired concentration ratio decreases and induction may be prolonged
- decrease in cardiac output causes increase in alveolar/inspired concentration ratio, but distribution to tissues hindered.

Peyton PJ, Horriat M, Robinson GJ, *et al*. Magnitude of the second gas effect on arterial sevoflurane partial pressure. *Anesthesiology* 2008; 108: 381–7.

20. Answers: T T F T T

The distribution of arterial blood supply to the spinal cord is quite variable. The arterial blood supply to the spinal cord is divided into three anatomic regions:

1. The cervicothoracic region receives segmental blood vessels from the vertebral arteries and the great vessels of the neck.
2. In the midthoracic region, the aorta provides segmental blood vessels. This region of the spinal cord receives the majority of the blood supply from the collateral superior and inferior arteries and therefore is susceptible to infarction as a watershed area. An aortic dissection or aortic atherosclerotic disease can send emboli to the anterior spinal artery. These patients present with a sudden onset of painless lower-extremity paralysis, with intact sensation.

The spinal cord infarction affects the anterior motor portion because the anterior spinal artery supply is lost but the posterior spinal arteries still perfuse the posterior spinal cord and sensory tracts.

3. The thoracolumbar region receives segmental vessels from the abdominal aorta and the iliac arteries. The largest segmental vessel, the artery of Adamkiewicz, is on the left side of the vertebral column in 78% of patients and is variably located between segments T8 and L4, usually T9–11.

The anterior spinal artery is formed by the branches of the vertebral artery. The posterior spinal artery (dorsal spinal artery) arises from the vertebral artery and it can also originate from the posterior inferior cerebellar artery.

Hunningher A, Calder I. Cervical spine surgery *Contin Educ Anaesth Crit Care Pain* 2007; 7(3): 81–84.

21. Answers: T T T F T

Central post-stroke pain (CPSP) is a neuropathic pain syndrome that can occur after a cerebrovascular accident. It can relate to spinal cord or brain injury. It may cause extreme discomfort and distress, limiting recovery of function following a stroke. CPSP develops in 8% of stoke patients. It usually presents within 2 months of stroke; occasionally after many years. CPSP is often associated with ischemic lesions within the thalamus. This syndrome is characterized by pain and sensory abnormalities in the body parts that correspond to the brain territory that has been injured by the cerebrovascular lesion. The presence of sensory loss and signs of hypersensitivity in the painful area in patients with CPSP might indicate the dual combination of deafferentation and the subsequent development of neuronal hyperexcitability. The exact prevalence of CPSP is not known, partly owing to the difficulty in distinguishing this syndrome from other pain types that can occur after stroke (such as shoulder pain, painful spasticity, persistent headache, and other musculoskeletal pain conditions). Future prospective studies with clear diagnostic criteria are essential for the proper collection and processing of epidemiological data. Although treatment of CPSP is difficult, the most effective approaches are those that target the increased neuronal hyper-excitability.

Klit H, Finnerup NB, Jensen TS; Central post-stroke pain: clinical characteristics, pathophysiology, and management. *Lancet Neurol* 2009; 8(9): 857–68.

22. Answers: T T T T T

Limitations of resting transthoracic echocardiography

The interposition of air-filled lung between body surface and heart limits access, particularly for:

- patients with COPD
- patients in ICU on IPPV
- patients in ICU who cannot be rotated into a lateral position
- patients in ICU with (recent) chest incisions that limit access to precordial or apical windows.

Relatively poor quality images are obtained in very obese individuals.

Ejection fraction is a relatively poor index of myocardial contractility; it is heavily influenced by afterload.

The pressure gradient across a stenosed aortic valve is deceivingly low if poor ventricular function (measure valve area instead or use stress echo).

In valve regurgitation, the jet area is affected by other factors than regurgitant jet flow rate (e.g. chamber constraint, blood pressure).

Diastolic function is difficult to quantify.

TTE is unlikely to improve management of patients at low risk of cardiac complications; it may even provoke further unnecessary investigation or intervention.

Hillis GS, Bloomfield P. Basic transthoracic echocardiography, *BMJ* 2005; 330: 1432.

23. Answers: F F F T F

Therapeutic components and goals of early goal-directed therapy (EGDT) are:

- give antibiotics (after multiple cultures)
- crystalloid infusion titrated to achieve CVP 8–12 mmHg; usually 6–10 L
- If MAP <65 mmHg, give inotrope (DB)
- If MAP >90 mmHg, give vasodilator (GTN)
- If $ScvO_2$ <70%, give RBCs to keep HCt >30%
- If $ScvO_2$ <70% and HCt >30%, add another inotrope and/or vasopressor
- EGDT does not mention IPPV, PEEP, or oxygen therapy
- nevertheless, oxygen delivery to tissues can be improved by increasing the oxygen content of arterial blood
- macrocirculatory oxygenation is not usually deranged in the first 6 h of sepsis, although it may become so following infusion of 10 L of Hartmann's.

Dellinger RP, Levy MM, Carlet JM, et al. Surviving Sepsis Campaign: International Guidelines for Management of Severe Sepsis and Septic Shock. Crit Care Med 2008; 36(1): 296–327.

24. Answers: T F F T F

Heparin is a negatively charged mixture of acid mucopolysaccharides: glycosaminoglycan, which is endogenously present in high concentration in the liver and granules of mast cells, and basophils. Its Mw is 3000–60 000 Da.

Commercially, it is extracted from bovine lung or porcine intestinal mucosa. It binds reversibly to antithrombin-III, causing enhanced inhibition of XIII, XII, XI, X, IX, and thrombin.

Adverse effects of heparin therapy include:

- heparin-induced thrombocytopaenia
  - ◆ occurs within 6–14 days of starting therapy; more quickly if previous exposure
  - ◆ caused by shortened platelet survival time
  - ◆ IgG binds to platelet surface causing activation, aggregation, and removal
  - ◆ associated with thrombosis, not bleeding
- thrombocytopaenia caused by direct effect of heparin on platelet activation
- long-term H therapy suppresses aldosterone production and causes hyperkalaemia
- long-term H therapy suppresses osteoblast formation and activates osteoclasts that promote bone loss.

Oranmore-Brown C, Griffiths R. Anticoagulants and the perioperative period. Contin Educ Anaesth Crit Care Pain 2006; 6(4): 156–59.

25. Answers: T T F T F

Serum sodium concentration is maintained by a homeostatic mechanism that involves thirst, anti-diuretic hormone (ADH) secretion. and the renal handling of sodium. This is defined as a serum sodium < 135 mmol/L. A level of less than 120 mmol/L is considered severe.

Acute hyponatraemic encephalopathy

Acute hyponatraemic encephalopathy (AHE) is four times more common in women (due to an unknown oestrogen effect).

The main cause of brain damage in patients with symptomatic hyponatraemia is hypoxia.

High concentrations of ADH (vasopressin):

- reduce cerebral blood flow by up to 80%
- reduce ATP and phosphocreatine production in brain by up to 80%.

Elderly males are resistant to AHE (ratio of brain size to skull size relatively small).

Children are particularly susceptible to AHE (ratio of brain size to skull size relatively large).

A low serum Na^+ causes water to flow into brain interstitium and thence into brain cells (so that osmolar balance is maintained).

Increase in brain water is less than expected because of compensatory mechanisms:

- cell swelling activates K^+ and Cl^- channels, resulting in loss of electrolytes from cells into interstitium and then into CSF (water follows); the process starts within minutes
- loss of intracellular organic osmolytes, e.g. myoinositol, AAS; the process starts within hours.

The brain cannot increase volume by >10% without herniation.

Upadhyay A, Jaber BL, Madias NE. Incidence and prevalence of hyponatremia. *Am J Med* 2006; 119 (7 suppl 1): S30–5.

26. Answers: T T T T T

All normobaric drugs given intrathecally are distributed rapidly within the CSF and are detectable within the cisterna magna within 20–30 min of injection. The extent of spread outside the CSF varies depending on the lipid solubility of the drug:

- lipophilic drugs penetrate the spinal cord and traverse the duramater to enter the epidural space
- rostral spread of lipophilic drugs is short-lived because take-up from the CSF is so rapid.

Lipophilic opioids, once they have penetrated the spinal cord, bind to both non-specific sites within white matter and opioid receptors in the dorsal horns. They eventually are cleared from the spinal cord to enter the systemic circulation.

Lipophilic opioids traverse the dura, initially to be sequestered in epidural fat, before eventually entering the systemic circulation.

Morphine is more hydrophilic than fentanyl, and it binds less to fat within the epidural space and to non-specific sites in the white matter of the spinal cord. Therefore, transfer to the systemic circulation is slower than for more lipophilic drugs.

Concentrations of morphine in the CSF decline more slowly, accounting for the greater degree of rostral spread, delayed respiratory depression, and more extensive dermatomal analgesia.

For intrathecal morphine, analgesia distribution is relatively unaffected by site of injection.

For more lipophilic drugs, such as fentanyl, however, even if given by prolonged infusion, analgesia is usually limited to a relatively narrow band surrounding the anatomical site of injection.

Stienstra R. Factors affecting the subarachnoid spread of local anesthetic solutions. *Reg Anesth* 1991; 16(1): 1–6.

27. Answers: T T F F F

Critical illness myopathy (CIM) presents in ICU patients as generalized weakness, failure to wean from IPPV, or paresis. Muscle biopsy characteristically shows a diffuse non-necrotizing myopathy accompanied by fibre atrophy, fatty degeneration of muscle fibres, and fibrosis. Myosin loss is evident, while actin and Z discs are preserved. Nerve histology is normal. It may occur together with critical illness polyneuropathy (CIP). Myopathy resolves over weeks/months without long-term sequelae. Usually there is no evidence of sensory neuropathy. EMG studies show the muscle unexcitable by direct stimulation and markedly decreased compound muscle action potentials. The nerve conduction is normal in CIM.

Risk factors for CIM include:

- sepsis
- prolonged NMBD; controversial
- prolonged IPPV
- SIRS
- high-dose prolonged steroid therapy
- severe asthma
- female gender.

Chawla J, Gruener G. Management of critical illness polyneuropathy and myopathy. *Neurol Clin* 2010; 28(4): 961–77.

28. Answers: T F T F T

Antiretroviral drugs fall into three categories according to the retrovirus life-cycle that they inhibit:

- NRTIs (nucleoside reverse transcriptase inhibitors) inhibit synthesis of DNA by reverse transcriptase by acting as a false nucleotide (e.g. zidovudine, didanosine); may cause gastrointestinal upset and, less commonly, neurological or hepatic impairment.
- NNRTIs (non-nucleoside reverse transcriptase inhibitors) bind to reverse transcriptase and inhibit enzyme activity (e.g. nevirapine).
- PIs (protease inhibitors) prevent the processing of viral proteins into functional forms (e.g. indinavir, ritonavir); may have the same side effects as NRTIs.

NRTIs may also cause inhibition of hepatic cytochrome p450 and thus cause interaction with other drugs.

A typical therapeutic regimen comprises three agents: two NRTIs combined with one PI or NNRTI. It is also called the highly active antiretroviral therapy (HAART), and the aim is to achieve an undetectable viral load and prolong duration and quality of life. HAART is recommended for individuals with WHO stage III or IV disease, irrespective of CD4 counts, and should be considered in asymptomatic individuals with CD4 counts of 350 cells/mm.

Prout J, Agarwal B. Anaesthesia and critical care for patients with HIV infection. *Contin Educ Anaesth Crit Care Pain* 2005; 5: 153–6.

29. Answers: F F T F F

Common peroneal nerve (L4–S2)

The common peroneal nerve separates from the tibial nerve behind and above the knee and descends around the neck of the fibula. Just below the head of the fibula, the common peroneal nerve divides into its terminal branches: the deep peroneal and superficial peroneal nerves.

Deep peroneal nerve (L4–S2)

At ankle level, the deep peroneal nerve is usually 'sandwiched' between the tendons of the anterior tibial and extensor digitorum longus muscles. At this point, the nerve divides into two terminal branches for the foot: the medial and the lateral branches. The medial branch passes to the first interosseous space, where it divides into two dorsal digital branches for the nerve supply to the first web space between the big toe and the second toe. The lateral branch of the deep peroneal nerve terminates as the second, third, and fourth dorsal interosseous nerves.

Superficial peroneal nerve (L4–S2)

The superficial peroneal nerve is a branch of the common peroneal nerve. After piercing the deep fascia covering the muscles, the nerve eventually emerges from the anterolateral compartment of the lower part of the leg and surfaces from beneath the fascia 5–10 cm above the lateral malleolus. These branches carry sensory innervation to the dorsum of the foot.

Tibial nerve (L5–S3)

The tibial nerve separates from the common popliteal nerve at various distances from the popliteal fossa crease and joins the tibial artery behind the knee joint. At the level of the medial malleolus, it is positioned laterally and posteriorly to the posterior tibial artery, and midway between the posterior aspect of the medial malleolus and posterior aspect of the Achilles tendon. Just beneath the malleolus, the nerve divides into lateral and medial plantar nerves. It carries the branches to the skin, subcutanous tissue, muscles, and bones of the sole.

Sural nerve (L5–S2)

The sural nerve courses between the heads of the gastrocnemius muscle and after piercing the fascia covering the muscles emerges on the lateral aspect of the Achilles tendon and descends 1–1.5 cm behind the lateral malleolus, anterolateral to the short saphenous vein. The sural nerve continues on the lateral aspect of the foot supplying innervation to the skin, subcutaneous tissue, fourth interosseous space, and sensory innervation of the fifth toe.

Saphenous nerve (L3,4)

The saphenous nerve is a terminal cutaneous branch (branches) of the femoral nerve. Its course is in the subcutaneous tissue of the skin on medial aspect of the ankle and foot.

- The saphenous nerve is the terminal branch of the femoral nerve, supplying sensation to the skin of the medial knee, calf and shin, and medial forefoot; the superficial peroneal nerve supplies the majority of forefoot sensation.
- The lateral cutaneous nerve of the thigh is a branch of the lumbar plexus (L2,3) supplying the lateral skin of the thigh.
- The deep peroneal nerve accompanies the anterior tibial vessels and lies lateral to the more medial dorsalis pedis artery in the foot.

The sural nerve arises in the popliteal fossa as a branch of the tibial nerve and runs with the short saphenous vein to lie behind the lateral malleolus, supplying sensation to the lower lateral aspect of the calf and lateral foot.

Shonfeld A, Harrop-Griffiths W. Regional anaesthesia: lower limb blocks. In: Allman KG, Wilson IH (eds), *Oxford Handbook of Anaesthesia*, 2nd edn. Oxford University Press, 2004: pp. 1086–93.

30. Answers: F T T F T

Mapleson classified modern breathing systems into A, B, C, D, and E. Mapleson F was added after a revision to the classification.

Mapleson A (Magill) is efficient for spontaneous ventilation (requiring a fresh gas flow (FGF) of 70–100 mL/kg/min) and inefficient for controlled ventilation (requiring an FGF three times per minute of alveolar ventilation). The coaxial Q1 version of Mapleson A is the Lack, which is also efficient for spontaneous ventilation. Mapleson D (Bain) is efficient for mechanical ventilation (FGF of 70–100 mL/kg/min), but requires FGF of 150–200 mL/kg/min for spontaneous ventilation. Mapleson B and C are used for remote locations or resuscitation and require a volume of 1.5–2 times per minute for spontaneous ventilation.

Al-Shaikh B, Stacey S. *Essentials of Anaesthetic Equipment*, 3rd edn. Churchill Livingstone, 2007.

31. Answers: T T F F T

Long QT syndrome is a familial condition associated with recurrent syncope and sudden cardiac death resulting from ventricular arrhythmias. A variety of conditions cause prolongation of the QT interval. There is impaired ventricular repolarization, and it predisposes to torsades de pointes, a polymorphic ventricular tachycardia.

The causes of QT syndrome are:

- congenital
  - ◆ autosomal dominant inheritance
  - ◆ genetic mutation in cardiac ion channels
- acquired
  - ◆ drugs
  - ◆ metabolic abnormalities—starvation, electrolyte imbalance, neurological injury.

$$QTC = QT/RR$$

In Jervell–Lange–Nielsen syndrome there can be deafness.

Romano–Ward syndrome is autosomal-dominant but Jervell–Lange–Nielsen syndrome is inherited as an autosomal recessive.

Hypokalaemia prolongs the QT and may cause VT.

It has been reported in intensive weight-reduction regimes and in anorexia nervosa.

Abrams DJ, Perkin MA, Skinner JR. Long QT syndrome. *BMJ* 2010; 340: b4815.

Hunter JD, Sharma P, Rathi S. Long QT syndrome. *Cont Educ Anaesth Crit Care Pain* 2007; 8(2): 67–70.

32. Answers: F F T F T

The most common congenital heart defect is ventricular septal defect.

The ostium secundum is the most common type of atrial septal defect.

Eisenmenger's syndrome is a right-to-left shunt associated with pulmonary hypertension and cyanosis.

The spontaneous closure of VSD occurs in 30–50% patients.

The Ebstein's anomaly is a congenital defect of the tricuspid valve in which the opening of the tricuspid valve is displaced towards the apex of the right ventricle of the heart.

Burns J, Mellor J. Anaesthesia for non-cardiac surgery in patients with congenital heart disease. *BJA CEPD Rev* 2002; 2(6): 165–169.

33. Answers: T T T T F

In 2003 the Budapest Group made consensus recommendations regarding the definition and diagnostic criteria for CRPS.

CRPS describes an array of painful conditions that are characterized by a continuing regional pain that is seemingly disproportionate in time or degree to the usual course of any known trauma or other lesion. The pain is not in any specific nerve territory or dermatome, but may spread and have a distal predominance.

CRPS is associated with abnormal osteoporosis and is less common in athletes.

Budapest criteria for clinical diagnosis of CRPS

1. Continuing pain, which is disproportionate to any inciting event.
2. Must report at least one symptom in three of the four following categories:
   - sensory: reports of hyperesthesia and/or allodynia
   - vasomotor: reports of temperature asymmetry and/or skin colour changes and/or skin colour asymmetry
   - sudomotor/oedema: reports of oedema and/or sweating changes and/or sweating asymmetry
   - motor/trophic: reports of decreased range of motion and/or motor dysfunction (weakness, tremor, dystonia) and/or trophic changes (hair, nail, skin).

3. Must display at least one sign at time of evaluation in two or more of the following categories:
   - sensory: evidence of hyperalgesia (to pinprick) and/or allodynia (to light touch and/or deep somatic pressure and/or joint movement)
   - vasomotor: evidence of temperature asymmetry and/or skin colour changes and/or asymmetry
   - sudomotor/oedema: evidence of oedema and/or sweating changes and/or sweating asymmetry
   - motor/trophic: evidence of decreased range of motion and/or motor dysfunction (weakness, tremor, dystonia) and/or trophic changes (hair, nail, skin).

4. There is no other diagnosis that better explains the signs and symptoms.

Sumitani M, Shibata M, Sakaue G, et al. Development of comprehensive diagnostic criteria for complex regional pain syndrome in the Japanese population. *Pain* 2010; 150(2): 243–9.

34. Answers: F T F F F

Xenon is the only noble gas that has anaesthetic properties under normal atmospheric conditions. It is colourless, odourless, and tasteless. It is manufactured by fractional distillation of liquefied air. It is non-flammable and non-explosive. It has seven stable, 20 unstable, and two radioactive isotopes. It has a critical temperature of 17°C. Its density is 3.2 times that of air and its viscosity is 1.7 times that of air. Due to this high viscosity and density it increases airway resistance. Xenon has a MAC of 63%. It can be used for inhalation induction. Xenon has an inhibitory action on NMDA receptors and competitively blocks the $5HT_{3A}$ receptor, which has been implicated in postoperative nausea, vomiting, and nociception. Xenon has neuroprotective effects and has minimal effects on the cardiovascular system. It produces ischemic preconditioning like other volatile agents. The main drawback of this agent is its production cost. Also it requires a closed system and scavenging. Other uses of xenon include its uses in gamma cameras and MRI imaging of lungs. It is also used in xenon phototherapy in dermatology and xenon CT imaging of lung and brain functions, and assessment of cerebral BF.

Jordan BD, Wright EL. Xenon as an anaesthetic agent. *AANA J* 2010; 78(5): 387–92.

35. Answers: F F T F F

Compartment syndrome (CS) is a serious limb-threatening and, rarely, life-threatening condition that can cause significant disability if not treated early.

The diagnosis is challenging, necessitating a high index of suspicion and should be anticipated after any limb injury or surgery that predisposes to CS. Despite clinical signs being unreliable, such assessments remain the key trigger to considering further investigations or interventions. It requires prompt diagnosis and urgent management as delays in treatment can result in limb damage, amputation, and even death.

Clinical features of CS are as follows:

- There is severe pain over the affected compartment, often disproportionate to the apparent injury, and aggravated by passive stretching of the involved muscles.
- Paraesthesia, especially loss of two-point discrimination in the distribution of the nerves traversing the compartment, is cited as characteristic.
- Weakness or paralysis of the limb is a late sign.
- Pain is subjective and variable, so may be an unreliable symptom, and may be absent in an established compartment syndrome.

Clinical signs of CS

The clinical signs of CS include tense and tender swelling over the compartment and dysfunction of the nerves traversing the compartment. Pulselessness is uncommon and implies a late stage, as by the time compartment pressures have risen to occlude the traversing arteries, extensive muscle and nerve injury will have occurred. A high index of suspicion is needed, and repeated assessment and observation are required. It should be appreciated that not all of these signs are required for the diagnosis to be made, and the clinical findings can change as the syndrome progresses.

The diagnosis is mainly by clinical suspicion, although compartmental pressure monitoring has been recommended for use in high-risk patients. The normal pressure in the muscle compartments is 10–12 mmHg. Compartmental pressure monitoring can be performed by using a pressure transducer attached to a needle or cannula that is placed into the suspect compartment. The transducer is zeroed to the level of the needle.

The recommendation is that the diagnosis is confirmed, and fasciotomy is required if the compartmental perfusion pressure is <30 mmHg.

Compartment syndrome must be treated as a matter of urgency and surgical decompression is the mainstay of therapy. The goals of treatment are to decrease tissue pressure, restore blood flow, and minimize tissue damage and related functional loss.

Farrow C, Bodenham A, Troxler M. Acute limb compartment syndromes. *Contin Educ Anaesth Crit Care Pain* 2011; 11(1): 24–28.

36. Answers: F T F T T

Patients with propofol infusion syndrome usually would have received a propofol infusion for more than 48 h. The infusion rates are usually greater than 4 mg/kg/h.

Propofol infusion syndrome should be suspected when patients present with acute refractory bradycardia leading to asystole in the presence of one or more of the following:

- metabolic acidosis
- rhabdomyolysis
- hyperlipidaemia
- enlarged/fatty liver

Probable mechanisms for this condition include an impaired mitochondrial respiratory chain function, mediated by either an unidentified metabolite or an underlying neuromuscular defect. Long-term propofol infusion is associated with increase in malonylcarnitine, which inhibits a mitochondrial transport protein. The entry of long-chain acylcarnitine esters into myocytes is impaired. The respiratory chain is impaired in the mitochondria, resulting in a failure of ATP production. This results in a build-up of fatty-acid metabolic by-products. The soya bean solvent increases the fat load and hampers oxidation of fatty acids, which, together with cellular hypoxia, worsens acidosis.

Predisposing factors for propofol infusion syndrome include young age, steroids, and/or catecholamine administration. Inadequate carbohydrate consumption and subclinical mitochondrial disease in critically ill patients also increases the risk of this condition.

Kam PC, Cardone D. Propofol infusion syndrome. *Anaesthesia* 2007; 62: 690–701.

37. Answers: F F F F F

All the above are indications for temporary pacing after cardiac surgery. About 2.6% of low-risk adults having uneventful cardiac surgery will require postoperative pacing. Therefore it is advisable that all patients having cardiac surgery have at least right ventricle temporary pacing wires. In addition, right atrial wires should also be placed in patients with low ejection fraction, a perioperative arrhythmia of any kind, and in patients having surgery near conduction pathways.

Reade MC. Temporary epicardial pacing after cardiac surgery: a practical review. Part 1: general considerations in the management of epicardial pacing. *Anaesthesia* 2007; 62: 264–271.

38. Answers: F F T F F

Tetanus is caused by a gram-positive bacillus, *Clostridium tetani*, which is commonly found in soil, but may also be isolated from animal or human faeces. It is a motile, spore-forming, obligate anaerobe. Spores are not destroyed by boiling but are eliminated by autoclaving at 120°C for 15 min (at 1 atm pressure).

Tetanus is usually diagnosed clinically, as the bacterium is rarely cultured.

Pathophysiology

Under the anaerobic conditions found in infected or necrotic tissue, the bacillus secretes two toxins: tetanospasmin and tetanolysin.

- Tetanolysin damages the surrounding viable tissue and optimizes conditions for bacterial multiplication.
- Tetanospasmin causes the clinical syndrome of tetanus, by entering peripheral nerves and travelling via axonal retrograde transport to the central nervous system. Tetanospasmin disables release of neurotransmitters from presynaptic vesicles.
- High toxin load results in diffusion of the toxins via the blood to nerves throughout the body.

Clostridium tetani is anaerobic bacterium. The drug of choice is metronidazole.

The respiratory failure can be of type 1 and 2.

Respiratory failure is observed in the developing world, autonomic dysfunction in the developed world.

Common complications are:

- cardiovascular: cardiac arrhythmias, cardiac failure, hypertensive crises, pulmonary oedema
- complications of mechanical ventilation
- SIADH
- bedsores
- bone fractures
- DVT.

Prevention

All patients with tetanus require active immunization with tetanus toxoid, as infection does not confer immunity. In the UK, a course of five injections is recommended: a primary course at the age of 2, 3, and 4 months and boosters at 5 and 15 years.

Cook IM, Protheroe RT, Handel JM. Tetanus: a review of the literature. *Br J Anaesth* 2001; 87: 477–87.

Beeching NJ, Crowcroft NS. Tetanus in injecting drug users. *BMJ* 2005; 330(7485): 208–209.

39. Answers: T F F T T

The transdermal drug delivery route is chosen for its convenience and simplicity. It does not necessitate intravenous access. This route bypasses the first-pass hepatic metabolism and can be used after surgery in the presence of PONV, dysphagia, gastric stasis, etc. The passive diffusion through the stratum corneum is gradual and the rate of drug absorption is slow. The physiochemical characteristics of a drug required for passive transdermal diffusion include low molecular weight, high lipophilicity, and low melting point. The drugs are delivered into circulation even after patch removal.

Power I. Fentanyl HCl iontophoretic transdermal system (ITS): clinical application of iontophoretic technology in the management of acute postoperative pain. *Br J Anaesth* 2007; 98: 4–11.

40. Answers: T F T F F

Croup is caused by parainfluenza virus type I, which can be recovered in 60% of cases, and causes most cases of croup. Parainfluenza types II, III, and IV, influenza A and B, adenovirus, and respiratory syncytial virus are also implicated in croup.

Clinical presentation of croup is as follows:

- distinctive, barking cough
- onset more gradual than that of epiglottis (prodromal fever, hoarse voice, URTI)
- do not have dysphagia with the attendant drooling
- most are infants and not toddlers or school-age children.

Management: humidification, nebulizers, steroids, racemic adrenaline.

Epiglottitis is caused by infection with:

- Group A B-haemolytic streptococcus
- H influenzae type B
- *Staphylococcus aureus*.

Epiglottitis is distinguished from croup by its fulminant onset and the toxic appearance of its victims. It occurs usually in children aged 2–6 years, with a peak incidence at 3 years.

Clinical presentation of epiglottitis is as follows. The most common symptoms are dysphagia, an intensely sore throat, and fever.

- there is sudden onset with a rapid progression
- the tripod position
- dyspnea, toxicity (most cases involving HIB include bacteremia)
- stridor, dysphonia, or muffled voice
- drooling, because of inability to swallow
- tachycardia and tachypnea
- lethargy or restlessness.

People with depressed immune systems may be more likely than others to be affected. The patient usually has no history of an upper respiratory infection.

Maloney E, Meakin GH. Acute stridor in children. *Contin Educ Anaesth Crit Care Pain* 2007; 7(6): 183–86.

41. Answers: T F F T F

The recurrent laryngeal nerve is a branch of the tenth cranial nerve. It innervates the larynx and has motor and sensory innervations. It first descends into thorax before it rises into the neck between the trachea and the oesophagus. The left recurrent laryngeal nerve is longer than the right. The left hooks round the arch of aorta and the right around the subclavian artery and gives off several fibres, which contribute to the deep part of cardiac plexus. However, non-recurrence and other variations can occur. This predisposes the nerve to injury during neck surgeries.

It provides motor supply to all the laryngeal muscles except the cricothyroid. (The cricothyroid is innervated by the external branch of superior laryngeal nerve.) The intrinsic muscles of the larynx are also innervated by the recurrent laryngeal, which is responsible for controlling the movements of the vocal folds.

Malhotra S, Sodhi V. Anaesthesia for thyroid and parathyroid surgery. *Contin Educ Anaesth Crit Care Pain* 2007; 7(2): 55–58.

42. Answers: T T F F T

Carbon dioxide narcosis is seen when $PaCO2$ is greater than 25 kPa, resulting in profound acidosis. When CO_2 exceeds 13 kPa there is depression of the central nervous system. This corresponds to CSF pH less than 7.1. Another feature of hypercapnia is flushed skin, which is an early sign. There is bounding pulse and a respiratory rate increase associated with respiratory distress, which rises as the level of carbon dioxide rises. Cardiac manifestations include various arrhythmias, including extrasystoles. The cardiac output is increased. The jugular venous pressure and blood pressure are increased.

Central nervous system signs include headache, confusion lethargy, muscle twitches, hand flaps, and depression of the central nervous system. Severe hypercapnia can result in seizures, which may progress to loss of consciousness and death.

Reid PT, Innes JA. In: Bouchier E, Chilvers H. (eds), *Davidson's Principles and Practice of Medicine*, 21st edn. Churchill Livingstone, 2010: p. 640.

43. Answers: F F T T T

Finger clubbing is deformity of the finger nail (and fingers) and is seen in a broad range of diseases. The first sign is fluctuation of the nail bed, followed by loss of the normal angle between the nail bed and the cuticula. If there is further worsening of clubbing, the increased convexity of the nail fold results in a parrot-beak appearance of the nail. Causes of clubbing include the following:

- respiratory system: malignancy, tuberculosis, broncheictasis, empyema, fibrosing alveolitis, lung abscess, cystic fibrosis, mesothelioma
- cardiovascular system: congenital cyanotic heart conditions, subacute bacterial endocarditis, atrial myxoma
- gastrointestinal and liver disease: inflammatory bowel disease, malabsorption syndrome, primary biliary cirrhosis, cirrhosis, hepatopulmonary syndrome
- miscellaneous: hyperthyroidism, thalassemia.

Swash M, Glynn M. *Hutchison's Clinical Methods*, 22nd edn. WB Saunders, 2006: Section 4, Chapter 11 p 251.

44. Answers: T T F F T

Physiological factors affecting induction include:

- hyperventilation increases speed of equilibration between inspired gas and alveoli, so speeds up induction (clinically insignificant for SEVO)
- reduced FRC (e.g. obese patients) associated with smaller intrapulmonary distribution space, which accelerates equilibrium between inspired and alveolar concentrations
- V/Q mismatch (e.g. atelectasis) decreases rate of increase of arterial concentration; induction time prolonged
- increase in cardiac output accelerates anaesthetic uptake and transport to brain, but alveolar-inspired concentration ratio decreases and induction may be prolonged
- decrease in cardiac output causes increase in alveolar/inspired concentration ratio, but distribution to tissues hindered.

Peyton PJ, Horriat M, Robinson GJ, et al. Magnitude of the second gas effect on arterial sevoflurane partial pressure. *Anesthesiology* 2008; 108: 381–7.

45. Answers: F F T F T

The vibration and position sense are transmitted via the posterior columns, which are supplied by the posterior spinal artery. Unlike the anterior spinal artery the posterior spinal artery is a plexus of vessels with extensive anastomosis. The anterior spinal artery is more vulnerable and ischaemia is more severe in its distribution. The spinothalamic tract, which transmits the pain, temperature, and the two-point discrimination sensation, is more vulnerable to injury than the posterior columns.

Cheshire WP, Santos CC, Massey EW, Howard JF. Spinal cord infarction: etiology and outcome. *Neurology* 1996; 47(2): 321.

46. Answers: F F T F T

The confidence interval indicates the reliability of the statistical estimate. In a study the confidence interval along with the confidence level gives assurance about the correctness of the statistical model that is employed. It describes the range of value around a mean, odds ratio, p-value, or a standard deviation. The true value lies within this range. The narrower the confidence interval the more significant is the result. If the confidence interval is very wide then more data need to be collected and the sample size needs to be increased.

Rees DG. *Essential Statistics*, 4th edn. Chapman and Hall/CRC, 2001.

Campbell MJ, Machin D, Walters SJ. *Medical Statistics: A Textbook for the Health Sciences.* Wiley-Blackwell, 2007.

47. Answers: F F F F T

Mean, median, and mode are measures of central tendency. These are the characteristics around which a set of values are distributed.

Mean is average of the observed values. It is obtained by adding all the values and dividing the sum by the number of observations. Median is the centrally occurring value when the observations are placed in ascending or descending order. It is shifted to the right when the distribution is negatively skewed and shifted to left when the distribution is positively skewed. Mode is the most frequently occurring value. Normal distribution is a continuous frequency distribution that is symmetrical and with tails extending to infinity. All the indices of central tendency are identical in a normal distribution, and the standard deviation along with the mean completely determine the shape of the distribution curve.

Rees DG. *Essential Statistics*, 4th edn. Chapman and Hall/CRC, 2001.

Campbell MJ, Machin D, Walters SJ. *Medical Statistics: A Textbook for the Health Sciences.* Wiley-Blackwell, 2007.

48. Answers: T T F T T

Tricyclic antidepressants (TCAs), such as amitriptyline and imipramine, can widen QRS and prolong QT interval, with a risk of precipitating arrhythmias. They reduce seizure threshold, have anticholinergic side effects, can cause postural hypotension (α-adrenergic blocking effect), and potentiate the effects of indirectly acting sympathomimetics such as ephedrine.

Selective serotonin reuptake inhibitors (SSRIs), such as venlafaxine and fluoxetine, work by inhibiting the presynaptic re-uptake of serotonin. Tramadol and pethidine increase the levels of serotonin, which can lead to serotonin syndrome (hyperpyrexia, agitation, and hyper-reflexia), if they are used in patients on SSRIs and TCAs. SSRIs interfere with platelet function, which increases the risk of bleeding in patients taking NSAIDs and warfarin.

Lithium prolongs the duration of depolarizing neuromuscular block and reduces the MAC of volatile agents. It has a narrow therapeutic window and causes cardiac arrhythmia, gastrointestinal disturbances, tremor, ataxia, coma, and renal failure.

Typical antipsychotics, such as haloperidol and chlorpromazine, can precipitate all kinds of extrapyramidal side effects, such as akathisia, Parkinsonism, dyskinesia, and occulogyric crisis. Atypical antipsychotics are less likely to produce extrapyramidal effects, but all antipsychotics can produce α-adrenergic blocking effects and neuroleptic malignant syndrome.

Peck A, Wong A, Norman E. Anaesthetic implications of psychoactive drugs. *Cont Educ Anaesth Crit Care Pain* 2010: 10(6): 177–81.

49. Answers: T T F T T

Autonomic neuropathy is a nerve disorder that affects either sympathetic or parasympathetic nervous system functions, including heart rate, blood pressure, perspiration, and digestion. This damage disrupts signals between the brain and portions of the autonomic nervous system, such as the heart, blood vessels, and sweat glands, resulting in decreased or abnormal performance of one or more involuntary body functions. Autonomic neuropathy can be a complication of a number of diseases and conditions.

The severity of the signs and symptoms has wide variability.

The causes of autonomic neuropathy are:

- central
  - ◆ primary: Shy–Drager syndrome
  - ◆ secondary: cerebrovascular accident, CNS infection, drugs
- peripheral
  - ◆ diabetes mellitus
  - ◆ Guillain–Barré syndrome
  - ◆ amyloidosis
  - ◆ etc.

These patients are at risk of developing severe hypotension with neuraxial blockade of any kind and with positive pressure ventilation.

Blanshard, H. Endocrine and metabolic disease. In: Allman KG, Wilson IH (eds), *Oxford Handbook of Anaesthesia*, 2nd edn. Oxford University Press, 2004; p 150–155.

Marks JB. Perioperative management of diabetes. *Am Fam Physician* 2003; 67(1): 93–100.

Jermendy G. Clinical consequences of cardiovascular autonomic neuropathy in diabetic patients. *Acta Diabetol* 2003; 40(Suppl 2): S370–4.

Weimer LH. Autonomic testing: common techniques and clinical applications. *Neurologist* 2010; 16(4): 215–22.

50. Answers: F F F F T

Bias is the deviation from the truth of the results that are obtained from a study. Precision is the ability of the test to measure something consistently. This indicates the reliability of the test. Accuracy indicates the validity of the test, which is the ability of the test to measure that which it was intended to measure.

It is possible to have bias in a study and obtain precise results. Precision is the ability of the repeated observations to agree with one another when repeated. It is measured by sampling error. It is possible to be very precise and still have a bias. The results are not accurate when there is a bias in the study.

Types of bias include:

- selection bias or sampling bias, where the study population is not representative of the population and hence the results of the study are not valid for the population
- measurement bias, where the methodology of gathering information itself distorts the data
- experimenter expectancy, where the beliefs of the researcher affect the outcome of the study
- Lead-time bias, when early detection of a condition is confused for increased survival
- recall bias, which is common when subjects give an inaccurate recollection of information
- late-look bias, which is introduced when individuals with severe disability are not uncovered in a survey, perhaps because they die early
- confounding bias, which is due to the presence of other unanticipated factors.

Rees DG. *Essential Statistics*, 4th edn. Chapman and Hall/CRC, 2001.

Campbell MJ, Machin D, Walters SJ. *Medical Statistics: A Textbook for the Health Sciences*. Wiley-Blackwell, 2007.

51. Answers: T T T T T

Hyponatraemia is defined as a serum sodium concentration of 135 mmol/L and occurs in up to 15% of the general adult inpatient population.

Hyponatraemia symptoms are:

- moderate
  - lethargy
  - nausea, vomiting, and anorexia
  - irritability
  - headache
  - muscle weakness/cramps
- severe
  - hyporeflexia
  - drowsiness and confusion
  - seizures
  - coma
  - death.

All the above conditions may be associated with demyelination within the pons. Rapid correction of sodium levels rather than the low concentration itself is thought to be the cause of the demyelination. The evidence regarding the optimal rate of correction of sodium levels is controversial. Rapid correction of the sodium levels is also associated with subdural haemorrhage and cardiac failure. The recommendation is that serum sodium should be increased by no more than 0.5 mmol/L/h or 8–10 mmol/L/day, with a maximum rate of up to 2 mmol/L/h. Treatment should always be targeted to the point of alleviation of symptoms rather than to an arbitrary serum sodium concentration.

Bradshaw K, Smith M. Disorders of sodium balance after brain injury. *Contin Educ Anaesth Crit Care Pain* 2008; 8(4): 129–133.

52. Answers: F T T F T

Cricothyroidotomy is the creation of an opening in the space between the anterior inferior border of the thyroid cartilage and the anterior superior border of the cricoid cartilage to gain access to the airway below the glottis.

Indications for cricothyroidotomy are:

- anticipated difficult airway: elective prophylactic cricothyroidotomy
- elective provision of oxygenation (+ventilation) by subglottic route
- 'can't intubate can't ventilate' (CICV) scenario: emergency oxygenation (+ventilation).

Cricothyroidotomy is an emergency procedure that is often life-saving and is usually performed as a last resort following failure to secure airway. The procedure involves incising the cricothyroid membrane. This should be considered only as a temporary measure until a more secure airway is established. The cricoid cartilage is at the level of the C6 vertebrae when the neck is extended.

Benumof JL, Scheller MS. The importance of transtracheal jet ventilation in the management of the difficult airway. *Anesthesiology* 1989; 71: 769–78.

Henderson JJ, Popat TM, Latto IP, Pearce AC. Difficult Airway Society guidelines for the management of the unanticipated difficult intubation. *Anaesthesia* 2004; 59: 675–94.

Greig HJ, Schnider T, Heidegger T. Prophylactic percutaneous transtracheal catheterisation in the management of patients with anticipated difficult airways: a case series. *Anaesthesia* 2005; 60: 801–5.

53. Answers: T T T T T

The diaphragm is a fibro-muscular structure that separates the thoracic and the abdominal cavities. It consists of a central tendon and a peripheral muscular structure, which consists of muscular fibres originating from the sternum, ribs, and the two crura originating from the upper lumbar vertebrae. The central tendon is attached to the pericardium above.

It has three main openings, which transmit various structures between the thorax and abdomen. The diaphragm is pierced by the splanchnic nerves and the left phrenic nerve, while the right phrenic nerve is transmitted through the opening for the inferior vena cava.

Downey R, Anatomy of the normal diaphragm. *Thorac Surg Clin* 2011; 21(2): 273–9.

54. Answers: F T F F T

Atlas is the first cervical vertebra and it lacks a body. It articulates with the skull and axis. Axis is the second cervical vertebra. All 12 thoracic vertebrae articulate with the corresponding ribs. Laminae extend between the transverse processes and the spinous processes and the pedicle extends between the vertebral body and the transverse processes. In children the spinal cord ends at L3, and hence lumbar puncture should be performed below this level. The spinal cord moves up as the children grow up and in adults the cord ends at L1.

Richardson J, Groen J. Applied epidural anatomy. *Contin Educ Anaesth Crit Care Pain* 2005; 5(3): 98–100.

55. Answers: T F T T F

A living will, or advance directive, is a legally binding statement made by an adult about the way that individual wishes to be treated in the event that he or she becomes incompetent in future to make a valid choice of treatment.

All competent adults have a right to refuse treatment and an advance directive is a way of prolonging this autonomy. However, a valid advance directive cannot request the treating physician to offer treatment that is not in the best interests of the patient.

For the advance directive to be valid it has to be made by a competent adult who is 18-years-old or above. The patient cannot be coerced into making this statement, irrespective of the circumstance, and the patient has to be sufficiently informed about the prognosis of his condition for the advance refusal to be respected. A person may refuse future treatment for any reason. She/he does not need to have access to any medical information to make this decision. A decision may be made for any reason the individual wishes. They need sufficient information, as defined by the individual making the decision and not the doctor.

If there is a doubt about the existence or validity of the statement emergency treatment should be provided until this doubt is clarified.

End-of-life Decisions: Views of the BMA. BMA, 2009. http://www.bma.org.uk/images/endlifedecisionsaug2009_tcm41-190116.pdf.

Treatment and Care Towards the End of Life. GMC, 2010. http://www.gmc-uk.org/guidance/ethical_guidance/end_of_life_care.asp.

Flew A. Advance directives are the solution to Dr Campbell's problem of voluntary euthanasia. *J Med Ethics* 1999; 25: 245–46.

Advance Statements about Future Medical Treatment. A Guide for Patients. The Patients Association, 1996. http://www.patients-association.com/Portals/0/public/files/AdvicePublications/LivingWills.pdf.

56. Answers: T T F T F

The Mental Capacity Act clearly states that the patient has the right to make an irrational decision that may not seem to be sensible to the professionals. However, a highly irrational choice based on misinterpretation of the information that is provided may indicate underlying mental illness; such an interpretation should probably be left to the courts. Refusal to accept any treatment by an adult is legally binding. The incapacity may be temporary and in such cases only emergency care should be provided until the patient is competent to make a choice. If incapacity is predictable as a natural course of the disease, the patient may choose to prepare an advance directive. In a case of incapacity to consent it is good practice to involve family, but no-one can consent on behalf of the patient without a power of attorney. A person may grant a lasting power of attorney to another individual. This enables that person to consent or refuse consent on behalf of the patient. The court of protection may appoint someone to perform the same task. The treatment offered should always be in the best interests of the patient. Assessment of best interest should include medical, personal, social, and financial factors. Except in exceptional circumstances the anaesthetic room is not where patient should be consented.

White SM. Consent for anaesthesia. *J Med Ethics* 2004; 30: 286–90.

Seeking Patients' Consent: the Ethical Considerations. General Medical Council, 1998. http://www.gmcuk.org/guidance/library/consent.asp.

57. Answers: F T T F T

Heparin, which is added to the blood to stop the sample from clotting, is acidic. It will increase the acidity of the sample and the pH of the sample will be lower because of increased hydrogen ion concentration. Atmospheric air has 21% oxygen, and an air bubble in the sample increases the partial pressure of oxygen. At room temperature there is metabolic activity of the cells in the blood. This consumes the oxygen and increases the acidity of the sample. The normal hydrogen ion concentration in blood is 40 nmol/L. Using a modified electrode (pH) the partial pressure of carbon dioxide can be measured in a sample.

Armstrong JAM, Guleria A, Girling K. Evaluation of gas exchange deficit in the critically ill. *Contin Educ Anaesth Crit Care Pain* 2007; 7(4): 131–34.

58. Answers: F F T T T

The face mask increases the dead space by about 200 mL. The effect on dead space is significant, especially when the wrong size is used and in children. The significance of the antistatic property of the carbon particles on the rubber mask has disappeared in the current practices of anaesthesia, as drugs are no longer used at concentrations at which they are flammable. It is essential that the face mask is snug-fitting to prevent leaks in the circuit and avoid application of excess pressure.

Sirian R, Wills J. Physiology of apnoea and the benefits of preoxygenation. *Contin Educ Anaesth Crit Care Pain* 2009; 9(4): 105–108.

59. Answers: T T F T T

Standard epidural catheters are 90 cm in length. The distal end of the catheter usually has two or more side ports with a rounded tip. They have lower incidence of causing trauma to the dura or the vessels than catheters with a single port. Radio-opaque catheters are available to aid accurate placement of catheter. It is recommended that length of the catheter in the epidural space is between 3 and 5 cm. There is increased chance of trauma to the dura and the vessels when the length of the catheter in the space is increased. It can also result in unilateral or segmental block. Ideally the filter should be changed every 24 h.

The epidural needle is typically 16–18G, 8 cm long, with surface markings at 1-cm intervals, and with a blunt bevel with a 15–30° curve at the tip. The most commonly used version of this needle is the Tuohy needle, and the tip is referred to as the Huber tip. Most commercially available needles have the Tuohy/Huber configuration and have wings attached at the junction of the needle shaft with the hub, which allow better control of the needle as it is advanced. The original winged needle was called the Weiss needle.

Portex 18G and Portex 19G epidural kits can be distinguished by the colour of the locking hub on the filter and the size and markings of the epidural catheter.

The catheter in the 18G Portex epidural kit has a single bold mark at 5 cm, then a mark every 1 cm up to the two bold lines indicating 10 cm. The 1-cm markings continue until there are three bold lines together, which indicate 15 cm. There are no further markings until four bold lines appear together, which indicates 20 cm. The catheter has a coloured closed tip and three lateral holes. The locking hub at the filter is blue.

The catheter in the 19G Portex epidural kit has a mark every centimetre from 2 cm, with a bold mark indicating 5 cm. There are two bold lines together indicating 10 cm. Markings continue every 1 cm up to three bold lines together, which indicate 15 cm. The catheter has a single end hole with a coloured tip. The locking hub at the filter is white.

Braun Perifx® Paed series epidural kits can be distinguished by the size and bold markings on the catheters. 18G Braun epidural kits have a solid mark at 9 cm and a clear tip (children). The 20G Braun epidural kit has a solid line at 12 cm and a clear tip (infants).

Al-Shaikh B, Stacey S. *Essentials of Anaesthetic Equipment*, 3rd edn. Churchill Livingstone, 2007.

60. Answers: T T F T F

There is a six-fold increase in the risk of thromboembolism during pregnancy. There are multiple factors responsible for this. Hypercoagulability of the blood is due to an increase in the concentration of most clotting factors, except XI and XIII. The levels of factor II and V usually remain unchanged.

These changes result in a state of hypercoagulability, are likely due to hormonal changes, and increase the risk of thromboembolism. The increase in clotting activity is greatest at the time of delivery with placental expulsion, when thromboplastic substances are released. These substances stimulate clot formation to stop maternal blood loss. As placental blood flow is up to 700 mL/min, considerable haemorrhage can occur if clotting fails. Coagulation and fibrinolysis generally return to pre-pregnant levels 3–4 weeks postpartum.

Platelets: the platelet count decreases in normal pregnancy possibly due to increased destruction and haemodilution, with a maximal decrease in the third trimester.

Coagulation factors: factors VIII (FVIII), von Willebrand factor (vWf), ristocetinco factor (RCoA) and factors X (FX) and XII (FXII) increase during pregnancy. Levels of factor VII (FVII) increase gradually during pregnancy and reach very high levels (up to 1000%) by term. Fibrinogen also increases during pregnancy, with levels at term 200% above pre-pregnancy levels.

Thornton P, Douglas J. Coagulation in pregnancy. *Best Pract Res Cl Obs* 2010; 24: 339–352.

Single Best Answers

1. Answer: A

Hyperextension of the spine in patients with degenerative spine changes, particularly in the elderly, is associated with central cord syndrome. The clinical features are due to selective damage to the central portion of the anterior cord, which carries the corticospinal tract and decussating fibres of the lateral spinothalamic tract. There is greater weakness of the upper limbs compared to the lower limbs. This is because the motor fibres of upper limbs in the corticospinal tract are nearer to the centre. In Brown–Séquard syndrome there is ipsilateral loss of vibration and proprioception along with ipsilateral spastic paresis. In posterior spinal cord syndrome there is bilateral loss of proprioception and vibratory sensation. Bilateral spastic paresis below the level of lesion is seen in anterior spinal cord syndrome.

Yan K, Diggan MF. A case of central cord syndrome caused by intubation. *J Spinal Cord Med*. 1997; 20(2): 230–32.

2. Answer: A

Hypotension and tachycardia following trauma is consistent with shock. The most common cause of shock in these settings is hypovolaemia. The PCWP is low in hypovolaemia.

Following a fluid challenge the PCWP increased with no corresponding change in blood pressure. These findings exclude the diagnosis of shock caused by hypovolaemia. Elevated CVP/PCWP with persistent hypotension after fluid bolus should suggest an alternative diagnosis. The clinical findings are not suggestive of pneumothoax in this patient. Pulmonary embolism is associated with high pulmonary artery pressure but normal PCWP. Myocardial contusion should be suspected in this patient, which can be confirmed with elevated cardiac enzymes and ECG changes.

Sybrandy KC, Cramer MJ, Burgersdijk C. Diagnosing cardiac contusion. *Heart* 2003; 89(5): 485–89.

3. Answer: E

This patient has developed postoperative atelectasis. Obstructive atelectasis occurs due to airway blockage, resulting in air retention distal to the occlusion. This affected lobe or segment collapses when the retained air is absorbed. Postoperative atelectasis usually sets in within 48 h of the procedure. The patient presents with hypoxaemia and respiratory alkalosis, as these patients usually hyperventilate to compensate for the drop in PaO_2. This condition can be prevented by initiating early chest physiotherapy and active breathing exercises. Use of broad-spectrum antibiotics or routine use of glucocorticoids is not useful for preventive respiratory complications in this setting. Patients should stop smoking at least 8–10 weeks prior to surgery to reduce the risk of pulmonary complications. This should be done carefully to prevent any complication associated with sudden cessation of smoking.

Pasquina P, Tramèr MR, Granier JM, et al. Respiratory physiotherapy to prevent pulmonary complications after abdominal surgery: a systematic review. *Chest* 2006; 130(6): 1887–99.

4. Answer: A

This patient has perforation of bowel and requires an emergency laparotomy. His INR of 2.1 must be corrected prior to the surgery. This warfarin-induced abnormal prothrombin time can be normalized by infusion of fresh frozen plasma (FFP), which restores vitamin-K-dependent clotting factors. This patient might require RBC transfusion later, but correction of the coagulation profile is a priority.

FFP is obtained from whole blood and contains all the clotting factors. It lasts for 12 months. It is also a source of cholinesterase. The activity of labile clotting factor is maintained, as FFP is stored at −30°C. Immediately before use it is thawed at 37°C.

Roback JD, Caldwell S, Carson J, et al. Evidence-based practice guidelines for plasma transfusion. *Transfusion* 2010; 50(6): 1227–39.

5. Answer: C

Brain parenchyma, CSF, and blood determine ICP, which is a function of volume and compliance. Brain parenchyma and CSF volume is usually constant unless there is a mass lesion or obstruction to CSF flow. The brain autoregulates cerebral blood flow and cerebral perfusion pressure. In traumatic brain injury autoregulation may be hampered. Cerebral blood flow increases with hypercapnia and it is important to maintain $PaCO_2$ at the lower end of normal values in patients with brain injury. Elevation of head end decreases ICP by increasing venous outflow. Adequate sedation in these patients is essential in order to decrease metabolic demands and control blood pressure. Mannitol may be used to extract free water out of brain tissue. Hyperventilation washes out CO_2 leading to cerebral vasoconstriction. Current guidelines encourage normocapnoea.

Head Injury: Triage, Assessment, Investigation and Early Management of Head Injury in Infants, Children and Adults. NICE guidelines, 2007. http://www.nice.org.uk/CG56.

Rangel-Castilla L, Lara LR, Gopinath S, *et al*. Cerebral hemodynamic effects of acute hyperoxia and hyperventilation after severe traumatic brain injury. *J Neurotrauma* 2010; 27(10): 1853–63.

6. Answer: E

Congenital diaphragmatic hernia (CDH) is a congenital anomaly consisting of a defect in the diaphragm. It is also known as a Bochdalek hernia. The incidence is between about 1 in 2000 and one in 3000 newborns. It is usually associated with pulmonary hypoplasia (PH) and persistent pulmonary hypertension (PPH). Newborns with CDH have high rates of mortality and morbidity, which is attributed to severe respiratory failure secondary to PH and PPH. Initial treatment includes achieving adequate peripheral and central venous access for drugs. Ideally, monitoring should include CVP, IABP, $EtCO_2$, pre- and postductal SpO_2, core and peripheral temperatures, and hourly urine output.

The stomach should be deflated using an orogastric tube, which reduces lung compression. Enteral nutrition should be commenced early. Adequate sedation with fentanyl or midazolam usually obviates need for paralysis.

While ventilating these patients, minimize mean airway pressures and allow (permissive) hypercapnia, as aggressive ventilatory support damages the vulnerable lungs. High-frequency ventilation may help reduce shear forces and volutrauma in these children. Inhaled NO may be of short-term benefit in selected patients with severe pulmonary hypertension (PHT). ECMO has only marginal effects on long-term survival. About 30% of affected babies receive ECMO in the USA. Use of surfactant has shown no benefits in term babies. Surgery should be delayed until the patient is stable, with no PHT crises and when ECMO and/or NO have been discontinued. Surgery will not improve oxygenation/lung function.

Keijzer R, Puri P. Congenital diaphragmatic hernia. *Semin Pediatr Surg* 2010; 19(3): 180–5.

7. Answer: C

The differential diagnosis of this condition includes central diabetes insipidus, drug-induction (diuretic therapy, use of hypertonic saline, ingested alcohol), and cerebral salt-wasting syndrome.

Central diabetes insipidus

There is a disproportionate loss of water over sodium:

- urine osmolality < 200 mOsmol/kg
- urinary Na concentration 20–60 mmol/L (normal)
- plasma osmolality >305 mOsmol/kg
- serum Na concentration > 145 mmol/L
- urinary specific gravity < 1.005.

Drug-induced polyuria

Mannitol-induced diuresis

- serum Na concentration <135 mmol/L
- serum osmolality > 305 mOsmol/kg.

Loop diuretics

- dose-dependent polyuria and natriuresis (urinary Na concentration > 20 mmol/L)
- serum Na concentration < 135 mmol/L
- serum osmolality < 280 mOsmol/kg.

Administration of hypertonic saline:

- high serum Na concentration (>145 mmol/L)
- high urinary Na concentration (>50 mmol/L).

Prior ingestion of alcohol

- suggestive history
- blood alcohol concentration high
- large serum osmolar gap.

Cerebral salt wasting syndrome

- causes polyuria and hyponatraemia 2° to excessive urinary Na excretion
- serum Na concentration < 135 mmol/L
- serum osmolality < 280 mOsmol/kg
- urinary Na concentration > 20 mmol/L
- patient is hypovolaemic.

Tisdall M, Crocker M, Watkiss J, et al. Disturbances of sodium in critically ill adult neurologic patients: a clinical review. *J Neurosurg Anesthesiol* 2006; 18: 57–63.

Makaryus AN, McFarlane SI. Diabetes insipidus: diagnosis and treatment of a complex disease. *Clev Clin J Med* 2005; 73: 65–71.

8. Answer: C

Hypoxia, confusion, and petechial rash following fracture of femur are suggestive of pulmonary embolism. This is caused when fat enters the venous circulation after fracture of long bones. Usually this presents between 12 and 36 h following the trauma. Pulmonary embolism has a longer latent period and does not cause petechial rash.

Fat embolism is caused by dispersion of fat droplets into the circulation. This occurs after trauma or surgery involving major bones. It is also associated with major burns, acute pancreatitis, cardiopulmonary bypass, and transplantation of bone marrow.

Clinical features include confusion and restlessness. Patients may present with reduced consciousness or seizures. Respiratory manifestations include dyspnoea, cough, and haemoptysis. 'Snowstorm' appearance on X-ray is characteristic of this condition. It is common to find reduced platelet count in these patients.

Management includes oxygen therapy and respiratory support.

Akhtar S. Fat embolism; *Anesthesiol Clin* 2009; 27(3): 533–50.

9. Answer: A

The clinical picture is suggestive of hypertrophic pulmonary osteopathy (HPO), which is characterized by clubbing, arthritis, and periosteal new bone formation. Conditions that may present with HPO include malignancy, lung abscess, congenital heart disease, etc. Bilateral osteomyelitis of wrist is very unlikely. Periosteal new bone formation and clubbing is not a feature of rheumatoid arthritis. Therefore, methotrexate or wrist aspiration is not the right choice of treatment. Chest X-ray should be performed to look for signs of infection of malignancy. Antibiotic treatment is not empirically recommended. HPO without clubbing may go unrecognized.

Vascular endothelial growth factor, platelet-derived growth factor, and platelets are involved in the pathogenesis of this condition. HPO may present without clubbing and about 20% of cases have hypertrophic osteoarthropathy without detectable malignancy.

Yao Q, Altman RD, Brahn E. Periostitis and hypertrophic pulmonary osteoarthropathy. *Semin Arthritis Rheum* 2009; 38(6): 458–66.

10. Answer: D

Pulmonary embolism (PE) results from introduction of blood clots, air, foreign material, etc. into the venous system. Clots from the lower limbs (usually above the knee) and pelvis are usually responsible. They can also originate from right side of the heart. Pulmonary embolus increases dead space and vascular resistance. There is loss of surfactant, and within 48 h the affected segment can become atelectatic. Embolus in a large pulmonary vessel can result in infarction. In the event that the patient survives acute PE the thrombus resolution usually begins within 2 weeks.

In patients with a high risk of developing PE, warfarin is recommended for prophylaxis. It should be started preoperatively to maintain INR between 2 and 3. Low-molecular-weight heparin given subcutaneously twice daily is also an option. Pneumatic boots, elastic stockings, and early ambulation also reduce the risk of PE but are not adequate in high-risk patients. In this setting warfarin is more effective than low-dose subcutaneous heparin.

Vaughan-Shaw PG. Thromboprophylaxis in trauma: a review of methods, evidence and guidelines. *Acta Orthop Belg* 2011; 77(1): 1–8.

11. Answer: D

The clinical findings are suggestive of right side pleural effusion. A large pleural effusion can push the trachea to the opposite side.

Atelectasis on the right side pulls the trachea to the right side. This occurs secondary to volume loss on the affected side. When the lower lobe is affected by atelectasis, the diaphragm is elevated on that side.

In consolidated pneumonia there will be increased tactile vocal fremitus and no tracheal deviation.

COPD will not cause tracheal deviation by itself and the signs are bilateral.

Reid PT, Innes JA. In: Bouchier E, Chilvers H. *Davidson's Principles and Practice of Medicine*, 21st edn. Churchill Livingstone, 2010: Chapter 19.

12. Answer: B

The air-fluid level is suggestive of pulmonary abscess, which is characteristic of infection by anaerobes. Pulmonary abscess is characterized by necrosis of lung tissue, resulting in formation of cavities. Primary lung abscess is usually caused by aspiration of oral anaerobic bacteria into the lungs. Other mechanisms of lung abscess include septic emboli to the lung, usually originating from the heart valves and septic thrombophlebitis.

Patients usually have a history of loss of consciousness. Infection in the superior segment of the right lower lobe suggests aspiration. Anaerobic infections cause a necrotizing process in the lungs. Streptococcus pneumonia can cause cavitations but it is rare.

Common anaerobes causing lung abscess include:

- peptostreptococcus species
- bacteroides species
- fusobacterium species
- microaerophilic streptococci.

Bartlett JG. The role of anaerobic bacteria in lung abscess. *Clin Infect Dis* 2005; 40(7): 923–25.

13. Answer: B

This patient has developed pulmonary oedema due to severe MR. His cardiac output is determined by after-load and the resistance to flow across the abnormal mitral valve. A large fraction of stroke volume will flow into the left atrium, which is the cause of pulmonary oedema in this patient. Reducing afterload in this patient is necessary to reduce pulmonary oedema. ACE inhibitors, nitroprusside, and hydralazine can be used to treat the cause of pulmonary oedema in this patient. On the other hand, IABP will worsen the patient's condition. β-blockers do not reduce afterload. The patient will need to be optimized before mitral valve replacement surgery.

Sinclair M, Evans R. Cardiac surgery. In: Allman KG, Wilson IH. *Oxford Handbook of Anaesthesia.* Oxford University Press, 2006: p. 338.

14. Answer: C

Control and prevention of seizures is a priority in patients with eclampsia. This patient has eclampsia and requires caesarean section. Magnesium sulphate ($MgSO_4$) is the treatment of choice for preventing further seizures. A loading dose of $MgSO_4$ is administered, followed by continuous infusion for prophylaxis. Randomized control trials have shown magnesium sulphate to be better than diazepam or phenytoin in seizure prophylaxis.

Systolic pressure greater than 160 mm Hg and diastolic pressure more than 110 mmHg is an indication for treatment with antihypertensive medication to prevent stroke. Hydralazine and labetalol are commonly used.

Calcium and aspirin have been used to prevent preeclampsia.

Magnesium plays a important role in many cellular functions, and there is increasing interest in its role in medicine. There is now clear evidence of magnesium's benefit to patients with eclampsia or torsades de pointes arrhythmias. There is some suggestion that magnesium has antinociceptive and anesthetic properties as well as neuroprotective effects.

Herroeder S. Magnesium—essentials for anesthesiologists. *Anesthesiology.* 2011; 114(4): 971–93.

Duley L, Henderson-Smart DJ, Walker GJ, *et al.* Magnesium sulphate and other anticonvulsants for women with pre-eclampsia. Cochrane Database Syst Rev 2010; 11: CD000025.

15. Answer: D

Failure of the uterus to contract following delivery is the most common cause of postpartum haemorrhage in obstetrics. Uterine atony accounts for about 75% of postpartum haemorrhage.

Oxytocin and ergot alkaloids represent the cornerstone of uterotonic therapy. Prostaglandin therapy has been studied more recently as an attractive alternative.

Newer medical therapies aimed at achieving uterine tamponade include recombinant factor VII and hemostatic agents, and adjunctive nonsurgical methods.

Terbutaline is a tocolytic agent and is contraindicated in uterine atony. All other agents can be used in this patient to increase the uterine tone.

Breathnach F, Geary M. Uterine atony: definition, prevention, non-surgical management, and uterine tamponade. *Semin Perinatol* 2009; 33(2): 82–7.

16. Answer: C

Aspiration is the most common cause of maternal anaesthesia-related mortality. The risk of aspiration pneumonitis can be decreased by reducing the volume and acidity of the gastric contents. The gastric emptying time is prolonged in labour. Extubation should be performed with the patient fully awake. Patients who aspirate may develop clinical signs and symptoms several hours after the incident. Aspiration is potentially a risk in all patients with reduced consciousness.

The treatment is mainly supportive. It includes oxygen therapy and bronchodilators. It may often be necessary to remove large particulate matter using bronchoscopy. Use of prophylactic antibiotics is controversial. CPAP or intermittent positive pressure ventilation with PEEP may be necessary in severe cases.

Paranjothy S, Griffiths JD, Broughton HK, *et al.* Interventions at caesarean section for reducing the risk of aspiration pneumonitis. *Cochrane Database Syst Rev* 2010; 20(1): CD004943.

17 Answer: D

Cerebrovascular accident with lesions involving the cerebellum usually results in decreased muscle tone. This decreased tone and diminished deep tendon reflex is due to decreased activity in gamma efferents.

Lesions of the pyramidal tract caused by spasticity and lesions in the extrapyramidal pathways result in rigidity. Disorders of basal ganglia produce rigidity. This is also seen in conditions such as Parkinsonism.

Cerebrovascular accident involving the cerebellum is an important cause of stroke. It often presents with common and non-specific symptoms, such as dizziness, nausea, and vomiting, gait disorder, and headache. Careful attention to patients' coordination, gait, and eye movements are required for accurate diagnosis.

The differential diagnosis includes many common and benign causes. Insufficient examination and imaging can result in misdiagnosis. Some of the complications can be fatal. These include brainstem compression and obstructive hydrocephalus.

Edlow JA, Newman-Toker DE, Savitz SI. Diagnosis and initial management of cerebellar infarction. *Lancet Neurol* 2008; 7(10): 951–64.

18. Answer: C

The ulnar nerve (C8–T1) is the nerve for finger abduction and adduction. It supplies all the interossei, the lumbrical muscles of the little and ring fingers, and the adductor of the thumb. Patients with chronic ulnar nerve palsy show weakness of opposition of the little finger.

The median nerve innervates the thenar muscles, which are responsible for opposition of the thumb to the index finger.

All the extensors of the wrist are supplied by the radial nerve. Flexor carpi ulnaris is responsible for flexion of the wrist. The nerve supply to this muscle arises from the ulnar nerve, high in the forearm.

Yentis SM, Hirsch NP, Smith GB. *A–Z of Anaesthesia and Intensive Care*, Butterworth Heinemann, 2004: p. 547.

19. Answer: A

The brachial plexus (Fig. 3.1) is formed by ventral rami of C5 to C8, with contributions from C4 and T2 in some. It provides nerve supply to the upper limb.

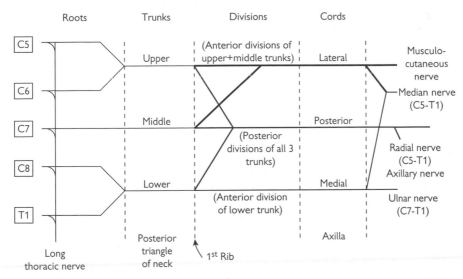

Figure 3.1 The brachial plexus.

Reproduced from Catherine Spoors and Kevin Kiff, Training in Anaesthesia, 2010, Figure 6.19, p. 119, with permission from Oxford University Press

It is composed of:

- roots: C5–C8 and TI (ventral rami)
- trunks: upper, middle, and lower
- divisons: anterior and posterior
- cords: medial, lateral, posterior.

The radial nerve innervates the supplies the triceps, brachioradialis, and most of the extensors of the wrist. Injury to the radial nerve results in wrist drop.

Shonfeld A, Harrop-Griffiths, W. Regional anaesthesia. In: Allman KG, Wilson IH (eds), *Oxford Handbook of Anaesthesia*, 2nd edn. Oxford University Press, 2004: pp. 1076–85.

20. Answer: E

Trigeminal neuralgia is an intermittent, usually unilateral, severe neuropathic pain, which can come on spontaneously or by stimulation of the trigger zone. There is an abnormality in the trigeminal sensory system. There is a significant female preponderance (2:1). Magnetic resonance imaging is recommended in these patients.

Classification is as follows:

- Type 1 is primary or idiopathic
- Type 2 is secondary to irritation or compression of the trigeminal nerve by tumour or disease, including multiple sclerosis.

Medical treatment

Response to carbamazepine is almost diagnostic of this condition. Gabapentine, baclofen, and sodium valproate have also been used.

Surgical treatment

Surgery should be considered if secondary causes are detected or medical therapy fails. This includes microvascular decompression (MVD), which has shown to be curative in patients in whom the condition has resulted from vascular compression of the trigeminal nerve. Teflon sponges are placed between dissected blood vessel and neural tissue. Compression is usually caused by a branch of the superior cerebellar artery, which should not be divided. Other procedures include glycerol rhizotomy, percutaneous balloon compression, retrogasserian rhizotomy, and gamma knife radio surgery.

Fisher A, Zakrzewska JM, Patsalos PN. Trigeminal neuralgia: current treatment and future developments. *Expert Opin Emergency Drugs* 2003; 8(1): 123.

Waldman SD. *Pain Management.* Saunders Elsevier, 2006.

21. Answer: B

The most common cause of coma in patients who have suffered traumatic brain injury without a mass-occupying lesion is diffuse axonal injury. The incidence of diffuse axonal injury in severe brain injury is more than 50%. More than 90% of these patients might not regain consciousness. There is characteristic axonal swelling, which affects the susceptible subcortical white matter, brain stem, and the corpus callosum. The lesions are haemorrhagic and are due to the shearing forces in the susceptible regions of the brain. The lesions are diffuse and not focal. Diffuse axonal injury is also seen in shaken baby syndrome. Uncontrolled blood pressure, ischemic infarction, and coagulopathies are unlikely to present with this picture. Amyloid angiopathy is seen in elderly patients.

Hijaz TA, Cento EA, Walker MT. Imaging of head trauma. *Radiol Clin North Am* 2011; 49(1): 81–103.

22. Answer: A

Intubated patients have a very high risk of having pneumonia. Selective digestive tract decontamination aims to prevent secondary colonization with Gram-negative bacteria, *Staphylococcus aureus*, and yeast. Selective digestive tract decontamination aims to maintain anaerobic intestinal flora through selective use of antibiotics. This is done by application of a non-absorbable antimicrobial agent in the oropharynx and gastrointestinal tract. Pre-emptive treatment of infections caused by respiratory tract bacteria with systemic cephalosporins through the first 4 days in intensive care is also done.

Maintenance of anaerobic intestinal flora is achieved through selective use of antibiotics. Meta-analyses and three randomized control trials have shown improved survival.

de Smet AM, Kluytmans JA, Cooper BS, *et al.* Decontamination of the digestive tract and oropharynx in ICU patients. *NEJM* 2009; 360: 1.

23. Answer: D

Spinal cord stimulation (SCS) has been used since 1967 for the treatment of refractory chronic pain, particularly failed back surgery syndrome. Simultaneous use of spinal cord stimulators and a permanent pacemaker is feasible. The presence of permanent pacemakers is not considered a general contraindication for neuromodulation therapy.

Patients with medtronic spinal cord stimulators (SCS) can be subjected to MRI of the brain provided the guidelines prescribed by the manufacturer are followed.

Neurostimulators have been reported to cause high-frequency artefacts on ECG.

A randomized control trial by North *et al.* has shown that patients with failed back surgery syndrome treated with spinal chord stimulators did better than those who had re-operation.

Ooi YC, Falowski S, Wang D, Jallo J, Ho R, Sharn A. Simultaneous use of neurostimulators in patients with a preexisting cardiovascular implantable electronic device. *Neuromodulation* 2011; 14: 20–26.

North RB, Kidd DH, Farrokhi F, *et al.* Spinal cord stimulation versus repeated lumbosacral spine surgery for chronic pain: a randomized, controlled trial. *Neurosurgery* 2005; 56: 98–106.

24. Answer: B

The priority in management of any patient remains maintenance of airway, breathing, and circulation. It is vital to resuscitate the patient before conducting diagnostic procedures. Assessment of coagulation profile is essential but not the first step. Caesarean section can be organized if necessary after resuscitation is commenced. Vaginal examination is contraindicated in this patient as it can aggravate the bleeding from placenta previa, which can be excluded after an ultrasound examination.

Postpartum Haemorrhage, Prevention and Management. Royal College of Obstetricians and Gynaecologists Guidelines, 2009 (Green-top 52). http://www.rcog.org.uk/files/rcog-corp/GT52PostpartumHaemorrhage0411.pdf.

25. Answer: A

Epidural and spinal anaesthesia as well as sedation administered in latent phase of labour prolong this stage of labour. This patient is experiencing a prolonged latent phase, which is highly variable in length. Causes of prolonged labour include cephalo-pelvic disproportion (CPD), hypotonic uterine contractions, and early or excessive use of labour anaesthesia. The uterus resumes its normal activity when the drug responsible is eliminated. The pelvis in this case has been tested by previous normal vaginal delivery, making CPD very unlikely. False labour is not accompanied by the cervical changes. Also the changes suggest that the cervix is responding appropriately, making cervical dysfunction unlikely. Review of the literature suggests that effective labour analgesia does not increase the rate of caesarean section, even when administered early in labour.

Cambic CR, Wong CA. Labour analgesia and obstetric outcomes. *Br J Anaesth* 2010; 105(Suppl 1): i50–60.

26. Answer: D

Rib fractures are associated with high mortality. Pain relief is extremely important in these patients to allow adequate ventilation and to prevent atelectasis and pneumonia. This condition is associated with severe pain. Oral analgesics and opiates are commonly used. Intercostal nerve block or paravertebral block or even an epidural are effective in providing effective pain relief and reduce the mortality associated with this condition.

Ziegler *et al.* reported that patients with one or two rib fractures had a 5% mortality rate, and patients with seven or more fractures had a 29% mortality rate.

Sirmali M, Türüt H, Topçu S, et al. A comprehensive analysis of traumatic rib fractures: morbidity, mortality and management. *Eur J Cardiothorac Surg* 2003; 24(1): 133–38.

Ziegler DW, Agarwal NN. The morbidity and mortality of rib fractures. *J Trauma* 1994; 37(6): 975–79.

27. Answer: B

The picture is suggestive of trauma to the spleen. The treatment of this condition depends on the patient's haemodynamic status and the response to intravenous fluids. Emergency laprotomy is indicated if the patient is unresponsive to fluid resuscitation and remains unstable. If the patient shows good response to fluid and does not require blood transfusion for resuscitation it is important to perform a CT scan.

Davies RH, Rees BI. Abdominal trauma. *BMJ* 2011; 342: d882.

28. Answer: C

This patient is presenting with massive atraumatic haemoptysis. The first step in the management of this condition is to perform bronchoscopy to locate and control the intrapulmonary bleeding. Rigid bronchoscopy offers control and protection of the patient's airway. The patient is at risk of asphyxiation due to airway flooding with blood. CT scan will aid in diagnostic work-up and planning of management of this patient. Endoscopy is indicated in gastrointestinal bleeding. In haemoptysis caused by vascular lesions, angiography and embolization may be necessary.

Sakr L, Dutau H. Massive hemoptysis: an update on the role of bronchoscopy in diagnosis and management. *Respiration* 2010; 80(1): 38–58.

29. Answer: D

Functional residual capacity (FRC) is the volume of air present in the lung at the end of passive expiration. It is the sum of the expiratory reserve volume and the residual volume. FRC and vital capacity can fall significantly following upper abdominal surgery. This patient is also at risk of developing alveolar atelectasis. Sitting the patient up can increase FRC by up to 35%. Increasing FRC also offers some protection against postoperative atelectasis. Bronchodialators do not have a significant role in improving FRC in patients who do not have a history of chronic obstructive airway devices.

Hedenstierna G, Edmark L. Mechanisms of atelectasis in the perioperative period. *Best Pract Res Clin Anaesthesiol* 2010; 24(2): 157–69.

30. Answer: C

The incidence of ischaemia of the bowel following aneurysm repair is about 1–7%. This is usually due to compromised flow through the inferior mesenteric artery during graft placement in the aorta. There are inadequate collaterals to the colon on the left and to the sigmoid colon. These patients present with abdominal pain and distension. The onset of *C. difficile* diarrhoea typically takes about 5 days after treatment with antibiotics. These patients present with watery diarrhoea initially. Invasive and infectious diarrhoea are uncommon in this setting. Formation of fistula is a rare and late complication due to erosion of duodenum into the proximal part of the graft in aorta.

Djavani K, Wanhainen A, Valtysson J, Björck M. Colonic ischaemia and intra-abdominal hypertension following open repair of ruptured abdominal aortic aneurysm. *Br J Surg* 2009; 96(6): 621–27.

True/False

1. **Which of the following statements regarding ketamine are true?**
   A. Ketamine is a phencyclidine derivative.
   B. It antagonizes the excitatory neurotransmitter glycine at NMDA receptors.
   C. It is a potent bronchodilator.
   D. It increases cardiac work.
   E. It increases cerebral metabolic oxygen requirement.

2. **Which of the following drugs are associated with the development of torsades des pointes?**
   A. Cisapride.
   B. Droperidol.
   C. Amiodarone.
   D. Methadone.
   E. Haloperidol.

3. **A 35-year-old African-American man with sickle cell disease presents for an open reduction and internal fixation of his fractured ankle. On admission his Hb is 9 g/dL and his haematocrit is 0.3. Which of the following statements are true?**
   A. Pre-operatively transfuse 2 units of packed red cells.
   B. Let him cool passively to low/normal temperature.
   C. Spinal is safe.
   D. Avoid thiopentone.
   E. Tourniquet is absolutely contra-indicated.

4. **Which of the following are seen as a consequence of right recurrent laryngeal nerve palsy following thyroid surgery?**
   A. The right vocal cord in midline position: partial.
   B. Dysphonia.
   C. The left vocal cord is immobile.
   D. Increased risk of aspiration.
   E. The left vocal cord moves to the opposite side.

5. **The common complications of coeliac plexus block are:**
    A. Erectile dysfunction.
    B. Constipation.
    C. Hypertension which resolves spontaneously.
    D. Paralysis.
    E. Hypotension.

6. **A patient is on your list for fracture neck of femur. He has aortic stenosis. Which of the following signs, symptoms, and investigations indicate that the lesion is severe?**
    A. Thrill in aortic area.
    B. Murmur in lower left sternal edge.
    C. LV–aortic gradient 40 mmHg.
    D. History of ischaemic heart disease or coronary artery disease.
    E. History of angina/syncope.

7. **Severe hypertension can affect women in pregnancy. What drug treatments should *not* be used routinely in pregnancy?**
    A. Hydralazine.
    B. Nifedipine.
    C. Labetalol.
    D. Metoprolol.
    E. Sodium nitropusside.

8. **Which of the following are appropriate management for post management of post-dural puncture headaches?**
    A. Prophylactic bed rest.
    B. Catheter in intrathecally.
    C   Allow patient to mobilize.
    D   Prophylactic blood patch.
    E   Give synthetic ACTH.

9. **NICE and the RCOG recommend magnesium sulphate as the drug of choice for the management of severe pre-eclampsia and eclampsia in the acute clinical setting. What factors should be routinely monitored to ensure that the magnesium levels are not too elevated?**
    A. Urinary magnesium levels to 2–3.5 mmol/L.
    B. Therapeutic serum drug level monitoring.
    C. Respiratory rate.
    D. Deep tendon reflexes.
    E. Urine output.

10. **Regarding the condition autonomic dysreflexia:**
    A. 50% of patients have injury level below T6.
    B. Unlikely if injury is below T10.
    C. Can be prevented.
    D. Can be precipitated by light touch.
    E. Is a medical emergency.

11. **Venous thromboembolism is a significant cause of morbidity and mortality in patients during the perioperative period. The British Thoracic Society has published guidelines for the identification of risk factors. Which of the following are major risk factors?**
    A. Dehydration.
    B. Factor V Leiden mutation.
    C. Pregnancy.
    D. Varicose veins.
    E. Malignancy.

12. **Diastolic heart failure can manifest in the perioperative course as:**
    A. Hypotensive crisis.
    B. Acute onset pulmonary oedema.
    C. Heart failure with abnormal LV function.
    D. Acute onset renal failure.
    E. Reduced cardiac output.

13. **Which of the following statements are true regarding foetal haemoglobin (HbF)?**
    A. Consists of two α and two γ chains.
    B. Binds 2,3-DPG less avidly than HbA.
    C. Has a P50 of 2.4 kPa.
    D. Forms 50% of circulating haemoglobin at birth.
    E. May persist.

14. **Regarding phaeochromocytoma:**
    A. Tumours arising from chromaffin cells in adrenal medulla.
    B. Tumour secretes only noradrenaline.
    C. Sustained hypotension is common presenting feature.
    D. Hypoglycemia is a common feature.
    E. Diagnosis is confirmed by measuring catecholamine metabolites in 24-h urine collection.

15. **Concerning heat loss in the operating theatre for a neonate, which of the following statements is correct?**
    A. Can be reduced by reducing the theatre temperature.
    B. The use of a foil blanket reduces convection loss.
    C. The use of a warming blanket reduces radiation loss.
    D. Increasing the humidity reduces convection loss.
    E. Most heat loss is via convection.

16. **The anterior branch of the femoral nerve supplies everything except:**
    A. Pectineus.
    B. Rectus femoris.
    C. Skin overlying medial thigh.
    D. Skin overlying anterior thigh.
    E. Sartorius.

17. **The body composition and metabolism are altered by advancing old age. Which of the following statements are true?**
    A. Body fat mass declines progressively.
    B. Total body water increases.
    C. Thyroid hormone production decreases.
    D. Glucocorticoid secretion is reduced.
    E. Glucose tolerance is reduced.

18. **In the otherwise normal elderly person, which of the following statements regarding cardiovascular physiology are true?**
    A. Ventricular compliance is decreased.
    B. Diastolic ventricular filling is more dependent on atrial contraction than in the young adult.
    C. The arterial pulse is widened.
    D. Baroreceptor function is impaired.
    E. Augmentation of cardiac output is more dependent on the Frank–Starling mechanism than in the young adult.

19. **Regarding lung functions in the otherwise normal elderly person, which of the following statements are true?**
    A. Tissue elasticity is the lung property most affected by aging.
    B. Total lung compliance is increased.
    C. Small airways may close during tidal breathing.
    D. The ventilatory response to hypoxia is maintained as in youth.
    E. There is a higher incidence of episodic breathing than in the young adult.

20. **Regarding the drug salbutamol, which of the following statements are true:**
    A. It is a selective $\beta2$ receptor agonist.
    B. It undergoes extensive first pass metabolism.
    C. It reduces the release of histamine from mast cells.
    D. The IV route is more effective in severe asthma.
    E. It is useful to improve cardiac output in low-output states.

21. **Regarding pharmacokinetics in the geriatric age group:**
    A. Intestinal absorption of most drugs decreases with age.
    B. Skin absorption of fentanyl is considerably increased in the elderly.
    C. Drugs that are relatively water soluble have a larger volume of distribution.
    D. The free plasma concentration of highly protein-bound drugs is often increased.
    E. Lipid-soluble drugs have a larger volume of distribution.

22. In brain stem death:

A. The definition requires the loss of capacity to breathe or the irreversible loss of capacity for consciousness.

B. Potentially reversible causes must be excluded.

C. The patient must be unconscious and apnoeic as preconditions.

D. Formal brain-stem testing must be undertaken by two independent clinicians, one of whom must have been fully registered with the General Medical Council for at least five years.

E. Time of death is recorded as the time at which the second set of brain-stem death tests are completed.

23. Serotonin (5-HT) is a monoamine neurotransmitter that is involved in a number of physiological systems of relevance to the anaesthetist. Which of the following statements about serotonin are true?

A. Serotonin is synthesized in enterochromaffin cells, serotonergic neurones in the central nervous system, and in monocytes.

B. Serotonin exerts its action specifically at 5-HT receptors by the action of magnesium flux.

C. The main metabolic product is 5-hydroxyindole acetic acid.

D. All 5-HT receptor interactions involve cyclic AMP and G-proteins.

E. Anaesthesia in patients taking selective serotonin reuptake inhibitors (SSRIs) can cause hypotension, arrhythmias, altered thermoregulation, and postoperative confusion.

24. The following are derived units:

A. Kelvin.

B. Newton.

C. Ampere.

D. Joule.

E. Kilogram.

25. Regarding the drug benzatropine mesylate, which of the following statements are true?

A. It is an anticholinergic drug.

B. It is used to treat acute dystonic reactions.

C. It is not effective for drug induced parkinsonism.

D. It can be given orally.

E. It has no sedative effects.

26. Regarding enoximone, which of the following statements are true?

A. It is an imidazole derivative.

D. It is a selective phosphodiestrase II inhibitor.

C. It undergoes substantial first-pass metabolism.

D. It can cause hypotension due to vasodilatation.

E. It improves myocardial function at the expense of increasing myocardial oxygen extraction.

27. Regarding pharyngeal pouch:

A. It is associated with recurrent lung infection.
B. It causes herniation of the posterior wall of the oesophagus.
C. Aspiration can be controlled by cricoid pressure.
D. It can be assessed by barium swallow.
E. It is caused by uncoordinated movement of the thyropharyngeus and cricopharyngeus.

28. Maxillary nerve block at pterygopalatine fossa causes anaesthesia of:

A. Upper molar.
B. Lower molar (mandibular).
C. Hard palate.
D. Anterior two-thirds of tongue (lingual/mandibular).
E. Anterior part of nasal septum (ophthalmic).

29. Concerning absorption of carbon dioxide in circle systems:

A. Soda lime granules are sized 4–8 mesh.
B. Baralyme contains calcium hydroxide as well as barium hydroxide.
C. Soda lime produces more compound A at low fresh gas flows.
D. Dry soda lime absorbs more carbon dioxide.
E. Carbon dioxide first reacts with sodium and potassium hydroxide in soda lime.

30. The following are recognized causes of thrombocytopaenia:

A. Systemic lupus erythematosus.
B. Infectious mononucleosis.
C. Cirrhosis of the liver.
D. Treatment with a thiazide diuretic.
E. Splenectomy.

31. Which of the following statements about carcinoid syndrome are true?

A. Ondansetron provides symptomatic relief.
B. It is caused by tumours originating from the enterochromaffin cells.
C. The tumours secrete prostaglandins, kinins, and serotonin.
D. Mediator release during surgery can cause profound hypertension.
E. Octreotide is a synthetic analogue of serotonin.

32. Concerning lymph drainage in the thorax:

A. The heart has no lymphatic system.
B. The thoracic duct passes through the aortic opening of the diaphragm.
C. The medial quadrants of the breast drain to the paraaortic nodes.
D. The thoracic duct drains all the lymph from the lower limbs and abdominal cavity.
E. A sentinel node is one that receives lymph drainage directly from a tumour.

33. **Complications associated with blood transfusion are commonly seen by anaesthetists. True statements regarding blood transfusion include:**
    A. Hypocalcaemia due to citrate is worse with the transfusion of packed red cells than FFP.
    B. Hypothermia occurs more commonly with platelets than with packed red cells.
    C. Transfusion-related acute lung injury (TRALI) presents within 6 h of transfusion.
    D. ABO incompatibility reactions occur 2–4 h after transfusion.
    E. In cases of true haemolytic transfusion reaction, the Coombs' test will be positive.

34. **Regarding Cushing's syndrome which following statements are true?**
    A. Results from excessive exogenous corticosteroids.
    B. Causes central obesity.
    C. Characterized by raised urinary cortisol.
    D. Causes hypernatremia with hyperkalemia.
    E. Diabetes is always present.

35. **NCEPOD published a report titled 'Adding insult to injury', which reviewed patients who died from acute kidney injury. The key recommendations included:**
    A. All patients admitted to the hospital should have urinalysis performed.
    B. All patients admitted to the hospital as an emergency should have their electrolytes routinely checked on admission.
    C. All emergency admissions should receive a consultant review within 12 h of admission.
    D. All level 3 units should have the ability to deliver renal replacement therapy.
    E. All acute admitting hospitals should have access to a renal ultrasound service 24 h a day, including weekends.

36. **Which of the following are recognized side effects of ondansetron?**
    A. Constipation.
    B. Tachycardia.
    C. Chest pain.
    D. Seizures.
    E. Transient blindness.

37. **Regarding statins, which of the following statements are true?**
    A. All selectively inhibit HMG-CoA-reductase.
    B. They lead to increased hepatic LDL-receptor expression.
    C. They lower LDL levels in a dose-dependent fashion.
    D. Therapy should be monitored with regular measurement of plasma creatine kinase (CK) levels.
    E. They are associated with development of rhabdomyolysis.

38. Regarding hyperbaric oxygen therapy, which of the following statements are true?

A. It is useful in treating arterial air emboli, as a application of Charles'law.
B. It increases the oxygen content of blood, based on Henry's law.
C. There is an increase in left ventricular afterload.
D. It is absolutely contraindicated in patients with a simple 'undrained' pneumothorax.
E. It is relatively contraindicated in patients with COPD.

39. Concerning renal replacement therapy:

A. Haemodialysis is more efficient.
B. Haemodialysis depends on the semi-permeable membrane.
C. Haemodialysis can be intermittent.
D. Convective transport is independent of solute concentration gradients.
E. Haemofiltration relies on the principle of diffusion.

40. The clinical condition botulism:

A. Is caused by an endotoxin from *Clostridium botulinum*.
B. Results in reversible binding of toxins to the neuromuscular junction.
C. Is characterized by a progressive ascending flaccid weakness.
D. Toxin binds irreversibly to the presynaptic membrane of cholinergic neurons.
E. Is most commonly food-borne.

41. In a patient who is not suffering acute myocardial infarction, elevated cardiac troponins may be encountered with which of the following:

A. Intracranial haemorrhage.
B. Poisoning.
C. Chemotherapy.
D. Pulmonary embolism.
E. Tachyarrhythmia.

42. A 78-year-old patient for carotid endarterectomy has deep cervical plexus block. What signs indicate the successive sympathetic blockade?

A. Meiosis.
B. Exopthalmos.
C. Tachycardia.
D. Nasal stuffiness.
E. Anhydrosis.

43. Regarding Down's syndrome which of the following are true.

A. Trisomy 21.
B. Recurrent respiratory tract infections are common.
C. Can have atlantoaxial instability.
D. Have enlarged jaws.
E. Have high arched, narrow palates.

44. Regarding diabetes mellitus.

A. Random blood glucose greater than 11.1 mmol/L is diagnostic.
B. Fasting blood glucose greater 7 mmol/L on two occasions is diagnostic.
C. It has a prevalence of about 3% in the UK population.
D. The risk of type 2 diabetes mellitus is two-fold in patients with BMI more than 30.
E. Tight glycaemic control does not affect microvascular complication rate.

45. Features of advanced liver disease include:

A. Increased prothrombin time with normal bleeding time.
B. Hyperglycemia.
C. Portal hypertension.
D. Hypoalbuminaemia.
E. Ecephalopathy.

46. Which of the following statements about electroconvulsive therapy are true?

A. Induces a tonic–clonic seizure.
B. Has a long parasympathetic phase.
C. Has a short sympathetic phase.
D. Should be preceded by administration of muscle relaxants.
E. Consists of a pulsatile sine wave of 35 J.

47. At the end of the total knee replacement, before closure of the wound, the tourniquet is deflated and tourniquet time was 145 min. The following will happen:

A. Increase in the serum lactate levels.
B. Rise in serum potassium levels, which peak after 30 min of deflation.
C. Rise in end-tidal CO_2 which peaks within 1 min.
D. No association with irreversible muscle damage.
E. Increased fibrinolysis.

48. The systemic effects of abdominal compartment syndrome are:

A. Reduced cardiac output.
B. Reduced pulmonary artery occlusion pressure (PAOP).
C. Hypercarbia.
D. Reduced glomerular filtration rate.
E. Increased intracranial pressure.

49. The indications for an interpleural block are:

A. Fractured rib.
B. Chronic pancreatitis.
C. Laparoscopic cholecystectomy.
D. Mastectomy.
E. Shoulder surgery.

50. Drugs safe to use in porphyria include:

    A. Nitrous oxide.

    B. Bupivacaine.

    C. Aspirin.

    D. Etomidate.

    E. Phenytoin.

51. Which of the following groups of patients are considered to be high risk for the development of delirium?

    A. Aged 65 or older.

    B. Dementia.

    C. Current humeral fracture.

    D. Severe intercurrent illness.

    E. Visual impairment.

52. With regard to the diagnosis of death.

    A. There is statutory law in the United Kingdom that defines death.

    B. During brain-stem testing the apnoea test should only be performed on one occasion, to minimize the hypoxic insult to the organs of the potential organ donor.

    C. In the event of death after cardiorespiratory arrest, the patient should be observed for no less than 5 min to establish that irreversible cardiorespiratory arrest has occurred.

    D. The absence of pupillary responses to light should be established prior to the confirmation of cardiorespiratory arrest.

    E. The time of the first brain-stem testing is recorded as the time of the death.

53. Radiofrequency procedures are used in the modulation of chronic pain syndromes to interrupt or alter nociceptive pathways. Which of the following statements are true?

    A. Low-energy, high-frequency direct current is used.

    B. Continuous radiofrequency techniques use current to produce a thermal lesion.

    C. Pulsed radiofrequency techniques use current to produce a thermal lesion.

    D. In continuous-wave radiofrequency procedures, greatest current density is produced distal to the tip of the insulated needle, leading to the needle being placed perpendicular to (against) the nerve.

    E. In pulsed-wave radiofrequency procedures, greatest current density is produced along the shaft of the insulated needle, leading to the needle being placed parallel to (alongside) the nerve.

54. With regard to mathematical relationships:

    A. $y = mx + c$ indicates a linear relationship.

    B. c represents the x-axis intercept.

    C. Linear functions only have two parameters, m and c, and this enables two-point calibration where a relationship is linear.

    D. A line that crosses an axis is called an asymptote.

    E. A decaying exponential decreases by a constant proportion each time period.

55. Transdermal drug delivery is improved if the drug:

    A. Has high melting point.

    B. Is non-ionic.

    C. Has low lipid solubility.

    D. Has molecular weight >500 Da.

    E. Has short half-life.

56. Regarding the critical temperature:

    A. The gas is in liquid form at this temperature.

    B. It is the temperature above which a gas cannot be liquefied by pressure alone.

    C. It is the temperature below which a gas does not vaporize.

    D. It is 36.5°C for nitrous oxide.

    E. It is different if a substance is in a mixture rather than on its own.

57. Regarding a subdural block:

    A. It occurs when an epidural catheter is misplaced between the duramater and ligamentum flavum.

    B. It is definitively diagnosed by a positive aspiration test.

    C. It may cause Horner's syndrome.

    D. It is characterized by a faster onset compared to intrathecal injection.

    E. It is typically dense and widespread.

58. You are presented with 58-year-old alcoholic patient with bleeding varices. Appropriate management includes:

    A. Administration of vasopressin.

    B. Application of a Sengstaken-type tube.

    C. Insertion of a large-bore nasogastric tube.

    D. Transjugular intrahepatic portosystemic stented shunting.

    E. Administration of propranolol.

59. On your list there is a 58-year-old patient with obstructed bowel. On examination of his pulse there is slow rising pulse and on auscultation he has loud ejection-systolic murmur. Your management during the peri-operative period would include:

    A. Maintain normal to high pulse rate.

    B. If there is hypotension administer isoprenaline.

    C. High-to-normal systemic vascular resistance (SVR)

    D. Low preload.

    E. Atropine administration for heart rates 60/min.

60. Regarding bioavailability of a drug:

    A. It is indicated by the area under the plasma concentration–time curve.

    B. Must be less than 100% for a drug injected intravenously.

    C. May be reduced by destruction of a drug in the gut.

    D. May be reduced by the destruction of a drug in the liver.

    E. It is greater by the sublingual route than by the enteral route.

Single Best Answers

1. **Acromegaly is a clinical syndrome causing the over-production and under-regulation of growth hormone. Which of the following features does not increase the difficulty on direct laryngoscopy?**
   A. Distorted facial anatomy.
   B. Macroglossia.
   C. Glottic stenosis.
   D. Prognathe mandible.
   E. Arthritis of the neck.

2. **Brachial plexus injury in the course of anaesthesia and critical care episodes is not an uncommon occurrence. Which of the following statements below is not correct?**
   A. Brachial plexus catheter insertion is associated with increased risk of injury.
   B. Arm abduction with lateral rotation of the head to the opposite side can cause excessive stretch.
   C. Lesions affecting the upper nerve roots are more common.
   D. Damage to the long thoracic nerve causes winging of the scapula.
   E. Upward movement of the clavicle and sternal retraction can cause a compression injury to the nerve.

3. **You are called to see a 32-year-old primiparous woman on the postnatal ward following caesarean section. The caesarean was done 8 h ago, under spinal anaesthesia as the top up epidural failed. The midwives in ward are now concerned that the patient is drowsy, with a respiratory rate of 6/min. What is the most likely cause?**
   A. Fentanyl 100mcg, administered via the labour epidural at the start of the caesarean section, acting on the local spinal receptors.
   B. Exhaustion due to long latent phase of labour.
   C. Diamorphine 300 mcg, administered via the spinal at the start of the caesarean section, acting by the cephalad spread of drug by the bulk flow of CSF.
   D. L-bupivacaine 0.5%, 20 mL, administered via the labour epidural at the start of the caesarean section, causing high regional anaesthetic block.
   E. Fentanyl 100 mcg, administered via the labour epidural at the start of the caesarean section, acting by the lipophilic systemic absorption of opioid.

4. The report by the UK's Centre for Maternal and Child Enquiries, entitled 'Saving mothers' lives', was published in 2010, and highlighted the leading causes of maternal death. Which of the complications below was the leading cause of direct maternal deaths?

A. Venous thromboembolism.
B. Genital tract sepsis.
C. Haemorrhage.
D. Amniotic fluid embolism.
E. Pre-eclampsia and eclampsia.

5. Trigeminal neuralgia is a chronic facial pain syndrome. Select the most reliable initial treatment from the list below.

A. Pregabalin.
B. Carbamazepine.
C. Gabapentin.
D. Amitriptyline.
E. Lamotrigene.

6. You are working on the trauma list and an 11-year-old boy presents to the anaesthetic room for an ORIF of his radius. You notice that he has bruising on his arms that looks like finger prints, scratches to his face, and is very withdrawn. He comes to theatre alone with a paediatric nurse. During the preparation for anaesthesia you ask him what happened and he bursts into tears and says that he is too frightened to go home as his mother's boyfriend was beating him up. What is your next action?

A. Proceed with the anaesthesia as quickly as possible.
B. Postpone the operation and send the patient back to the ward.
C. Ask the nurse to talk to the patient and report back to the ward.
D. Briefly explain to the surgeon that there will be a short delay and listen to and observe the child, allowing him to talk and document the conversation. Proceed with surgery.
E. Briefly explain to the surgeon that there will be a short delay and listen to and observe the child, allowing him to talk and document the conversation. Postpone surgery.

7. A 41-year-old man has been induced for a laparoscopic cholecystectomy with fentanyl 100 mcg, propofol 200 mg, and atracurium 40 mg. On direct laryngoscopy it is not possible to pass the back of the tongue and no epiglottis is seen. The patient is oxygenated with 100% oxygen, repositioned, and a further attempt at direct laryngoscopy is made with no improvement in the view. What is the next management strategy?

A. One further attempt at direct laryngoscopy with a McCoy blade laryngoscope.
B. One further attempt at direct laryngoscopy with a bougie.
C. Abandon further direct laryngoscopy and insert a laryngeal mask airway.
D. Abandon further direct laryngoscopy and intubate with asleep fibreoptic technique.
E. Abandon further direct laryngoscopy and establish an airway with an emergency cannula cricothyroidotomy.

8. **The recovery nurse calls you to see a 35-year-old African-American woman who has had an ORIF for a fractured medial malleolus. She is known to have a positive Sickledex test. The patient is complaining of severe abdominal pain, which is not resolving with morphine intravenously. She has Hb 10.4 g/dL, oxygen saturation 94% on air, HR 110 bpm, BP 138/62, tympanic temperature 36.9°C. What is the most appropriate initial management strategy?**

    A. Oxygen 2 L/min via nasal cannulae.
    B. Oxygen 4 L/min via Hudson mask.
    C. Oxygen 15 L/min via non-rebreathe mask.
    D. Morphine 5 mg bolus IV.
    E. Diclofenac 7 5mg IV.

9. **A fit and well 71-year-old man has undergone total knee replacement under a general anaesthetic, spontaneously ventilating on a laryngeal mask and with opioid analgesia combined with a femoral nerve block. Before closure of the wound, the surgeon requests that you release the surgical tourniquet, which has been inflated for 68 min. What is the first clinical parameter that you will see change?**

    A. An increase in the respiratory rate.
    B. A decrease in the blood pressure.
    C. A decrease in the heart rate.
    D. An increase in the serum potassium.
    E. An increase in the end-tidal carbon dioxide.

10. **A 60-year-old is diagnosed with sciatica. Which of the following do not increase or decrease the risk of having this condition?**

    A. Gender.
    B. Age.
    C. Genetic predisposition.
    D. Smoking.
    E. Height.

11. **A young female patient presents with recurrent severe right side pulsating headache. The attacks last for about 5 h. These are accompanied by photophobia and nausea. Which of the following is true about this condition?**

    A. Must occur with aura.
    B. NSAIDs are not useful in its treatment.
    C. Triptans (5-HT agonists) are the most potent abortive agents in migraine attacks.
    D. Triptans should be taken on daily basis to prevent recurrent migraine attacks.
    E. Sumatriptan can be safely used in patients suffering from ischaemic heart disease.

12. **A 17-year-old male is admitted for elective scoliosis surgery to insert Harrington rods. The procedure is undertaken in the prone position. Which of the following methods of intra-operative monitoring of neurological function should be used to aid in the instrumentation of the spine?**
    A. Bispectral index.
    B. Somato-sensory evoked potentials.
    C. Wake the patient from general anaesthesia.
    D. Peripheral nerve stimulation.
    E. Invasive blood pressure monitoring.

13. **A 62-year-old man presents to A&E with an acute onset of severe central upper abdominal pain. It radiates through to his back, and he has been vomiting all day. He is known to have gallstones and has had a recent course of oral antibiotics and steroids for an infective exacerbation of COPD. On examination he is found to have rebound epigastric tenderness, pyrexia, and discolouration of his flanks. Which of the following blood tests is most specific for the diagnosis of acute pancreatitis?**
    A. Serum transaminases.
    B. Serum trypsinogen.
    C. Serum amylase.
    D. Serum lipase.
    E. Serum calcium.

14. **A 67-year-old male is undergoing minimally invasive oesophagectomy, requiring one-lung anaesthesia. Which of the following is least likely to occur during one-lung anaesthesia?**
    A. Hypoxia.
    B. Hypercarbia.
    C. Hypoxic pulmonary vasoconstriction.
    D. Ventilation-perfusion mismatch.
    E. Intrapulmonary shunt.

15. **A 27-year-old male motorcyclist is admitted to the orthopaedic ward following a road traffic collision involving a lorry. He suffered a crush injury and tibia/fibula fracture to his right leg and is admitted for observation. The nurses are concerned that he may be developing acute limb compartment syndrome. What is the earliest cardinal feature of compartment syndrome?**
    A. Pain disproportionate to the injury in the affected compartment.
    B. Paralysis of the limb.
    C. Pain aggravated by passive stretching of the involved muscles.
    D. Pulselessness of the vessels in the affected compartment.
    E. Paraesthesia to two-point discrimination in the nerves of the affected compartment.

16. **A 44-year-old woman had a laparotomy and interval debulking surgery for ovarian cancer 3 days ago. You are asked by the acute pain nurse to review the patient on the ward. She has a temperature of 38.2°C, pain in her lower back, and, on further questioning, admits to some increasing numbness in her legs over the last 4 h. The pain nurse reports that she turned the epidural off 8 h ago, as the patient's blood pressure had been low and pulse was rising. What is your next action?**

   A. Arrange for an MRI scan of the spine and start multimodal oral analgesia.
   B. Give an epidural top up of 20 mL of 0.125% bupivacaine to improve the analgesia from the epidural.
   C. Arrange for urgent MRI scan of the spine and start broad-spectrum intravenous antibiotic.
   D. Request a surgical review as an emergency.
   E. Remove the epidural catheter and start intravenous antibiotics.

17. **A 29-year-old teacher presents to the pain clinic with burning pain in her right forearm, associated with muscular spasms, fluctuant discolouration, fluctuant temperature, and occasional swelling. She reports that she had a fracture of her radius at the age of 9, which was treated conservatively. It was complicated by compartment syndrome caused by a tight cast, causing a neurological deficit, which fully recovered. The most likely diagnosis is:**

   A. Post-surgical pain due to nerve damage.
   B. Complex regional pain syndrome type 1.
   C. Venous thrombosis to the upper limb.
   D. Complex regional pain syndrome type 2.
   E. Peripheral nerve injury sustained at time of injury due to tight cast.

18. **A 66-year-old man has been admitted to the intensive care unit following a craniectomy and resection of a right-sided tumour. He has a residual left-sided weakness. A fine-bore nasogastric (NG) tube has been inserted in the intensive care unit for commencement of entral feeding. Which of the following tests is the best for confirming the correct placement of the feeding tube?**

   A. Checking the pH of any aspirated fluid.
   B. Portable chest X-ray.
   C. Injection of 50 mL of air down the NG tube whilst auscultating over the stomach.
   D. Abdominal X-ray.
   E. Aspiration of greater than 10 mL of fluid up the NG tube.

19. **A 58-year-old woman is admitted to the intensive care unit from A&E. She is known to have mild asthma, but is otherwise fit and well. She had a 2-day history of a productive cough, high fever, and worsening breathlessness. She was intubated and ventilated due to type 1 respiratory failure and worsening severe sepsis with rapid deterioration. What is the most likely causative organism?**

    A. *Legionella pneumophilia.*
    B. *Staphyloccus aureus.*
    C. *Streptococcus pneumoniae.*
    D. *Haemophilus influenzae.*
    E. *Mycoplasma pneumoniae.*

20. **A 33-year-old woman underwent an emergency laparotomy and hysterectomy for massive primary post-partum haemorrhage. The estimated blood loss during the vaginal delivery and subsequent hysterectomy was 8 L. She was transfused 10 units of packed red cells during the procedure and received an additional 2 L colloid and 2 L crystalloid. Once transferred to critical care the patient is noted to be bleeding from the abdominal wound and drain. Which of the following tests supports the diagnosis of disseminated intravascular coagulation (DIC) rather than dilutional coagulopathy?**

    A. INR.
    B. Platelet count.
    C. Bleeding time.
    D. D-dimer.
    E. Haemoglobin.

21. **The Clarke polarographic sensor is used to analyse oxygen in blood samples. Which of the following best describes the components of the Clarke sensor?**

    A. Gold cathode, lead anode, potassium hydroxide solution.
    B. Gold cathode, silver/silver chloride anode, potassium chloride solution, electrical source.
    C. Glass pH electrode, H^+ selective Teflon membrane, hydrogen carbonate buffer.
    D. Calomel reference electrode, silver/silver chloride electrode, potassium chloride solution.
    E. Gold cathode, lead anode, potassium hydroxide solution, electrical source.

22. **You attend the coronary care unit on a peri-arrest call. A 52-year-old man is experiencing chest pain. He is a tablet-controlled diabetic, overweight, hypertensive, and a smoker. You notice that his heart rate is 120 bpm, blood pressure is 88/50, and the cardiac monitor is showing ventricular tachycardia. You confirm that the patient does have a pulse. What is your next treatment action?**

    A. Take blood samples for electrolytes and troponin.
    B. Metoprolol 50 mg IV over 5 min.
    C. Amiodarone 300 mg IV over 20 min.
    D. Amiodarone 900 mg IV over 24 h.
    E. Synchronized DC cardioversion.

23. **Venous thromboembolism is a major cause of morbidity and mortality in hospital and in the community. Anti-embolism stockings (AES) are an effective mechanical method of reducing the risk of venous thromboembolism. Which of the following patients should *not* have anti-embolism stockings?**

    A. A 29-year-old primigravida for elective lower-segment caesarean section.
    B. A 17-year-old man with asthma for open reduction and internal fixation of clavicle.
    C. A 71-year-old woman with ischaemic heart disease, admitted with acute coronary syndrome.
    D. A 66-year-old woman with pneumonia and mild varicose veins without symptoms.
    E. An 83-year-old man who is bedbound following an acute stroke.

24. **A 41-year-old woman (gravida 4, para 3) is delivered of a 4.1 kg baby girl by vaginal delivery with a forceps lift out after a prolonged second stage. Despite three previous normal vaginal deliveries it has been 8 years since her last baby. In this pregnancy she had gestational diabetes mellitus and essential hypertension. In post-partum stage, 4 h after delivery of the placenta, she had primary post-partum haemorrhage of 900 mL. What is the most likely cause?**

    A. Coagulopathy.
    B. Retained membranes.
    C. Atonic uterus.
    D. Ruptured uterus.
    E. Vaginal wall tear.

25. **A 63-year-old lady is scheduled for total abdominal hysterectomy and bilateral salpingo-oophrectomy under general anaesthesia. She is an insulin-dependent diabetic and has Parkinson's disease, treated with levodopa. What would be the most appropriate combination of antiemetics for this patient?**

    A. Dexamethasone and ondansetron.
    B. Ondansetron and domperidone.
    C. Droperidol and prochlorperazine.
    D. Metoclopramide and dexamethasone.
    E. Prochlorperazine and ondansetron.

26. **A 52-year-old man presents for an inguinal hernia repair. His BMI is recorded at 43. On further questioning he reports that he snores and keeps his wife awake, falls asleep at work, and wakes in the morning feeling tired. On examination, he has HR 75/min sinus rhythm, BP 172/93, fine bibasal crackles at lung bases, and bipedal pitting oedema. His pre-operative blood gas shows $PaCO_2$ of 6.8 kPa. What is your next action?**

    A. Postpone the surgery until he loses weight and is commenced on diuretic.
    B. Postpone surgery until investigated and treated by local sleep unit along with treatment of hypertension.
    C. Postpone the surgery until his blood pressure is controlled and he has commenced on a diuretic.
    D. Proceed with the surgery under regional anaesthesia.
    E. Proceed with the surgery under judicious general anaesthesia.

27. **You are called to the orthopaedic theatre to assist with an emergency. A 78-year-old man, with a known history of difficult intubation due to rheumatoid arthritis in his neck, is scheduled for open reduction and internal fixation of radius and ulna under a brachial plexus block. The block was performed via the supraclavicular approach, infiltrating 25 mL 0.5% laevo-bupivacaine.-bupivacaine. Shortly after the injection was completed he began convulsing. What is your immediate medical strategy?**

    A. Rapid sequence induction and intubation.
    B. Intralipid 20% 1.5mL/kg.
    C. 3 min of preoxygenation and then RSI and intubation.
    D. Midazolam 50 mg.
    E. ABC and oxygenation.

28. **A 29-year-old male undergoes a rapid sequence induction to secure his airway for emergency trauma surgery to fix multiple limb fractures following a serious motorcycle accident. He is very cold and venous access was very difficult in A&E. As the thiopentone is injected into his left hand, the patient cries out in pain and his arm becomes suddenly very pale and cyanosed. What is the most suitable analgesic method to control this situation?**

    A. Intra-arterial injection of lignocaine.
    B. Stellate ganglion block.
    C. Intra-arterial methylprednisolone.
    D. Interscalene brachial plexus block.
    E. Intra-arterial papaverine.

29. **A 72-year-old lady is brought into the A&E resuscitation bay complaining of light-headedness on standing and severe lethargy. She has had intermittent chest heaviness over the last 3 days but no chest pain at present. Her initial observations reveal a heart rate of 37/min and a blood pressure on 96/42. Her ECG shows complete heart block. Which of the following is the most appropriate initial therapy?**

    A. Atropine.
    B. Adrenaline.
    C. Dopamine.
    D. Glucagon.
    E. Isoprenaline.

30. **A 33-year-old man requires an open reduction and internal fixation of his radius, which he fractured falling off his bicycle during an elite triathlon competition. During your preoperative visit you notice that his initial haemoglobin on admission to A&E was 8.0 g/dL. The haematologist has commented on the blood film that there was a 10% reticulocyte count. What is the most likely clinical diagnosis?**

    A. Untreated pernicious anaemia.
    B. Aplastic anaemia.
    C. Acute lymphocytic leukaemia.
    D. Anaemia of chronic disease.
    E. Hereditary spherocytosis.

1. Answers: T F T T T

Ketamine is a phencyclidine derivative that antagonizes the excitatory neurotransmitter glutamate at NMDA receptors. It produces a state of dissociative anaesthesia, profound analgesia, and amnesia. It is also a potent bronchodilator. Ketamine is not commonly used as a sedative infusion due to sympathetic nervous system stimulation resulting in increased cardiac work and a rise in cerebral metabolic oxygen consumption. Hallucinations, delirium, nausea, and vomiting frequently follow its use, but it still has a role in the management of status asthmaticus.

Rowe K, Fletcher S. Sedation in the intensive care unit. *Contin Educ Anaesth Crit Care Pain* 2008; 8(2): 50–55.

2. Answers: T T T T T

Torsade de pointes is a well-recognized side effect of any anti-arrhythmic drug that prolongs cardiac repolarization. However, it appears that patients with drug-induced long QT interval may have some underlying genetic susceptibility to arrhythmias. Recent research has identified the human ether-a-go-go-related gene (HERG) as responsible for drug-induced QT prolongation. HERG regulates iKr channels to cause cardiac cell repolarization. Virtually all drugs that prolong the QT interval and cause torsade de pointes also block iKr channels. However, this finding is not specific, as many drugs that block this current and prolong the QT interval do not cause torsades. It is postulated that torsadogenic drugs may be arrhythmogenic by preferentially affecting M-cell repolarization dynamics, thereby increasing transmural dispersion of repolarization (TDR). Females seem especially prone to develop drug-induced LQTS.

Hunter JD, Sharma P, Rathi S. Long QT syndrome. *Contin Educ Anaesth Crit Care Pain* 2008; 8(2): 67–70.

3. Answers: F F T F F

Sickle cell disease is a congenital haemoglobinopathy that is associated with high incidence of perioperative complications. Traditional anaesthetic management, based largely on extrapolation from biochemical models, has emphasized the need to avoid red blood cells sickling and prevent exacerbations of the disease.

Sickle cell disease is characterized by deformed red blood cells, which changes the rheology and blocks capillaries. This results in sickle cell crisis, leading to acute episodic attacks of pain, pulmonary compromise, widespread organ damage, and early death.

The central pathological event has traditionally been assumed to be an increase in sickling or deformation of erythrocytes, as a result of the insolubility of the deoxygenated mutant sickle haemoglobin, haemoglobin S.

The factors that need to be looked at during the perioperative period to prevent sickling include good oxygenation and hydration, but avoiding hypercarbia, pain, and hypothermia. There is no evidence at the moment to advise avoiding tourniquet in patients with the sickle cell gene.

Firth PG. Anaesthesia for peculiar cells—a century of sickle cell disease. *BJA* 2005; 95(3): 287–99.

4. Answers: T T F T T

Recurrent laryngeal nerve (RLN) palsy can be unilateral or bilateral, which present with either respiratory difficulty or stridor. If there is a unilateral palsy or partial cord paralysis, the patient may simply complain of hoarseness of voice or have difficulty in phonation. Because of difficulty with apposition of vocal cords in unilateral RLN palsy, patients are at an increased risk of aspiration. The normal vocal cord will also try to compensate and move to the opposite side.

RLN injury may result from ischaemia, contusion, traction entrapment, or actual transaction. The laryngeal mask airway and fibrescope can be been used to observe the vocal cords during surgery. Increasingly, electrophysiological monitoring of the recurrent laryngeal nerves has been found to be useful, particularly when the identification of the nerve is expected to be difficult.

Malhotra S, Sodhi V. Anaesthesia for thyroid and parathyroid surgery. *Cont Educ Anaesth Crit Care Pain* 2007; 7(2): 55–57.

5. Answers: T F F T T

Anatomy

The coeliac plexus is also known as the solar plexus. It is the largest sympathetic plexus and is the main junction for autonomic nerves supplying the upper abdominal organs (liver, gall bladder, spleen, stomach, pancreas, kidneys, small bowel, and two-thirds of the large bowel).

Sympathetic supply is via the greater splanchnic nerve (T5/6 to T9/10), the lesser splanchnic nerve (T10/11), and the least splanchnic nerve (T11/12).

The upper abdominal organs receive their parasympathetic supply from the left and right vagal trunks, which pass through the coeliac plexus but do not connect there.

Each plexus lies on each side of L1 (aorta lying posteriorly, pancreas anteriorly, and inferior vena cava laterally).

The complications associated with coeliac plexus are:

- severe hypotension may result, even after unilateral block
- bleeding due to aorta or inferior vena cava injury by the needle
- intravascular injection (should be prevented by checking the needle position with radio-opaque dye)
- upper abdominal organ puncture with abscess/cyst formation
- paraplegia from injecting phenol into the arteries that supply the spinal cord (prevented by checking the needle position with radio-opaque dye)
- sexual dysfunction (injected solution spreads to the sympathetic chain bilaterally)
- intramuscular injection into the psoas muscle
- lumbar nerve root irritation (injected solution tracks backwards towards the lumbar plexus).

Menon R, Swanepoel A. Sympathetic blocks. *Contin Educ Anaesth Crit Care Pain* 2010; 10(3): 88–92.

6. Answers: F F F T T

Aortic stenosis is a fixed outlet obstruction to left ventricular ejection. Anatomic obstruction to left ventricular ejection leads to concentric hypertrophy of the left ventricular heart muscle. This reduces the compliance of the left ventricular chamber, making it difficult to fill. Contractility and ejection fraction are usually maintained until late stages. Atrial contraction accounts for up to 40% of ventricular filling.

There is a high risk of myocardial ischemia due to increased oxygen demand and wall tension in the hypertrophied left ventricle. Thirty per cent of patients who have aortic stenosis with normal coronary arteries have angina. The severity of the aortic stenosis is given in Table 4.1 showing the aortic valve area and the left ventricle pressure gradient.

Table 4.1 Severity of Aortic Stenosis

Aortic valve area	LV-aortic gradient
Normal 2.6–3.5 cm^2	Mild 12–25 mmHg
Mild 1.2–1.8 cm^2	Moderate 25–40 mmHg
Moderate 0.8–1.2 cm^2	Significant 40–50 mmHg
Significant 0.6–0.8 cm^2	Critical >50 mmHg
Critical <0.6 cm^2	

Brown J. Aortic stenosis and non-cardiac surgery. *Contin Educ Anaesth Crit Care Pain* 2005; 5(1): 1–4.

Evans R. Cardiac surgery. In: Allman KG, Wilson IH, (eds), *Oxford Handbook of Anaesthesia*, 2nd edn. Oxford University Press, 2006: pp. 332–33.

7. Answers: F F F T T

Severe hypertension is defined as systolic ≥160 mmHg or diastolic ≥110 mmHg. Based on maternal mortality reports, this degree of hypertension is associated with an increased risk of intracerebral haemorrhage if left untreated. Reducing severe levels of hypertension decreases the risk of death.

Drugs that can be safely used include labetalol, nifedipine, and hydralazine. There are different formulations of each of these and they change over time including availability for different routes of administration. The choice should be made based on clinician familiarity and experience with a particular agent. Particular care should be taken to avoid precipitous falls in blood pressure, which may induce maternal or foetal complications as a result of falling below critical perfusion thresholds. Blood pressure should be lowered to levels of SBP 140–150/DBP 90–100 at a rate of 10–20 mmHg every 10–20 min. Consideration should also be given to the extent of placental transfer of the administered drug and the direct effect of the agent and any metabolites.

There is extensive evidence of the safety and efficacy of intravenous hydralazine. This is usually administered by intermittent bolus of 5 mg IV or IM, and repeated as necessary; it has an onset of action time of 10–15 min. Continuous infusion of 0.5–10.0 mg/h is typically employed in more refractory cases. The use of hydralazine is often accompanied by maternal tachycardia. It has been noted, however, that there is an absence of robust trials comparing hydralazine with intravenous labetalol or oral nifedipine. These latter agents may be preferable due to reduced maternal and foetal complications. Labetalol should be avoided in women with severe asthma. Continuous foetal heart-rate monitoring should be employed until the BP is stable. Sodium nitroprusside is rarely used in pregnancy and cannot be recommended for routine use due to known adverse effects of hypotension, paradoxical bradycardia in women with severe pre-eclampsia, and the unknown risk of foetal cyanide toxicity. It should be viewed as a last resort, to be used in situations of life-threatening hypertension immediately prior to delivery and in circumstances where clinicians are very familiar with its use.

Hypertension in Pregnancy. NICE guideline CG107, 2010. http://www.nice.org.uk/cg107.

8. Answers: F T T F F

There is no evidence that either bed rest or additional IV fluids reduce the likelihood of a headache developing following accidental dural puncture. Both the gauge and type of spinal needle tip do affect the risk of headache. Small-gauge spinal needles with a non-traumatic (pencil-point) tip should be used so as to minimize post-dural puncture headache (PDPH) after spinal anaesthesia.

Although PDPH cure rates of 90% were originally reported following epidural blood patch, more recent studies suggest the success rate is much lower (around 50%). The incidence of headache after spinal anaesthesia is related to the needle type and gauge. Rates of PDPH of around 0.5% may be achieved with very fine pencil-point needles, but higher rates can be expected with larger needles.

Synthetic ACTH was first reported to be effective for treating PDPH in the 1990s. Postulated mechanisms include CSF retention through increased mineralocorticoid-mediated sodium reabsorption, and a direct analgesic effect via its glucocorticoid activity. Most reports of its effectiveness stem from case reports and case series, but a randomized controlled trial in 2004 found no effect of a single intramuscular injection of synacthen compared with an intramuscular injection of normal saline.

Sudlow CLM, Warlow C. Posture and fluids for preventing post-dural puncture headache. *Cochrane Database of Systematic Reviews*, 2001. http://www2.cochrane.org/reviews/en/ab001790.html.

Apfel CC. Prevention of postdural puncture headache after accidental dural puncture: a quantitative systematic review. *Br J Anaesth* 2010; 105(3): 255–63.

9. Answers: F F T T T

The MAGPIE study has demonstrated that administration of magnesium sulphate to women with pre-eclampsia reduces the risk of an eclamptic seizure. Women allocated magnesium sulphate had a 58% lower risk of an eclamptic seizure (95% CI 40–71%). The relative risk reduction was similar regardless of the severity of pre-eclampsia. More women need to be treated when pre-eclampsia is not severe (109) to prevent one seizure when compared with severe pre-eclampsia (63). If magnesium sulphate is given, it should be continued for 24 h following delivery or 24 h after the last seizure, whichever is the later, unless there is a clinical reason to continue. When magnesium sulphate is given, regular assessment of the urine output, maternal reflexes, respiratory rate, and oxygen saturation is important. Somnolence, slurred speech, and blurred vision are also features of magnesium toxicity.

Magnesium toxicity is unlikely with these regimens and routine level check is not recommended. Magnesium sulphate is mostly excreted in the urine. Urine output should be closely observed and if it becomes reduced below 20 mL/h the magnesium infusion should be halted. Magnesium toxicity can be assessed by clinical assessment as it causes a loss of deep-tendon reflexes and respiratory depression. If there is loss of deep-tendon reflexes, the magnesium sulphate infusion should be halted. Calcium gluconate 1 g (10 mL) over 10 min can be given if there is concern over respiratory depression.

Hypertension in Pregnancy. NICE guideline CG107, 2010. http://www.nice.org.uk/cg107.

10. Answers: T T F T T

Autonomic hyper-reflexia is now more commonly called *autonomic dysreflexia*. Autonomic dysreflexia (AD) is a syndrome of massive imbalanced reflex sympathetic discharge above the splanchnic sympathetic outflow (T5-T6), occurring in patients with spinal cord injury (SCI). Anthony Bowlby first recognized this syndrome in 1890 when he described profuse sweating and erythematous rash of the head and neck initiated by bladder catheterization in an 18-year-old patient with SCI. Guttmann and Whitteridge completed a full description of the syndrome in 1947. This condition represents a medical emergency, so recognizing and treating the earliest signs and symptoms efficiently can avoid dangerous sequelae of elevated blood pressure.

Hambly PR, Martin B. Anaesthesia for chronic spinal cord lesions. *Anaesthesia* 1998; 53(3): 273–89.

11. Answers: F F T T T

Venous thromboembolism (VTE), comprising deep vein thrombosis (DVT) and pulmonary embolism (PE), has an annual incidence in Europe of 60–70 per 1 000 000 inhabitants. Half of these occur in hospitalized patients or those in care homes, and 25% in people with no recognized risk factors. The risk in the postoperative population is higher still, with the incidence of subclinical DVT after total knee arthroplasty or hip fracture surgery between 40% and 60%, and an incidence of PE in the same group of 4–10%. In the UK, patients with a PE who receive treatment have 14- and 90-day mortality rates of approximately 10% and 20%, respectively. The House of Commons Health Committee reported in 2005 that an estimated 25,000 people in the UK die from preventable hospital-acquired VTE every year. It is our duty to do what we can to reduce the incidence of VTE by both understanding the mechanism of formation and ensuring correct prophylaxis is received.

Thrombogenesis is a normal mechanism by which the body maintains haemostasis is response to injury. Venous thromboembolism, however, is the abnormal development and propagation of a clot. The thrombus itself can cause local problems relating to mechanical obstruction to blood flow. In this situation, fragments of the thrombus can break off and cause further harm by similar means. The formation of a thrombus and its subsequent embolization was first described by Rudolph Virchow in 1856. He subsequently described the eponymously named Virchow's triad. In an environment where one or more of the following conditions are met, there is a risk of thrombogenesis, venous stasis, damage or dysfunction of the endothelium, and hypercoagulability.

The British Thoracic Society has published guidelines for the identification and management of patients at risk of venous thromboembolism. They have identified a significant number of risk factors of which malignancy, bone fracture, major abdominal or pelvic surgery, hip or knee replacement, pregnancy, puerperium, caesarean section, post-operative intensive care, varisose veins, previous VTE, and age >60 years constitute the major risk factors. NICE have incorporated these into their VTE guidelines.

Ross N. Venous thromboprophylaxis Part I and II. *Anaesthesia Tutorial of the Week*, May 2011. http://www.aagbi.org/sites/default/files/244%20Thromboprophylaxis%20part%202[2].pdf.

12. Answers: F T F T T

Diastolic heart failure is an underestimated pathology, with a high risk of acute decompensation during the perioperative period. Diastolic heart failure involves heart failure with preserved left ventricular (LV) systolic function, but LV diastolic dysfunction. This may account for acute heart failure and is associated with hypertensive crisis, sepsis, and myocardial ischaemia. Symptomatic treatment focuses on the reducing pulmonary congestion and the improving LV filling.

There is no specific treatment, but encouraging data is emerging on the use of renin–angiotensin–aldosterone axis blockers, nitric oxide donors, and new agents specifically targeting actin–myosin cross-bridges.

Pirracchio R, Cholley B, De Hert S, Solal AC, Mebazaa A. Diastolic heart failure in anaesthesia and critical care. *Br J Anaesth* 2007; 98(6): 707–21.

13. Answers: T T T F T

Most types of normal haemoglobin, including haemoglobin A, haemoglobin A2, and haemoglobin F, are tetramers composed of four protein subunits and four heme prosthetic groups. Whereas adult haemoglobin is composed of two α and two β subunits, foetal haemoglobin is composed of two α and two γ subunits, commonly denoted $\alpha_2\gamma_2$. Because of its presence in foetal haemoglobin, the γ subunit is commonly called the foetal haemoglobin subunit.

Foetal haemoglobin (HbF) consists of two α and two γ chains. Lower 2,3-DPG (diphosphoglycerate) levels result in a leftward shift of the oxyhaemoglobin dissociation curve, which results in a decreased PO_2 and favours O_2 transfer from mother to foetus. HbF forms 80% of circulating Hb at birth and is replaced by HbA within 3–5 months. It may persist in haemoglobinopathies.

At birth, red cells contain 70–90% HbF until about 2–4 months of age. β-chain production begins just after birth and γ-chain production begins to decline, resulting in an adult profile by age 4 months.

Foetal haemoglobin (also haemoglobin F) is the main oxygen transport protein in the foetus during the last 7 months of development in the uterus and in the newborn until roughly 6 months old. Functionally, foetal haemoglobin differs most from adult haemoglobin in that it is able to bind oxygen with greater affinity than the adult form, giving the developing foetus better access to oxygen from the mother's bloodstream.

Murphy PJ. The fetal circulation. *Contin Educ Anaesth Crit Care Pain* 2005; 5(4): 107–12.

14. Answers: T F F F T

Phaeochromocytoma is a catecholamine-secreting tumour of chromaffin cells. Most commonly it occurs within the adrenal gland, but 10% of tumours occur at other ganglia of the sympathetic chain, 10% are bilateral, 10% malignant, and 10% familial. A minority are associated with multiple endocrine neoplasia (MEN I or II), neurofibromatosis type I, or von Hippel–Lindau syndrome. They can secrete noradrenaline, adrenaline, and dopamine.

Classically phaeochromocytomas present with episodic severe hypertension, headaches, drenching sweats, palpitations, anxiety, tremor, and chest pain. Sustained hypertension with other symptoms may be a more common presentation, and may occur in as many as 85% of presenting cases. Hyperglycaemia may occur due to increased glycogenolysis and impaired insulin secretion. Diagnosis is usually made via urinary VMA levels and plasma catecholamines, with later MRI to localize the tumour and MIBG (meta-iodobenzyl guanidine) scan to assess the functionality.

Pace N, Buttigieg M. Phaeochromocytoma. *Cont Educ Anaesth Crit Care Pain* 2003; 3(1): 20–23.

15. Answers: F F F F F

The loss of heat is caused by:
- radiation (60% of total heat loss)
  - increases as fourth power of temperature difference between body and surroundings
  - reduced by forced air warming and maintaining a warm theatre environment
  - reducing the theatre temperature will increase the heat loss
  - the foil blanket reduces heat lost via radiation
- convection (25% of total heat loss)
  - reduced by preventing passive air movements around patient, e.g. blanketing, forced air warming
- respiration (10% of total heat loss)
  - due to warming and humidification (latent heat of evaporation of water lost)
  - reduced by use of heat and moisture exchange filter
- conduction (1–2% total losses)
  - reduced by warming mattress, forced air warming (forms insulating layer of air)
- evaporation (normally small contribution, may be significant is patient wet)

- thermodilution
  - due to infusion of cold fluid
  - prevented by fluid warming.

Gormley SMC, Crean PM. Basic principles of anaesthesia for neonates and infants. *BJA CEPD Rev* 2001; 1(5): 130–33.

16. Answers: T T F T T

The femoral nerve, the largest branch of the lumbar plexus, arises from the dorsal divisions of the ventral rami of the second, third, and fourth lumbar nerves. It descends through the fibres of the psoas major muscle, emerging from the muscle at the lower part of its lateral border, and passes down between it and the iliacus muscle, behind the iliac fascia; it then runs beneath the inguinal ligament, into the thigh, and splits into an anterior and a posterior division. Under the inguinal ligament, it is separated from the femoral artery by a portion of the psoas major.

Femoral nerve blocks are commonly used for hip and knee surgery, and a thorough working knowledge of the regional anatomy is considered core for all anaesthetists. Femoral nerve block alone can be used for femoral shaft fractures, osteotomies, and superficial skin-grafting procedures.

Al-Haddad MF, Coventry DM. Major nerve blocks of the lower limb. *Contin Educ Anaesth Crit Care Pain* 2003; 3(4): 102–105.

17. Answers: F F T F T

Body fat increases in middle years but declines in extreme old age. There are gender differences as well.

Total body water decreases and there is significant intracellular fluid which decreases. Glucocortoid secretion remains at similar levels to young people. The response to stress differs slightly but the clinical significance is questioned.

Hornick T. Effects of advanced age on body composition and metabolism. In: Fleisher LA, Prough DS, (eds). *Management of the Elderly Surgical Patient*. Lippincott-Raven, 1997; pp. 461–70.

18. Answers: T T T T T

As people age, there are significant changes in their cardiovascular physiology. Essentially these manifest as globally reduced physiological reserve and subsequent, more rapid deterioration in the event of physiological derangement.

Ventricular wall thickness increases, and myocardial fibrosis and valvular fibro-calcification occur. Ventricular elasticity is reduced and diastolic filling is slower. This is partly due to increased systolic pressure and partly due to a lesser rise in diastolic pressure. Both are due to age-related changes in the vascular tree. Baroreflex responses to blood-pressure changes are retained but less able to respond to extremes.

Murray D, Dodds C. Perioperative care of the elderly. *Br J Anaesth/CEPD Rev* 2004; 4(6): 193–196.

Rooke G, Robinson B. Cardiovascular and autonomic nervous system ageing. In: Fleisher LA, Prough DS, (eds), *Management of the Elderly Surgical Patient*, Lippincott-Raven, 1997: pp. 482–97.

19. Answers: T F T F T

Lung function

As people age, there are significant changes in their respiratory physiology. Essentially this manifest as globally reduced physiological reserve and subsequent, more rapid deterioration in the event of physiological derangement.

Total compliance is little altered because chest wall compliance decreases as lung compliance increases. The elderly have a marked reduction in the ventilatory response to both hypoxia and hypercarbia. This has clinical relevance, especially in the recovery room.

Muravchick S. Anesthesia for the elderly. In: Miller RD (ed.), *Anesthesia*, 5th edn. Churchill Livingstone, 2000: pp. 2149–50.

20. Answers: F T T T

Salbutamol is a β-adrenergic agonist mainly used a bronchodilator. It is relatively selective for β2 receptors, but has some β1 action as well, and the latter is mainly responsible for its principal side effect of tachycardia. There is some evidence that it reduces release of histamine and other inflammatory mediators from mast cells.

It is given mainly by the inhalational route although IV is more effective in severe bronchospasm (250–500 mcg slow infusion over 30–60 min). The oral route is ineffective due to extensive first-pass metabolism.

It is also used for tocolysis and for chronic heart failure states where there is upregulation of β2 receptors.

British National Formulary, 61st edn. British Medical Association and Royal Pharmaceutical Society of Great Britain, 2011: Section 3.1.1.1.

Yentis SM, Hirsch NP, Smith GB. *A–Z of Anaesthesia and Intensive Care*, 3rd edn. Butterworth Heinemann, 2004: p. 461.

21. Answers: F T F T T

Pharmacokinetics is altered in the elderly due to reduced hepatic and renal blood flow and a reduction in total body water. There is decreased lean body mass as well as reduced plasma proteins, which results in reduced protein binding of drugs and metabolites, thereby increasing free drug levels and possible toxic effects. Absorption is minimally affected because most drugs are absorbed from the small intestine by passive non-ionic diffusion.

Pharmacodynamics may also be altered, with increased sensitivity to many agents, especially CNS depressants. Minimum alveolar concentration (MAC) decreases steadily with age by 4–5% per decade after 40 years. For example, the MAC of isoflurane is approximately 0.92 at 80 years of age.

Dodds C, Murray D. Preoperative assessment of the elderly. *BJA CEPD Rev* 2001; 1(6): 181–84.

22. Answers: F T T F F

The diagnosis and confirmation of death is required in a number of different situations, both as a result of a natural process and also in situations where artificial interventions are sustaining cardiorespiratory function in the absence of a patient's ability to breathe independently. Death entails the irreversible loss of those essential characteristics that are necessary to the existence of a living human person and, thus, the definition of death should be regarded as the irreversible loss of the capacity for consciousness, combined with irreversible loss of the capacity to breathe.

When considering the criteria for brain-stem testing, the most important factor is the establishment of an unequivocal cause for the individual's unconsciousness. It is recognized that circulatory, metabolic, and endocrine disturbances (e.g. hypernatraemia, diabetes insipidus) are likely accompaniments of death as a result of cessation of brain-stem function. It is important to emphasize that these may be the effect rather than the cause of cessation of brain-stem function and do not preclude the diagnosis of death by neurological testing of brain-stem reflexes.

The diagnosis of death by brain-stem testing should be made by at least two medical practitioners who have been registered for more than 5 years and are competent in the conduct and interpretation of brain-stem testing. At least one of the doctors must be a consultant.

Testing should be undertaken by the nominated doctors acting together and must always be performed on two occasions. A complete set of tests should be performed on each occasion. If the first set of tests shows no evidence of brain-stem function there need not be a lengthy delay prior to performing the second set. Although death is not confirmed until the second test has been completed the legal time of death is when the first test indicates death due to the absence of brain-stem reflexes.

A Code of Practice for the Diagnosis and Confirmation of Death. Academy of Medical Royal Colleges, 2008. http://www.ics.ac.uk/intensive_care_professional/code_of_practice_08.

23. Answers: F F T T T

Serotonin is an endogenous monoamine neurotransmitter involved in vascular reactivity, bronchomotor tone, platelet aggregation, pain modulation, and nausea and vomiting. It is synthesized in enterochromaffin cells, serotonergic neurones in the central nervous system, and in platelets. It is unclear exactly where and how serotonin exerts its effect. It has multiple actions, and this is reflected in the wide variety of clinical uses for serotonin-related drugs.

Chinniah S, French JLH, Levy DM. Serotonin and anaesthesia. *Contin Educ Anaesth Crit Care Pain* 2008; 8(2): 43–45.

24. Answers: F T F T F

The seven base SI units are: the metre, second, kilogram, ampere, Kelvin, candela and mole.

Derived units include the newton, pascal, joule, watt and hertz.

Al-Shaikh B, Stacey S. *Essentials of Anaesthetic Equipment,* 3rd edn. Churchill Livingstone, 2007.

25. Answers: T T F T F

Benzatropine is an anti-muscarinic agent used in acute treatment of drug-induced dystonic reactions (except tardive dyskinesia). It is mainly used for drug-induced Parkinsonism. It is used IV/IM in a dose of 1–2 mg, repeated as needed, but can be given orally as well in a dose of 1–4 mg. Side effects are dry mouth, blurred vision, urinary retention, and sedation.

O'Donnell A. Drug formulary. In: Allman KG, Wilson IH, (eds), *Oxford Handbook of Anaesthesia,* 2nd edn. Oxford University Press, 2006: p. 1110.

Yentis SM, Hirsch NP, Smith GB. *A–Z of Anaesthesia and Intensive Care,* 3rd edn. Butterworth Heinemann, 2004: p. 59.

26. Answers: T F T T F

Enoximone is an imidazole derivative, which is a selective phosphodiesterase III (PDE III) inhibitor. There is therefore increased cGMP, leading to an increase in NO and smooth muscle relaxation. Milrinone is a bipyridine derivative. It is absorbed from the gut. Enoximone undergoes substantial first-pass metabolism. It is metabolized to a sulfoxide compound, an active metabolite, which is then excreted via the kidneys. All PDEs can cause hypotension as they are potent arterial, coronary, and venodilators. They improve myocardial function and this occurs without increasing myocardial oxygen extraction due to improved coronary artery perfusion. Enoximone may cause abnormal heartbeats or (less commonly) low blood pressure, headache, insomnia, nausea, vomiting, and diarrhoea.

Aitkenhead A, Rowbotham D, Smith G. *Textbook of Anaesthesia,* 4th edn. Churchill Livingstone: p. 77.

Robinson S, Zincuk A, Strøm T, Larsen TB, Rasmussen B, Toft P. Enoxaparin, effective dosage for intensive care patients: double-blinded, randomised clinical trial. *Crit Care* 2010; 14(2): R41.

27. Answers: **T F T T F**

Pharyngeal pouches occur most commonly in elderly patients (over 70 years), and typical symptoms include dysphagia, regurgitation, chronic cough, aspiration, and weight loss.

The aetiology remains unknown, but theories centre upon a structural or physiological abnormality of the cricopharyngeus.

A diagnosis is easily established using barium studies.

These patients should be treated as full stomach and cricoid pressure should be applied.

Treatment is surgical, via an endoscopic or external cervical approach, and should include a cricopharyngeal myotomy. Unfortunately pharyngeal pouch surgery has long been associated with significant morbidity, partly due to the surgery itself and also to the fact that the majority of patients are elderly and often have general medical problems.

External approaches are associated with higher complication rates than endoscopic procedures. Recently, treatment by endoscopic stapling diverticulotomy has becoming increasingly popular, as it has distinct advantages, although long-term results are not yet available.

Siddiq MA, Sood S. Current management in pharyngeal pouch surgery by UK otorhinolaryngologists. *Ann R Coll Surg Engl* 2004; 86(4): 247–52.

28. Answers: **T F T F F**

Maxillary nerve block

The maxillary nerve block provides good local anaesthesia in order to perform operative treatment in the upper oral cavity. There are three basic techniques with the maxillary nerve block. The greater palatine canal approach is the technique used most frequently, and with greatest success.

The pterygopalitine, or greater palatine foramen, is located adjacent to the second molar on the hard palate. The branches are divided into four groups, depending upon where they branch off: in the cranium, in the pterygopalatine fossa, in the infraorbital canal, or on the face.

In the cranium:

* middle meningeal nerve in the meninges.

From the pterygopalatine fossa:

* infraorbital nerve through infraorbital canal
* zygomatic nerve (zygomaticotemporal nerve, zygomaticofacial nerve) through inferior orbital fissure
* nasal branches (nasopalatine) through sphenopalatine foramen
* superior alveolar nerves (posterior superior alveolar nerve, middle superior alveolar nerve)
* palatine nerves (greater palatine nerve, lesser palatine nerve)
* pharyngeal nerve.

In the infraorbital fissure:

* anterior superior alveolar nerve
* infraorbital nerve.

On the face:

* inferior palpebral nerve
* superior labial nerve.

Amsterdam JT, Kilgore KP. Regional anesthesia of the head and neck. In: Roberts JR, Hedges JR, (eds), *Clinical Procedures in Emergency Medicine*, 4th edn. WB Saunders, 2004: pp. 552–66.

29. Answers: **T T T F T**

Soda-lime is used in breathing systems to absorb expired CO_2 during anaesthesia. It can be incorporated in a Mapleson C system or a circle system. CO_2 in solution reacts with sodium hydroxide to form the respective carbonates, which then react with calcium hydroxide to produce calcium carbonate, replenishing sodium hydroxide. Heat and water are produced during the reaction. Exhaustion of its activity is indicated by dyes; the most common one changes from pink to white. The size of the soda-lime granules is 4–8 mesh (i.e. will pass through a mesh of 4–8 strands per inch in each axis—about 2.36–4.75 mm).

The reaction is explained as four stages:

1. $H_2O + CO_2 \rightarrow H_2CO_3$

     high pH

2. $H_2CO_3 + 2NaOH \rightarrow Na_2CO_3 + 2H_2O$

     high pH

3. $Na_2CO_3 + Ca(OH)_2 \rightarrow CaCO_3 + 2NaOH$

     high pH

also

4. $H_2CO_3 + Ca(OH)_2 \rightarrow CaCO_3 + 2H_2O$

     high pH

Nunn G. Low-flow anaesthesia. *Contin Educ Anaesth Crit Care Pain* 2008; 8(1): 1–4.

30. Answers: **F F T T F**

Causes, incidence, and risk factors for thrombocytopenia are often divided into three major causes of low platelets:

1. low production of platelets in the bone marrow
2. increased breakdown of platelets in the bloodstream (called intravascular)
3. increased breakdown of platelets in the spleen or liver (called extravascular).

Disorders that involve low production in the bone marrow include:

- aplastic anemia
- cancer in the bone marrow
- cirrhosis (chronic liver disease)
- folate deficiency
- infections in the bone marrow (very rare)
- myelodysplasia
- vitamin B12 deficiency.

Use of certain drugs may also lead to a low production of platelets in the bone marrow. The most common example is chemotherapy treatment.

Disorders that involve the breakdown of platelets include:

- disseminated intravascular coagulation (DIC)
- drug-induced non-immune thrombocytopenia
- drug-induced immune thrombocytopenia
- hypersplenism
- immune thrombocytopenic purpura (ITP)
- thrombotic thrombocytopenic purpura.

Symptoms include:

- bruising
- nosebleeds or bleeding in the mouth and gums
- rash (pinpoint red spots called petechiae).

Other symptoms may be present as well, depending on the cause of the condition. Mild thrombocytopenia can occur without symptoms.

McMillan R. Hemorrhagic disorders: abnormalities of platelet and vascular function. In: Goldman L, Ausiello D, (eds), *Cecil Medicine*, 23rd edn. Saunders Elsevier, 2007: Chapter 179.

31. Answers: T F T F F

Carcinoid syndrome is caused by tumours originating in the endocrine argentaffin cells of the small bowel mucosa. These tumours secrete, variably, peptides, kinins, prostaglandins, and serotonin, resulting in flushing, hypotension, diarrhoea, and occasionally bronchospasm.

Ondansetron provides symptomatic relief (especially from diarrhoea) for patients with carcinoid syndrome. Surgical management may involve resection or debulking of primary or metastatic carcinoid tumours. The key anaesthetic consideration is prevention of mediator release. Octreotide, a synthetic analogue of somatostatin, is used before operation to counteract serotonin and kinin activity. 50–200 mcg is given by SC injection, 8-hourly. Small intravenous doses can be used to treat sudden bronchospasm or hypotension on handling of the tumour. A response is usually seen within 5 min.

Chinniah S, French JLH, Levy DM. Serotonin and anaesthesia. *Contin Educ Anaesth Crit Care Pain* 2008; 8(2): 43–45.

32. Answers: F T F T T

The thoracic duct drains all the lymph from the lower limbs, abdominal and pelvic cavities, left thorax, left head and neck, and left upper limb; it passes through the aortic opening in the diaphragm and drains the cisterna chyli. The medial breast drains into internal mammary nodes via intercostal spaces, while the lateral quadrants drain into anterior axillary nodes. The heart contains extensive networks of lymph vessels throughout the epicardium, myocardium, and endocardium.

Neas JF. The lymphatic system. In: Martini FH, Timmons MJ, Tallitsch B, (eds), *Human Anatomy*, 4th edn. Pearson Education/Benjamin Cummings, 2003: p. 613.

33. Answers: F F T F T

Over 3 million blood components are issued in the UK each year. Since 2005, reporting of all serious adverse reactions attributable to the safety or quality of blood is required by European Union Directive. In the United Kingdom this is not yet mandatory. The serious hazard of transfusion (SHOT) scheme collates the adverse events information in the United Kingdom.

Complications can be broadly divided into immune-related, iatrogenic, and infective causes. Although the immune-related form the largest proportion of complications seen in clinical practice, it is the iatrogenic errors that comprise 75% of the SHOT voluntary reports. Pathophysiology of the complication predicts the timescale for the development of symptoms. For example, the ABO incompatibility reaction is precipitated by an antigen–antibody complex, causing complement fixation, intravascular haemolysis, and destruction of the transfused blood. This immune-mediated reaction occurs within seconds to minutes of the blood-product transfusion.

Citrate is added to blood products to prolong storage time and is found in higher concentrations in FFP and platelet preparations than in packed red blood cells. Storage conditions are specific to individual blood products. Packed red cells are stored and issued at 4°C, whereas platelets are frozen and are warmed prior to issue.

Maxwell MJ, Wilson MJA. Complications of blood transfusion. *Contin Educ Anaesth Crit Care Pain* 2006; 6(6): 225–29.

34. Answers: F T T F F

Cushing's syndrome is due to excess plasma cortisol caused by iatrogenic steroid administration (most common), pituitary adenoma (Cushing's disease—80% of remainder), ectopic ACTH (15% of remainder—e.g. oat cell carcinoma of lung), adrenal adenoma (4% of remainder), or adrenal carcinoma (rare).

Clinical features of Cushing's syndrome include:

- moon face, central (truncal) obesity, proximal myopathy, and osteoporosis
- easy bruising and fragile skin, impaired glucose tolerance, diabetes
- hypertension, LVH, sleep apnoea
- high Na^+, HCO^-_3, and glucose; low K^+ and Ca^{2+}
- gastrointestinal reflux
- 60% of patients have diabetes or impaired glucose tolerance, and a sliding scale should be started before major surgery if glucose is >10 mmol/L.

Criteria for diagnosis include:

- high plasma cortisol and loss of diurnal variation (normal range 165–680 nmol/L; trough level at 24:00 hours, peak level at 06:00 hours).
- increased urinary 17-(OH) steroids
- loss of suppression with dexamethasone 2 mg
- ACTH level:
  - ◆ normal/high—pituitary
  - ◆ low—adrenal, ectopic cortisol administration
  - ◆ very high—ectopic ACTH.

Blanshard H. Endocrine and metabolic disease. In: Allman KG, Wilson IH, (eds), *Oxford Handbook of Anaesthesia*, 2nd edn. Oxford University Press, 2006: p. 168.

Yentis SM, Hirsch NP, Smith GB. *A–Z of Anaesthesia and Intensive Care*, Butterworth Heinemann, 2004: p. 146.

35. Answers: F T T T T

Acute kidney injury (AKI), formerly known as acute renal failure, is a prevalent and serious problem amongst hospitalized patients. Although no definitive studies have been undertaken in the UK, the prevalence amongst hospitalized patients in the USA is 4.9%. Associated mortality rates have been wide ranging. Clinically, AKI should be easily recognized by the onset of oliguria, anuria, and/or deteriorating biochemistry. However, if unrecognized and allowed to deteriorate, AKI will result in uraemia, acidosis, hyperkalaemia, and ultimately death. Strategies to reduce the risk of AKI are well known; they include identifying relevant risk factors, appropriate monitoring of blood biochemistry, rapid remedial action when AKI occurs, and appropriate referral of patients to specialist services. However, it is not known if these strategies are being implemented and many factors around patients with AKI, both amongst those admitted to and already within UK hospitals, remain unclear.

Despite the seriousness of this condition and its potential for treatment if detected early, it lacks a standard definition, and historically its treatment has been a matter of debate amongst clinicians. Recently, attempts have been made to classify AKI using a set of functional criteria that give perspective on the degree of injury. To this end the RIFLE classification (risk, injury, failure, loss of kidney function, end-stage kidney disease) was devised and then further refined by the Acute Kidney Injury Network.

All hospital patients, regardless of specialty, are at risk of AKI either through their presenting illness or subsequent iatrogenic injury. However, it is unknown whether potential deficiencies in the care of patients with AKI are predominantly due to clinical failure (risk assessment, recognition, and management) or whether organizational issues such as a lack of availability of expert advice and intensive support are equally culpable. In addition, there exist treatments for AKI that are the result of historical dogma rather than evidence-based therapeutics (e.g. diuretics/dopamine) and it is unclear to what extent these are still practiced.

Adding Insult to Injury – a Review of the Care of Patients who Died in Hospital with a Primary Diagnosis of Acute Kidney Injury (Acute Renal Failure). NCEPOD, June 2009. http://www.ncepod.org.uk/2009report1/Downloads/AKI_summary.pdf.

36. Answers: T F T T T

Ondansetron is a $5HT_3$ antagonist that is routinely used for antiemesis. The common side effects are constipation, headache, flushing, and injection-site reactions. Less commonly seen are hiccups, hypotension, bradycardia, chest pain, arrhythmias, movement disorders, and seizures. Rarely seen are dizziness and transient visual disturbances. Transient blindness is very rare.

British National Formulary, 61st edn. British Medical Association and Royal Pharmaceutical Society of Great Britain, 2011: Section 4.6.

37. Answers: T T T F T

Statins are one of the lipid-lowering agents, whose action is exerted by selective inhibition of HMGCoA-reductase, which is the rate-limiting enzyme in cholesterol biosynthesis. This leads to increased low-density lipoprotein (LDL) receptor expression, which increases LDL clearance and reduces levels in a dose-dependent manner. Studies have shown that lipid reduction with statin therapy in high-risk patients is beneficial regardless of baseline LDL levels. Severe myopathy and rhabdomyolysis have been reported associated with statin therapy, particularly in combination treatment with drugs interfering with the cytochrome p450 (3A4) metabolism of statins, but creatine kinase levels need not be monitored routinely.

Lipid modification (Cardiovascular risk assessment and the modification of blood lipids for the primary and secondary prevention of cardiovascular disease). NICE Clinical Guideline, May 2008.

British National Formulary, 61st edn. British Medical Association and Royal Pharmaceutical Society of Great Britain, 2011: Section 2.12.

38. Answers: F T T T T

The physics of hyperbaric oxygen therapy (HBOT) for treatment of gas emboli is based upon Boyle's law, where *PV* is a constant and hence as pressure (*P*) increases, volume (*V*) decreases if temperature remains constant.

Based on Henry's law, HBOT increases the dissolved oxygen content of blood, as haemoglobin will be fully saturated.

HBOT leads to vasoconstriction and thus an increase in afterload; it can also lead to a reduction in stroke volume and heart rate, leading to a fall in cardiac output.

Untreated pneumothoraces are an absolute contraindication to HBOT. This is because of the risk of driving gas emboli into the vascular system, causing a tension pneumothorax or pneumomediastinum.

COPD patients and pacemakers are a relative contraindication.

Pitkin AD, Davies JH. Hyperbaric oxygen therapy. *BJA CEPD Rev* 2001; 1(5): 150–56.

39. Answers: T T T T F

Renal replacement therapy can be provided with haemodialysis (HD), haemofiltration (HF), a combination of these, and peritoneal dialysis. The aim of the treatment is:

- clearance of solute and water
- correction of electrolyte and acid–base disturbances and
- removal of toxins.

Diffusion is the process of passive movement of substances along a concentration gradient and occurs across a semi-permeable membrane. The rate of diffusion is proportional to the concentration gradient that drives the process.

Haemofiltration depends on the principle of convective transport, where a solute is swept through a membrane by an ultrafiltrate (solvent drag). This is independent of solute concentrations and it is the membrane characteristics that determine solute removal and also transmembrane pressure, which serves to effectively push or pull a solute into the ultra filtrate. Solute removal occurs more quickly in HD, which can be intermittent, whereas HF is a continuous form of renal replacement.

Hall NA, Fox AJ. Renal replacement therapies in critical care. *Contin Educ Anaesth Crit Care Pain* 2006; 6: 197–202.

40. Answers: F F F T T

Botulism is a rare and lethal disease caused by the exotoxins of the Gram-positive anaerobe *Clostridium botulinum*, typically found in soil and dust. Toxins are classed from A to E. A, B, or E account for almost all human cases.

It can be transmitted in the following ways:

- food-borne (most common, especially with canned foods)
- by growth of the bacterium and production of toxin in traumatic wounds
- intestinal colonization (seen in infants)
- deliberate (bioterrorism)
- accidental (through therapeutic use).

The toxin binds irreversibly to the presynaptic membrane of cholinergic neurons. Symptoms include gastrointestinal disturbance, sore throat, fatigue, dizziness, paraesthesiae, cranial involvement. and a progressive descending flaccid weakness; parasympathetic symptoms are common.

Wenham T, Cohen A. Botulism. *Contin Educ Anaesth Crit Care Pain* 2008; 8(1): 21–25.

41. Answers: T T T T T

Cardiac muscle contains a contractile complex with contractile proteins (actin and myosin) and regulatory proteins (troponin and tropomyosin). Troponin complex consists of three single-chain polypeptides: troponin T, I, and C.

Cardiac troponins (cTn) have been recommended as the biomarker of choice in the diagnosis of myocardial infarction by the Joint European Society of Cardiology and the American College of Cardiology Committee. There are a variety of causes for a raised cTn in the absence of coronary artery disease:

- ischemia due to increased demand (mismatch between myocardial oxygen demand and supply, in the absence of flow-limiting coronary artery stenosis)
  - ◆ sepsis/systemic inflammatory response syndrome
  - ◆ hypotension
  - ◆ hypovolaemia
  - ◆ tachyarrhythmias

- ◆ left ventricular hypertrophy
- ◆ myocardial ischaemia
- ◆ Prinzmetal's angina (vasospasm)
- ◆ cerebrovascular accident (CVA), intracranial haemorrhage (over-activity of the autonomic nervous system)
- • direct injury to myocardial cell
  - ◆ trauma, myocarditis, pericarditis, toxins
- • myocardial conditions
  - ◆ congestive heart failure, pulmonary embolism, extreme exercise
- • chronic renal insufficiency
  - ◆ end-stage renal failure.

Wolfe Barry JA, Barth JH, Howell SJ. Cardiac troponins: their use and relevance in anaesthesia and critical care medicine. *Contin Educ Anaesth Crit Care Pain* 2008; 8: 62–6.

42. Answers: T F F T T

Carotid endarterectomy surgery is commonly performed under cervical plexus block. This offers advantages over general anaesthesia in terms of monitoring neurological function during cross-clamping of the carotid artery since, in conscious patients, speech, cerebration, and motor power provide early measures of inadequate cerebral perfusion. Some studies suggest lower shunting requirements, lower cardiovascular morbidity, and shorter hospital stay.

The common methods of cervical plexus block are termed 'deep' or 'superficial'. The deep block, as described by Moore or Winnie and colleagues, consists of identifying the transverse processes of upper cervical vertebrae C2–C4 and injecting local anaesthetic directly into the deep (prevertebral) cervical space. This may be achieved either as three separate injections or as a single injection. The superficial block incorporates a variety of procedures. The simplest is an SC infiltration of local anaesthetic along the posterior border of sternocleidomastoid muscle by either the surgeon or the anaesthetist. It is also possible to use a 'combined block', consisting of a deep injection and a superficial or intermediate injection.

The first sign of the blockade is the decreased sensation in the area of the distribution of the respective components of the cervical plexus. Horner's syndrome is caused by interruption of the sympathetic innervation to the head; it may be due to lesions along the pathway, intentional cervical sympathectomy, or inadvertent sympathetic blockade. It consists of partial ptosis, meiosis, apparent enophthalmos, lack of sweating (anhydrosis). and nasal stuffiness on the ipsilateral side.

Pandit JJ Satya-Krishna R, Gration P. Superficial or deep cervical plexus block for carotid endarterectomy: a systematic review of complications. *Br J Anaesth* 2007; 99(2): 159–69.

43. Answers: T T T F T

Down's syndrome is characterized by

- • extra chromosome 21 due to non-dysjunction of chromosomes during germ-cell formation—the most common congenital anomaly with incidence of 1.6 per 1000 births
- • recurrent respiratory tract infections due to relative immune deficiency and a degree of upper airway obstruction—tonsillar and adenoid hypertrophy
- • excessive secretions (common)
- • increased tendency for subluxation/dislocation due to bony abnormality and laxity of transverse atlantal ligament (up to 30%)
- • micrognathia
- • relatively large tongue/short broad neck/crowding of midfacial structures.

Allt JE, Howell CJ. Down's syndrome. *BJA CEPD Rev* 2003; 3(3): 83–86.

44. Answers: T T T F F

Diagnosis of diabetes mellitus requires random blood glucose greater than 11.1 mmol/L and or fasting blood glucose greater than 7.0 mmol/L on two occasions. The prevalence of diabetes mellitus in the UK is 3% (1.8 million sufferers). About 1% of the population live with undiagnosed type 2 diabetes. The risk of type 2 diabetes mellitus increases tenfold in patients with BMI greater than 30. Tight glycaemic control in diabetics decreases microvascular complication rate but does not affect incidence of macrovascular complications or the mortality rate.

Robertshaw HJ, Hall GM. Diabetes mellitus: anaesthetic management. *Anaesthesia* 2006; 61: 1187–90.

45. Answers: F F T T T

The clinical features of advanced liver disease include:

- clotting factors are reduced
- thrombocytopaenia is common, with defective platelet function bleeding more likely to be secondary to thrombocytopenia than due to clotting factor deficiency
- liver contains major stores of glycogen, which is precursor for glucose
- fibrotic changes in liver
- build up of toxic products, especially ammonia
- precipitated by sedatives, high protein diet, GI bleed, infection, surgery, trauma, hypokalemia, and constipation.

Park GR, Kang Y (eds). *Anesthesia and Intensive Care for Patients with Liver Disease.* Butterworth Heinemann, 1995.

46. Answers: T F F T F

The National Institute for Health and Clinical Excellence recommends that electroconvulsive therapy (ECT) is used to achieve short-term improvement of severe symptoms in individuals with severe depressive illness, catatonia, or a prolonged/severe manic episode, after an adequate trial of other treatment options or when the condition is potentially life-threatening.

ECT consists of a pulsatile square wave, which discharges at 35 J to one or both cerebral hemispheres. Following a brief tonic–clonic convulsion there is a short lived parasympathetic phase, which consists of vagal stimulation, which may in turn result in asystole. This is followed by a longer sympathetic phase, consisting of increased heart rate, blood pressure, and myocardial and cerebral oxygen consumption.

Uppal V, Dourish J, Macfarlane A. Anaesthesia for electroconvulsive therapy. *Contin Educ Anaesth Crit Care Pain* 2010; 10(6): 192–96.

Guidance for Electro-convulsive Therapy (ECT) Provided in Remote Sites. The Royal College of Anaesthetists, 2003. http://www.rcoa.ac.uk/docs/ECT-remote.pdf.

The Clinical Effectiveness and Cost Effectiveness of Electroconvulsive Therapy (ECT) for Depressive Illness, Schizophrenia, Catatonia and Mania. Appraisal TA59. NICE, London, 2003. http://www.nice.org.uk/TA059.

47. Answers: T F T F T

Tourniquets provide a bloodless surgical field, but can cause significant morbidity through tissue ischaemia distal to application and direct pressure injuries to underlying structures. Upon inflation, there is a progressive rise in PCO_2 and fall in PO_2 within muscle cells, with a decline in ATP and creatine phosphate stores. These are exhausted after 2 and 3 h, respectively.

The serum lactate rises (by 2 mmol/L) following deflation due to reperfusion of the ischaemic limb and serum potassium levels peak at 3 min (an increase of 0.3 mmol/L). There is increased finbrinolytic activity following deflation, due to the release and circulation of tissue plasminogen activator. Irreversible muscle damage can occur following inflation times of 2–3 h.

Deloughry JL, Griffiths R. Arterial tourniquets. Contin Educ Anaesth Crit Care Pain 2009; 9: 56–60.

48. Answers: T F T T T

Compartment syndrome develops when a compartment, defined by bony, muscular, or fascial layers, becomes subject to elevated pressure. Normal intra-abdominal pressure is between zero and slightly subatmospheric.

Abdominal compartment syndrome has been graded according to intra-abdominal pressure:

- Grade I: 10–15 mmHg
- Grade II: 16–25 mmHg
- Grade III: 26–35 mmHg
- Grade IV: >35 mmHg

Compartment syndrome causes a direct pressure injury, leading to reduced organ perfusion, tissue ischaemia, and organ dysfunction in:

- cardiovascular system:
  - reduced left ventricular afterload
  - reduced venous return leading to decreased cardiac output
  - reduced pulmonary and systemic vascular resistance leading to increased PAOP
  - reduced myocardial contractility
  - increased CVP
- respiratory system:
  - increased intrathoracic pressure
  - reduced PaO_2/FiO_2 ratio
  - reduced pulmonary and chest wall compliance
  - hypercarbia
- renal system:
  - reduced renal perfusion
  - increased ADH
- CNS:
  - increased intracranial pressure.

Hopkins D, Gemmell LW. Intra-abdominal hypertension and the abdominal compartment syndrome. Contin Educ Anaesth Crit Care Pain 2001; 1: 56–9.

49. Answers: T T F T F

Indications for interpleural block include:

- breast surgery
- upper abdominal surgery (open cholecystectomy)
- chronic pancreatitis
- fractured ribs.

Laparoscopic cholecystectomy may cause shoulder pain due to subdiaphragmatic gas, and thus is not effectively covered by this block.

For an intrapleural block, the patient is positioned laterally and a 16 G Tuohy needle is connected to a column of saline via a one-way valve. It is introduced at 45° to the skin at the posterior angle of the upper border of the fourth to the sixth rib, thus avoiding the neurovascular bundle. A loss of resistance technique is employed and free flow of saline indicates entry into the space between the parietal and visceral pleurae. Local anaesthetic is injected directly or via an epidural catheter, threaded 8–10 cm into the space, ensuring a closed system throughout. The effect is due to paravertebral spread.

Rucklidge R. General surgery; anaesthesia for breast surgery. In: Allman KG, Wilson IH, (eds), *Oxford Handbook of Anaesthesia*, 2nd edn. Oxford University Press, 2006: p. 536.

Dravid RM, Paul RE. Interpleural block–part 2. *Anaesthesia* 2007; 62(11): 1143–53.

50. Answers: T T T F F

Porphyria describes a heterogeneous group of diseases characterized by defects in the enzymes involved in the biosynthesis of haem, resulting in the overproduction and excretion of intermediate compounds (porphyrins). Barbiturates, phenytoin, and sulphonamides are definite precipitants. Etomidate, lignocaine, and chlordiazepoxide are implicated in laboratory studies.

A full list of unsafe drugs can be found in the *British National Formulary*.

British National Formulary, 61st edn. British Medical Association and Royal Pharmaceutical Society of Great Britain, 2011: Section 15.2.

51. Answers: T T F T F

Delirium, also known as acute confusional state, is a clinical syndrome characterized by disturbed consciousness, cognitive function, or perception, which has an acute onset and a fluctuating course. It can be hypo-active, hyper-active, or, rarely, mixed. It is common in secondary care, especially in the elderly, as there is disruption to the familiar routines and surroundings. NICE Clinical Guideline 103 states that the risk factors for the development of delirium are aged 65 and older, cognitive impairment/dementia, current hip fracture, and severe inter-current illness.

Delirium: understanding NICE guidance. Clinical Guideline 103. NICE, 2010. http://www.nice.org.uk/guidance/CG103/PublicInfo.

52. Answers: F F T F T

The diagnosis and confirmation of death is required in a number of different situations, both as a result of a natural process and also in situations where artificial interventions are sustaining cardio-respiratory function in the absence of a patient's ability to breathe independently.

Death entails the irreversible loss of those essential characteristics that are necessary to the existence of a living human person and thus the definition of death should be regarded as the irreversible loss of the capacity for consciousness, combined with irreversible loss of the capacity to breathe. There is no statutory law defining death, but the guidelines below have been developed to encourage consensus in the testing process. This is important with the increase in organ donation.

The diagnosis of death by brain-stem testing should be made by at least two medical practitioners who have been registered for more than 5 years and are competent in the conduct and interpretation of brain-stem testing. At least one of the doctors must be a consultant. Testing should be undertaken by the nominated doctors acting together and must always be performed on two occasions. A complete set of tests should be performed on each occasion. The tests, in particular the apnoea test, are therefore performed only twice in total

In cardiorespiratory arrest, the individual should be observed by the person responsible for confirming death for a minimum of 5 min to establish that irreversible cardiorespiratory arrest has occurred. After 5 min of continued cardiorespiratory arrest the absence of the pupillary responses to light, of the corneal reflexes, and of any motor response to supra-orbital pressure should be confirmed.

A Code of Practice for the Diagnosis and Confirmation of Death. Academy of Medical Royal Colleges, 2008. http://www.ics.ac.uk/intensive_care_professional/code_of_practice_08.

53. Answers: F T F F F

Radiofrequency (RF) techniques are commonly used in a broad range of chronic pain syndromes. The techniques utilize low-energy, high-frequency alternating current to generate thermal energy from the friction of oscillating tissue molecules.

Continuous-wave RF techniques generate significant current density around the shaft of the insulated needle. This thermal energy, when applied alongside (parallel) to the nerve, creates a thermal lesion, which is thought to interrupt conduction of nociceptive signals.

Pulsed-wave RF techniques generate less thermal energy, because of heat dissipation into the tissues during the pauses, and hence do not produce thermal lesions. In contrast to continuous RF, pulsed RF generates the greatest current density at the tip of the insulated needle, and the needle must therefore be placed on (perpendicular) to the nerve. The mechanism of action of pulsed RF is poorly understood.

Rea W, Kapur S, Mutagi H. Radiofrequency therapies in chronic pain. *Contin Educ Anaesth Crit Care Pain* 2011; 11(2): 35–38.

54. Answers: T F T F T

Understanding simple mathematical equations allows the anaesthetist to apply the natural world to the theoretical models. $y = mx + c$ represents a linear relationship, where c is the y-axis intercept. The points m and c on this line allow a crude, two-point calibration, although most systems modelling a linear relationship require more than two known points to calibrate. By definition, an asymptote is a line that approaches but never reaches the axis. A decaying exponential decreases by a constant proportion each time period, but not by a constant amount.

Ercole A, Roe P. Mathematical relationships in anaesthesia and intensive care medicine. *Contin Educ Anaesth Crit Care Pain* 2011; 11(2): 50–55.

55. Answers: F T F F T

Absorption rate is proportional to the diffusion coefficient, the constant concentration of drug in the patch, the partition coefficient between the skin and the bathing medium, and the skin thickness. It is improved with drugs of molecular weight < or less than 500 Da, affinity for both the lipophilic and hydrophilic phases, low melting point, non-ionic, high potency and short half-life.

Bajaj S, Whiteman A, Brandner B. Transdermal drug delivery in pain management. *Contin Educ Anaesth Crit Care Pain* 2011; 11(2): 39–43.

56. Answers: F T F T T

Critical temperature is that temperature above which a gas cannot be liquefied, no matter how much pressure is applied. The critical pressure is the pressure needed to liquefy the gas at the critical temperature.

A gaseous substance is termed as a gas when it is above its critical temperature and a vapour when it is below it.

The critical temperature of nitrous oxide is 36.5°C. Oxygen, nitrogen, and hydrogen are traditionally called permanent gases because it was thought they could not be liquefied. This is because each of these gases has a critical temperature below room temperature (oxygen −118°C, nitrogen −146°C, hydrogen −240°C).

Al-Shaikh B, Stacey S. *Essentials of Anaesthetic Equipment*, 3rd edn. Churchill Livingstone, 2007.

57. Answers: F F T F F

A subdural block is an uncommon complication of epidural anaesthesia/analgesia and occurs when the catheter is placed between the dura and the arachnoid mater. Incidence is 1:1000 and it can be diagnosed definitively only by radiological methods (X-ray/CT contrast). The block has a classically slow onset, and can be widespread, although patchy and asymmetrical, with sparing of the motor fibres of the lower limb.

A subdural block can have a variable presentation depending upon the extent of the spread of local anaesthetic. The onset of the block is intermediate between that of a subarachnoid and epidural block because the nerves in the subdural space are covered with pia and arachnoid maters, as compared to the subarachnoid space, where the nerves are sheathed by pia mater only, and the epidural space, where arachnoid, pia, and dura mater envelop the nerves.

The sensory block produced by subdural injection is usually high and disproportionate to the volume of drug injected, as the limited capacity of the space results in extensive spread. Sensory block may be inadequate or completely absent. There is usually sparing or minimal effect on sympathetic and motor functions, due to the relative sparing of the ventral nerve roots. Less hypotension is likely.

Features of subdural block include:

- development of motor weakness is slow and less profound, with progressive respiratory incoordination rather than sudden apnoea
- significant motor weakness in the intercostal muscles and upper extremities
- a faster than usual onset of block and a delayed onset of up to 30 min with unduly prolonged blockade have been reported
- significant hypotension has also been observed
- unilateral blocks are common
- on rare occasions, permanent neural damage can occur as a result of unintentional subdural injection due to the compression of nerve roots or the radicular arteries traversing the space, causing ischaemia of neural tissues.
- due to the subdural space extending intracranially, local anaesthetic block of the brainstem is also possible, and periods of unconsciousness and apnoea lasting several hours have been reported
- Horner's syndrome and trigeminal nerve palsy have been reported following subdural catheterization.

Eldridge J. Obstetric anaesthesia and analgesia. In: Allman KG, Wilson IH, (eds), *Oxford Handbook of Anaesthesia*, 2nd edn. Oxford University Press, 2006.

58. Answer: T T T T F

Varices are portosystemic venous collaterals developed as a result of elevated portal pressures (>12 mmHg). The vast majority of varices in the UK are a result of cirrhosis, but worldwide the main cause is schistosomiasis resulting in hepatic fibrosis. Management should initially follow an ABC approach. Following airway protection an endotracheal tube facilitates placement of a Sengstaken–Blakemore tube; this tube has oesophageal and gastric balloons that are inflated to provide tamponade to bleeding varices. Balloon tamponade stops the bleeding in about 90% of cases and is used as a bridging measure before more definitive management.

Pharmacological management consists of intravenous vasopressin or terlipressin to constrict mesenteric vessels; concurrent GTN administration counters coronary vasoconstriction. A nasogastric tube can be placed with reasonable safety and reduces the risk of aspiration via gastric decompression. If bleeding continues after 2–3 days following attempts at control with balloon tamponade or endoscopic sclerotherapy, a transjugular intrahepatic portosystemic stented shunt

(TIPSS) may be performed. Surgical management includes portocaval anastamosis, which carries a greater risk of encephalopathy or oesophageal transection. β-blockade is beneficial as primary prophylaxis to reduce cardiac output and blood flow within the splanchnic circulation, thereby reducing portal pressure. It is not indicated as treatment in the acute setting of bleeding varices.

McKay R, Webster NR. Variceal bleeding. *Contin Educ Anaesth Crit Care Pain* 2007; 7: 191–4.

Singer M, Webb AR. *Oxford Handbook of Critical Care*, 3rd edn. Oxford University Press, 2009.

59. Answers: F F T F F

The clinical signs indicate the patient has aortic stenosis (AS). As a result of AS there is a pressure gradient across the aortic valve; this is used to grade severity of the condition.

The aim of the haemodynamic management is divided into to preload, contractility and afterload.

- Preload: patients with AS have a fixed cardiac output (CO) and it is thus essential to maintain preload since they are less able to compensate by increasing stroke volume.
- Contractility: tachycardia reduces diastolic coronary filling time and thus can lead to myocardial ischaemia even with normal coronary arteries. This is compounded by increased VO_2 of the left ventricle, which undergoes hypertrophy as it ejects against a pressure gradient; low-to-normal heart rate is ideal and maintenance of sinus rhythm is paramount.
- Afterload: since CO is relatively fixed, maintenance of systemic vascular resistance is vital for coronary perfusion; as systolic pressure falls, the gradient driving coronary flow also falls.
- Isoprenaline is arrhythmogenic and, through β_1 effects, may also lead to a tachycardia; it should therefore be avoided.

Martin B, Sinclair M. Cardiac surgery. In: Allman KG, Wilson IH, (eds), *Oxford Handbook of Anaesthesia*, 2nd edn. Oxford University Press, 2006: p. 332.

60. Answers: T F T T T

Bioavailability

Bioavailability is the degree to which or rate at which a drug or other substance is absorbed or becomes available at the site of physiological activity after administration, i.e. the fraction of a dose that reaches the systemic circulation. It is a pharmacokinetic property of drugs that is important for calculating dosages for administration routes other than IV.

Calculation of bioavailability

A plasma drug concentration vs time curve is plotted for the drug after both IV and extravascular administration. Bioavailability is the dose-corrected area under curve (AUC) for the extravascular route divided by AUC for the intravenous route.

$$F=[AUC]po/[AUC]_{IV}$$

A drug given by the intravenous route will have an absolute bioavailability of 1 (F = 1). Drugs given by other routes usually have an absolute bioavailability of less than one.

Factors affecting the bioavailability

Drug factors include:

- solubility: lipid solubility favours passive diffusion through membranes
- ionization state: non-ionized state important in passive diffusion through membrane
- dose formulation: liquid or in solution, the latter being fastest; time-release forms dissolve at different rates; small particles favour dissolution over large particles; tablets can be enteric coated to protect drug from gastric acids.

Patient factors include:

- site-related factors affecting absorption: there is low absorption from intramuscular route
- pH (drugs with low pKa non-ionized in stomach and therefore absorbed better)
- surface area (intestines have a large surface area relative to stomach)
- gastric emptying time (autonomic neuropathy can result in slower gastric emptying)
- hepatic first-pass effect (degradation of the drug by hepatic metabolism prior to reaching system circulation): drugs that undergo significant first-pass metabolism include propranolol, morphine, and lidocaine and these drugs have a high extraction ratio
- first-pass metabolism can be bypassed by giving the drugs parenterally, submucosally, or rectally
- other sites of first-pass metabolism include intestinal mucosa following oral administration (e.g. of methyldopa, isoprenaline and chlorpromazine) and bronchial mucosa (e.g. following inhalation of isoprenaline).

Holford, NHG, Benet LZ. Pharmacokinetics and pharmacodynamics: dose selection and the time course of drug action. In: Katzung, BG, (ed), *Basic and Clinical Pharmacology*, Appleton-Lange, 1998: pp. 34–49.

Single Best Answers

1. Answer: C

Whilst glottic stenosis is a feature of acromegaly and increases the difficulty of tracheal intubation, it does not increase the difficulty of the process of direct laryngoscopy. Acromegaly is a rare clinical syndrome caused by the overproduction and under-regulation of growth hormone (GH) from the anterior pituitary. It can be an insidious and potentially life-threatening condition for which there is good, albeit incomplete, treatment that can augment life by many years of high-quality. It is often associated with a GH-secreting somatotroph pituitary tumour. Other causes of increased and unregulated GH production, all very rare, include increased growth hormone-releasing hormone (GHRH) from hypothalamic tumours, ectopic GHRH from non-endocrine tumours, and ectopic GH secretion by non-endocrine tumours.

In acromegaly the symptoms develop slowly, taking years to decades to become apparent and the mean duration of symptom onset to diagnosis is 12 years. Excess GH produces a myriad of signs and symptoms and significantly increases morbidity and mortality rates. Additionally, the mass effect of the pituitary tumour itself can cause symptoms.

Seidmann PA. Anaesthetic complications of acromegaly. *Br J Anaesth* 2000; 84(2): 179–82.

2. Answer: A

Injury to peripheral nerves is a recognized complication of surgery and anaesthesia. It is also largely preventable if careful attention is paid to high-risk positioning and measures are undertaken to minimize compression by padding the pressure areas. Brachial plexus injury varies in incidence between 1 in 15,000 and 1 in 30 000 patients having a brachial plexus block, and the incidences are, perhaps, under-reported. Broadly, injury to the brachial plexus can to avoided by ensuring that there is no stretching (due to contralateral twisting of the head with the arm in abduction), compression (particularly in the axilla in the prone position), and by the introduction of nerve-location techniques (ultrasound and peripheral nerve stimulation) to reduce injury to the plexus during regional anaesthesia. There is no evidence that nerve catheter techniques are associated with a specific increase in the risk of injury.

Jenkins K, Baker B. Consent and anaesthetic risk – peripheral nerve injury. In: Allman KG, Wilson IH, (eds), *Oxford Handbook of Anaesthesia*, 2nd edn. Oxford University Press, 2006: p. 15–37.

Saha S, Turner J. *Nerve Damage Associated with Peripheral Nerve Blockade*. Royal College of Anaesthetists patient information leaflets. Section 12. http://www.rcoa.ac.uk/docs/Risk_12nerve-peripheral.pdf.

3. Answer: C

Neuraxial anaesthesia describes the use of spinal, epidural, and caudal techniques. Neuraxial adjuvants are often used to decrease the adverse effects associated with high doses of a single local anaesthetic agent, increase the speed of onset of neural blockade, and improve the quality and prolong the duration of neural blockade. Neuraxial adjuvants include opioids, sodium bicarbonate, vasoconstrictors, α2-adrenoceptor agonists, cholinergic agonists, N-methyl-D-aspartate (NMDA) antagonists, and γ-aminobutyric acid (GABA) receptor agonists.

After epidural administration of opioids, variable quantities will diffuse across the dura and arachnoid mater into the subarachnoid space to bind opioid receptors in the dorsal horn of the spinal cord. Lipid solubility is the most important factor affecting the rate of diffusion and the subsequent onset and duration of analgesia. Lipophilic opioids such as fentanyl diffuse rapidly across the dura into the CSF to give rapid onset of action with relatively short acting analgesia. This is compared to hydrophilic opioids such as diamorphine, which have a slower onset of action but a prolonged duration of action.

Respiratory depression is potentially the most serious adverse effect caused by neuraxial opioids. The incidence after neuraxial administration is similar to that of parenterally administered opioids. Early respiratory depression generally develops within 2 h of epidural administration of lipophilic opioids such as fentanyl. It is due to systemic absorption from the epidural space. Delayed respiratory depression usually develops between 6–12 h after intrathecal administration of poorly lipid-soluble opioids such as diamorphine. This is due to cephalad migration of the opioid in the CSF, which reaches opioid receptors in the respiratory centre. It is uncommon with lipophilic opioids because they rapidly penetrate the spinal cord, leaving minimal free opioid in the CSF.

Khangure N. Adjuvant agents in neuraxial blockade. *Anaesthesia Tutorial Of The Week* 230, 2011. http://totw.anaesthesiologists.org/wp-content/uploads/2011/07/230-Neuraxial-adjuvants.pdf.

4. Answer: B

Overall, the latest triennial CMACE report has shown a reduction in maternal mortality. In the 2006–2008 report, it was concluded that genital tract sepsis, particularly from streptococcal A acquired in the community, was the leading cause of direct maternal death. This partly reflects the reduced incidence of venous thrombo-embolism and haemorrhage in the obstetric population, following increased awareness of the complications in the previous report.

Saving Mothers' Lives: Reviewing Maternal Deaths to make Motherhood Safer: 2006–2008. The Eighth Report of the Confidential Enquiries into Maternal Deaths in the United Kingdom. *BJOG* 2011; 118(Suppl. 1): 1–203.

5. Answer: B

Anticonvulsant drugs reduce the excitability of gasserian ganglion neurons, preventing anomalous discharges and related lancinating volleys of pain. Thus these agents may help control paroxysmal pain by limiting the aberrant transmission of nerve impulses and reducing the firing of nerve potentials in the trigeminal nerve.

Carbamazepine is the standard in the medical management of trigeminal neuralgia and is considered first-line therapy. Lamotrigine and baclofen are second-line therapy. Other treatments are third line and the evidence for their efficacy is scant.

Carbamazepine acts by inhibiting the neuronal sodium channel activity, thereby reducing the excitability of neurons. A 100-mg tablet may produce significant and complete relief within 2 h, and for this reason it is a suitable agent for initial trial, although the effective dose ranges from 600–1200 mg/day, with serum concentrations between 40–100 mcg/mL. Indeed, serum levels of carbamazepine (but not necessarily phenytoin) in ranges appropriate for epilepsy may be necessary, at least to control initial symptoms.

Anticonvulsants, tricyclic antidepressants, skeletal muscle relaxants, and botulinum toxin have all been trialled with, at best, moderate success.

Singh MK. Trigeminal neuralgia medication. Medscape Reference, 2011. http://emedicine.medscape.com/article/1145144-treatment.

Campbell FG, Graham JG, Zilkha KJ. Clinical trial of carbazepine (tegretol) in trigeminal neuralgia. *J Neurol Neurosurg Psychiatry* 1966; 29(3): 265–67.

6. Answer: D

It is the responsibility of all professionals who come into contact with children to be familiar with the guidelines produced by NICE, *When to suspect child maltreatment*. Online training modules are available and are a requirement if your practice involves the care of children. The process for dealing with suspected maltreatment is:

- Listen and observe: the child should be allowed to explain in their own words any obvious external signs such as bruising, burns, bite marks, and signs of neglect, which should be carefully documented.
- Seek an explanation from the parent/carer and the child in an open and non-judgemental manner; beware of unsuitable explanations, including those that are implausible, inadequate, inconsistent, or based on cultural practice.
- Record all areas of concern and report to the person nominated as responsible for child protection within your trust.

In this case postponing the surgery would potentially put the patient at more risk of harm, but the small amount of time needed to listen to the child's concerns is a justifiable delay.

When to Suspect Child Maltreatment. NICE Clinical Guideline 89, December 2009. http://www.nice.org.uk/CG89.

7. Answer: C

The Difficult Airway Society has produced guidelines on the management of failed intubation during routine laryngoscopy. Plan A involves the process of direct laryngoscopy and tracheal intubation. Should this not be possible, the patient should be ventilated manually to ensure adequate oxygenation. The position should then be optimized and a second attempt at direct laryngoscopy performed. If this is unsuccessful, plan B should involve the insertion of a laryngeal mask (LMA) or intubating laryngeal mask to establish a controlled airway and oxygenation maintained. As intubation is required in this setting, intubation via a fibreoptic technique through the LMA is indicated. Should intubation fail or LMA not establish an airway, plan C is followed with manual ventilation with a mask and waking the patient. Should ventilation not be achieved, plan D is activated, and ventilation is attempted with an LMA. If this is not achieved, an emergency technique such as a cannula or surgical cricothyroidotomy must be performed. All anaesthetists should be familiar with, and drilled in, emergency airway procedures.

Failed Intubation and Ventilation at Routine Intubation. Difficult Airway Society, 2009. http://www.das.uk.com/guidelines/ddl.html.

8. Answer: C

Sickle cell crises can be precipitated by a number of factors: hypoxia, pain, anaemia, cold, tourniquet use, incorrect positioning. Whilst analgesia is important in this case, it is possible that the mild degree of hypoxia suggested by the lowered oxygen saturation has precipitated an abdominal sickle-cell crisis.

Sickle-cell disease is a congenital haemoglobinopathy with a high incidence of perioperative complications. Traditional anaesthetic management, based largely on extrapolation from biochemical models, has emphasized avoidance of red cell sickling to prevent exacerbations of the disease.

Sickle-cell disease is characterized by deformed red blood cells, acute episodic attacks of pain and pulmonary compromise, widespread organ damage, and early death.

The central pathological event has traditionally been assumed to be an increase in sickling or deformation of erythrocytes, as a result of the insolubility of the deoxygenated mutant sickle haemoglobin, haemoglobin S. While acute pain and pulmonary complications often have no clearly identifiable triggers in the community setting, the perioperative period is a well-recognized and predictable time of disease exacerbations. As these problems occur in an environment of close patient management and observation, the perioperative period can offer a unique insight into the origins of acute and chronic complications of sickle cell disease.

Firth PG. Anaesthesia for peculiar cells – a century of sickle cell disease. *Br J Anaesth* 2005; 95(3): 287–99.

9. Answer: E

Arterial tourniquets are used to provide a bloodless field to the surgeon for operative procedures on the extremities. Inflation of the tourniquet renders the tissues beyond the tourniquet temporarily ischaemic and can cause direct pressure injuries to underlying structures. Release of the tourniquet will result in rapid reperfusion of the ischaemic limb, and result in physiological changes to counteract the subsequent release of anaerobic metabolic by-products, especially lactate, which rises by 2 mmol/L. The immediate consequence of this is a rapid increase in end tidal carbon dioxide (metabolic by-product) and a reduction in serum pH. This will initially cause a compensatory tachycardia and possibly a transient hypotension. The increase in carbon dioxide will cause an increase in the respiratory rate to aid in returning the blood pH to normal limits. Although the serum potassium levels do increase, these do not peak until 3 min (an increase of 0.3 mmol/L).

Deloughry JL, Griffiths R. Arterial tourniquets. *Contin Educ Anaesth Crit Care Pain* 2009; 9(2): 56–60.

10. Answer: A

Sciatic neuralgia is a chronic pain condition characterized by pain in the distribution of the sciatic nerve. Sciatica is associated with pathology of the sciatic nerve.

The main risk factors include:

- height: increasing height increases risk, especially in patients aged 50–64 years
- age: the peak incidence is seen between 50 and 64 years
- patients are thought to have a genetic predisposition
- walking and jogging increases the incidence in patients with history of this condition
- occupation: associated with driving or physical activity
- smoking.

Note: gender and body mass index have no influence.

Pinto RZ, Maher CG, Ferreira ML, *et al.* Drugs for relief of pain in patients with sciatica: systematic review and meta-analysis. *BMJ* 2012; 344: e497.

11. Answer: C

Migraine is one of the most common primary headache disorders, which presents as periodic unilateral headache. It invariably develops before the age of 30. It results from an overactivity and amplification in pain and sensory pathways. Neurovascular symptoms usually predominate in this condition.

Central sensitization of C-fibres in the trigeminal system is thought to take place. The C-fibres release calcitonin gene-related peptide (CGRP), substance P, glutamate, etc. This sensitization results in increased excitability of neurons.

Clinical presentation

Migraine has a female preponderance, with a female to male ratio of 3:1. It has a prevalence of approximately 18% in females and 5% males. The highest prevalence is between ages 25 and 55 years.

Migraine headache has the following characteristics:

- unilateral
- usually peri-orbital or retro-orbital

- headache is severe and pounding in nature
- headache may be associated with nausea, vomiting, and photophobia..

Aura

About one in five migraine sufferers experience aura before the onset of headache. Aura is mostly visual but can also be olfactory or auditory. Decrease in cerebral blood flow is thought to be the cause of the phenomenon. The aura typically precedes the headache by 30–60 min. Characteristically, the aura is completely reversible. Neurological symptoms usually last for less than 1 h. Aura followed by a headache that does not fulfil diagnostic criteria for migraine must be investigated for organic lesions like transient ischemic attack and multiple sclerosis. The aura symptoms may present as scotoma, an arc of zigzag scintillating lights. Aura may be associated with sensory symptoms like pins and needles, numbness, and dysphasia. Some elderly patients may present with typical aura but without the headache as the disease progresses.

Migraine can occur with or without aura.

Treatment

Pharmacological treatment includes abortive, preventive, and symptomatic treatment. Abortive medications should be taken at the earliest on the onset of the attack and should not be administered daily.

Triptans are the most potent drugs in this group. They are powerful vasoconstrictors and should not be given to patients with unstable hypertension and ischaemic heart conditions.

The anti-inflammatory effect of NSAIDs makes them useful in treatment of migraine attacks.

Prophylactic treatment includes treatment with non-selective β-blockers such as propranolol, calcium channel blockers such as verapamil, and antidepressants such as amitriptyline and anticonvulsants.

International Headache Society: international classification of headache disorders, 2nd edn. *Cephalalgia* 2004; 24(Suppl 1): 1.

Diamond S, *Diagnosing and Managing Headaches*, 4th edn. Professional Communications, 2001.

12. Answer: B

Although the 'wake-up' test was originally used in scoliosis surgery, it has been superseded by more modern techniques. It involved lightening the plane of anaesthesia for a short period of time so that the patient can complete simple tasks on command. This is impractical with modern anaesthetic techniques and with intubation. Bispectral index is a monitor of depth of anaesthesia and does not indicate neurological injury. Invasive blood pressure monitoring and peripheral nerve stimulation are important components of a safe anaesthetic technique, but, again, do not monitor for neurological injury.

Somato-sensory evoked potentials involve stimulating peripheral nerves and determining a response in scalp electrodes. It is required that the patient not be under the effects of neuromuscular blockade for this method to work. The introduction of remifentanil has made this a more acceptable technique in modern scoliosis surgery.

Gardner AC, Dunsmuir RA. What's new in spinal surgery? *Contin Educ Anaesth Crit Care Pain* 2008; 8(5): 37–40.

13. Answer: D

Classically it was taught that a raised serum amylase was consistent with acute pancreatitis, but it is also elevated in bowel perforation, obstruction and ischaemia, diabetic ketoacidosis, pneumonia, and neoplasms. Serum lipase levels are both more sensitive and specific in acute pancreatitis and remain elevated for up to 14 days.

Young SP, Thompson JP. Severe acute pancreatitis. *Contin Educ Anaesth Crit Care Pain* 2008; 8(4): 125–28.

14. Answer: B

Patients undergoing minimally invasive oesophagectomy are in the lateral decubitus position. During surgery non-dependent (upper) lung is collapsed on the dependent (lower) lung. Ventilation is ceased to the non-dependent lung. However, blood supply to the non-dependent lung is maintained, and therefore ventilation–perfusion mismatch, shunt, and subsequent hypoxia may occur. Carbon dioxide exchange is not affected to the same degree, so there is less of a problem with hypercarbia.

Rucklidge M, Sanders D, Martin A. Anaesthesia for minimally invasive oesophagectomy. *Contin Educ Anaesth Crit Care Pain* 2010; 10(2): 43–47.

15. Answer: A

Compartment syndrome is a serious limb-threatening, and potentially life-threatening, condition that requires a high index of suspicion for diagnosis. Acute limb compartment syndrome refers to acutely raised pressures in an osseofascial compartment of a limb, associated with injury or surgery to that compartment. It can be caused internally by an increase in tissue volume or externally by a compressive force. The most common cause is trauma, usually after a fracture, in male patients under 35 years of age. Severe pain that is disproportionate to the injury in the affected compartment is the cardinal symptom. Paralysis, pulselessness, and paraesthesia are later signs. Pain is aggravated by passive stretching of the involved muscles, but this is less specific.

Farrow C, Bodenham A, Troxler M. Acute limb compartment syndromes. *Contin Educ Anaesth Crit Care Pain* 2011; 11(1): 24–28.

16. Answer: C

The clinical triad of back pain, pyrexia, and worsening neurological deficit is suggestive of an epidural abscess formation. The symptoms often follow a sequential order—localized spinal pain, radicular pain, radicular paraesthesia, muscular weakness, sensory loss, sphincter dysfunction, and paralysis. With the introduction of guidelines suggesting strict aseptic technique, the occurrence of an epidural abscess is very rare. This is an emergency situation. Rapid assessment of the spine with an MRI, and emergency surgical decompression of the spinal cord and drainage of the abscess are indicated. Consultation with a senior spinal or neurosurgeon should be arranged as an emergency.

Grewal S, Hocking G, Wildsmith JA. Epidural abscesses. *Br J Anaesth* 2006; 96: 292–302.

17. Answer: B

Complex regional pain syndrome 1 consists of continuous pain in an extremity following trauma, especially fractures. Pain is worse with movement and not restricted to a dermatome. The patient often reports that the limb is cool and clammy, and it gradually becomes cold, stiff, pale, and muscular atrophied. This differs from complex regional pain syndrome 2, which involves similar symptoms, but in the presence of a partially damaged peripheral nerve. Although there was nerve damage in this case, there is a report that it fully recovered.

Wilson JG, Serpell MG. Complex regional pain syndrome. *Contin Educ Anaesth Crit Care Pain* 2007; 7(2): 51–54.

18. Answer: B

It is important to confirm correctly the placement of an NG tube prior to commencing feeding. It is possible to aspirate fluid up an NG tube from the oesophagus or the back of throat. The pH of the stomach contents is normally acidic, and this can guide the recognition of placement, but is not as accurate as a chest X-ray. The fine-bore feeding NG tube contains a guide wire, and this is left in situ once the tube is placed. This wire is radiolucent and allows location of the tube with a chest X-ray. If is often necessary to remove the wire in order to successfully aspirate up the fine-bore feeding tube.

Reducing the Harm caused by Nasogastric Tubes – Interim Advice for Healthcare Staff. Baxa Resources, 2005. http://www.npsa.nhs.uk/advice.

19. Answer: C

Community-acquired pneumonia can be caused by all of the above organisms, but the most common organism is *Streptococcus pneumoniae*. Patients with severe community-acquired pneumonia are at risk of secondary bacterial, viral, and fungal infections.

Varley AJ, Sule J, Absalom, AR. Principles of antibiotic therapy. *Contin Educ Anaesth Crit Care Pain* 2009; 9(6): 184–88.

20. Answer: D

Disseminated intravascular coagulation (DIC) is a complex systemic thrombo-haemorrhagic disorder involving the generation of intravascular fibrin and the consumption of pro-coagulants and platelets. The resultant clinical condition is characterized by intravascular coagulation and haemorrhage. It is an example of a consumptive coagulopathy. The subcommittee on DIC of the International Society on Thrombosis and Haemostasis has suggested the following definition for DIC:

> An acquired syndrome characterized by the intravascular activation of coagulation with loss of localization arising from different causes. It can originate from and cause damage to the microvasculature, which if sufficiently severe, can produce organ dysfunction.

Fibrinolysis is an important component of DIC. Breakdown products of fibrin—such as D-dimers—are therefore elevated. This is not a specific test for DIC as D-dimers are also raised in a number of other clinical circumstances (venous thrombo-embolism, trauma, recent surgery). However, D-dimers would not be elevated in a dilutional coagulopathy.

Becker JU. Disseminated intravascular coagulation in emergency medicine. Medscape eReference, April 2011. http://emedicine.medscape.com/article/779097-overview.

21. Answer: B

Analysis of respiratory gases can be formed with the gases in a gas mixture or as dissolved components in the blood. The Clarke polarographic sensor analyses oxygen dissolved in solution, and is the device used to measure the partial pressure of oxygen on the bench arterial blood-gas analyser. It uses a gold cathode, silver/silver chloride anode, potassium chloride solution as an electrolyte buffer between the electrodes, and requires an electrical source as a supply of electrons. Option A is the components of the oxygen fuel cell. This is a cheaper sensor, but the gold cathode is consumed in the analysis process, and no power source is required. Option D is the pH electrode, which measures the H^+ concentration. When this is added to option C, it forms the Severinghaus reference electrode for measuring carbon dioxide dissolved in a solution.

Langton JA, Hutton A. Respiratory gas analysis. *Contin Educ Anaesth Crit Care Pain* 2009; 9(1): 19–23.

22. Answer: E

The patient meets the criteria for unstable ventricular tachycardia due to the shock and myocardial ischaemia. ALS guidelines suggest that the next treatment action should be synchronized DC cardioversion.

Peri-arrest Algorithms – Tachyarrhythmias. Resuscitation Council, Adult Advanced Life Support Guidelines, 2010. http://www.resus.org.uk/pages/periarst.pdf.

23. Answer: E

Anti-embolism stockings (AES) exert graded circumferential pressure from distal to proximal regions of the leg. They increase blood velocity and promote venous return. They have been shown to be effective, are well tolerated by patients, and are relatively inexpensive. They are suitable for the majority of patients, but it important that they are appropriately fitted and applied. AES should not be used if the patient has peripheral vascular disease, arteriosclerosis, severe peripheral neuropathy, massive leg oedema, pulmonary oedema, oedema secondary to congestive cardiac failure, local skin diseases, local soft tissue diseases, or in patients with an acute stroke.

Barker RC, Marval P. Venous thromboembolism: risks and prevention. *Contin Educ Anaesth Crit Care Pain* 2011; 11(1): 18–23.

24. Answer: C

Uterine atony is the most common cause of primary postpartum haemorrhage in the first 24 h after delivery, and accounts for up to 70% of cases. Although the other causes are also possible, and must be excluded, it is unlikely that these would cause this degree of bleeding at this stage after delivery. Risk factors predisposing to an atonic uterus include: chorioamnionitis, prolonged labour, augmented labour (especially with syntocinon), and conditions predisposing to an abnormally distended uterus (multiple pregnancy, polyhydramnios, macrosomia, abnormal placentation).

Eldridge J. Obstetric anaesthesia. In: Allman KG, Wilson IH, (eds), *Oxford Handbook of Anaesthesia*, 2nd edn. Oxford University Press, 2006: p. 695.

25. Answer: B

Parkinson's disease is a neurological disease of the extrapyramidal system. It is thought to be due to loss of dopaminergic neurones in the substantia nigra, which causes an imbalance of acetyl choline and dopamine. It is treated with drugs to increase available dopamine substrate, using dopamine precursors (e.g. levodopa), dopamine agonists (e.g. apomorphine), and monoamine oxidase inhibitors (e.g. selegiline).

Anti-emetic drugs are designed to act at a number of receptors throughout the central nervous system, vomiting centres, vestibular centres, and on the gut. One subtype of antiemetic is the dopamine receptor antagonists. Metoclopramide, droperidol, and prochlorperazine all act as dopamine anatagonists, and can therefore worsen the symptoms of Parkinson's disease.

Dexamethasone is used as an antiemetic agent, although its mechanism of action remains unclear. However, in this case, using a steroid as an antiemetic may cause derangement of the blood glucose, and impair glycaemic control in the post-operative period. For that reason it is best avoided in the insulin dependent diabetic.

Errington DR, Severn AM, Meara J. Parkinson's disease. *Contin Educ Anaesth Crit Care Pain* 2002; 2(3): 69–73.

26. Answer: B

This patient has classic signs and symptoms of obstructive sleep apnoea (OSA). Predisposing conditions for OSA include obesity, age 40–70, male, excess alcohol intake, smoking, pregnancy, low physical activity, unemployment, neck circumference > 40 cm, surgical patient, tonsillar and adenoidal hypertrophy, craniofacial abnormalities, and neuromuscular disease. OSA is an independent risk factor for serious neuro-cognitive, endocrine, and cardiovascular morbidity and mortality in all age groups.

Patients at risk of, or with known OSA, should be comprehensively assessed and investigated for the associated risk factors. This man has evidence of congestive heart failure and hypercapnia. These would warrant postponing the elective surgery until he has been medically managed and received CPAP therapy for a preoperative period of 3 months. The CPAP should be continued during his hospital admission.

Martinez G, Faber P. Obstructive sleep apnoea. *Contin Educ Anaesth Crit Care Pain* 2011; 11(1): 5–8.

27. Answer: E

This is most likely to be an inadvertent intravascular injection. It could also be inadvertent intra-arterial injection; this is possible and in that setting a much smaller volume will result in convulsions. Intralipid is not immediately indicated here—this is for cardiovascular toxicity. In this case, once the immediate issue is under control, ECG monitoring and a 12 lead ECG would be useful.

The priorities are:

- Airway, Breathing, Circulation, and oxygenation
- prevention of injury to patient (and staff)
- drugs to terminate fitting (and facilitate ventilation).

The toxicity of local anaesthetic technique could be prevented by avoiding

- follow the monitoring guidelines as set out by the AAGBI
- identify the site to be blocked
- use the correct dose of local anaesthetic—the maximum dose varies depending on site to be anaesthetized, vascularity of the tissues, individual tolerance, and anaesthetic technique
- aspiration during regional techniques should be gentle, as the side wall of a small blood vessel is easily sucked on to the needle/catheter.

Calvey N, Williams N. *Principles and Practice of Pharmacology for Anaesthetists*, 4th edn. Wiley-Blackwell, 2001.

Management of Local Anaesthetic Toxicity. AAGBI safety guideline, The Association of Anaesthetists of Great Britain and Ireland, 2010. http://www.aagbi.org/publications/guidelines/docs/latoxicity07.pdf.

28. Answer: B

Intra-arterial injection of drugs is, thankfully, very rare. Where it occurs, it is as a result of inadvertent injection into an arterial line, or injection into a venous line that is inadvertently in an artery. It is more likely to occur in the hypotensive, cold, peripherally shut-down patient, such as the one in the question.

An early symptom is pain and discomfort on injection of an irritant drug. Patients with distracting injuries, sedation, anaesthesia, or depressed consciousness are at risk. The drug will fail to have its desired effect, and limb pain, paraesthesia, pallor, hyperaemia, and cyanosis can occur.

Damage is thought to occur due to arterial spasm, direct tissue destruction by the drug, subsequent chemical arteritis causing endothelial destruction, release of thromboxane, and drug precipitation and crystallization.

Management strategies aim to maintain perfusion distal to the injection. Elevation improves venous drainage, anticoagulation prevents thrombosis, and analgesia is imperative. Stellate ganglion block interrupts the sympathetic supply to the limb, producing arterial and venous vasodilation, and analgesia. Intra-arterial lignocaine may prevent reflex vasospasm, but can cause damage itself. Methylprednisolone and papaverine reverse tissue ischaemia, but do not immediately provide analgesia. Interscalene brachial plexus block will provide analgesia, but not sympathetic blockade.

Lake C, Beecroft CL. Extravasation injuries and accidental intra-arterial injection. *Contin Educ Anaesth Crit Care Pain* 2010; 10(4): 109–13.

29. Answer: A

All of the above drugs are appropriate for the management of severe bradycardia, but atropine is the most appropriate initial therapy as the patient fulfils the criteria for unstable bradycardia as defined in the Resuscitation Council's 2010 *Advanced Life Support Guidelines*. A patient is considered unstable if there are adverse features (shock, syncope, myocardial ischaemia, or heart failure) and the recommended initial therapy is atropine 500 mcg IV, repeated until clinical effect or maximum dose of 3 mg.

Periarrest Algorithms – Bradyarrhythmias. Resuscitation Council, Adult Advanced Life Support Guidelines, 2010. http://www.resus.org.uk/pages/periarst.pdf.

30. Answer: E

All of the conditions mentioned present with anaemia with a low reticulocyte count, except for hereditary spherocytosis, where the count is generally 6–20%. Hereditary spherocytosis (HS) is an autosomal dominant form of spherocytosis. It is a haemolytic anaemia characterized by the production of red blood cells that are sphere-shaped rather than doughnut-shaped, and therefore the red blood cells are more prone to haemolysis. The morphologic hallmark of HS is the microspherocyte, which is caused by loss of the membrane surface area, and an abnormal osmotic fragility *in vitro*. Investigation of HS has afforded important insights into the structure and function of cell membranes and into the role of the spleen in maintaining red blood cell integrity.

There is a marked heterogeneity of clinical features, ranging from an asymptomatic condition to fulminant haemolytic anaemia. The major complications are aplastic or megaloblastic crisis, haemolytic crisis, cholecystitis and cholelithiasis, and severe neonatal haemolysis. Haemolysis in HS results from the interplay of an intact spleen and an intrinsic membrane protein defect that leads to abnormal RBC morphology.

Purday J. Haematological disorder. In: Allman KG, Wilson IH, (eds), *Oxford Handbook of Anaesthesia*, 2nd edn. Oxford University Press, 2006: p. 208.

Single Best Answers—Mini Exam 1

1. **A 54-year-old man with a history of COPD undergoes left shoulder arthroscopic surgery under interscalene brachial plexus block. The operation was uneventful. In recovery after 30 min the nurse looking after the patient noticed he was looking pale, with heart rate of 110, BP of 110/70 mmHg, respiratory rate of 25/min, and saturation of 90% on room air. On auscultation there was no wheeze and air entry on left base was reduced. The chest X-ray in recovery appears normal. What is the most likely cause of his symptoms?**
    A. Local anaesthetic toxicity.
    B. Left phrenic nerve block/palsy.
    C. Exacerbation of COPD.
    D. Horner's syndrome.
    E. Recurrent laryngeal nerve block.

2. **A 54-year-old patient is having retinal detachment surgery under general anaesthetic. During the surgery the patient became bradycardic with heart rate of 40 beats per minute and blood pressure of 75/40. What is the first thing would you do?**
    A. Reduce the inspired inhalation concentration of isoflurane.
    B. Give intravenous glycopyrolate 200 mcg.
    C. Give intravenous atropine 600 mcg.
    D. Stop the surgeon operating and release the muscles of the globe.
    E. Give intravenous ephedrine 6–12 mg.

3. **A 65-year-old lady with BMI of 38 had a total knee replacement under general anaesthesia. Femoral nerve block was performed using ultrasound. She suffers from mild asthma and hypertension. The total tourniquet time was 1 h 40 min. Twenty-four hours postoperative, the patient complained of paraesthesia in the right foot and is found to have foot drop. Which of the following is the most likely cause?**
    A. Pressure injury from the long duration of operation.
    B. Ischaemic injury to the calf muscle.
    C. Deep vein thrombosis in the calf muscle.
    D. Compression injury to the sciatic nerve.
    E. Compartment syndrome in the thigh.

4. **An 8-year-old child is rescued 20 min after near-drowning and has a core temperature of 30°C and fixed dilated pupils. Along with the resuscitation what would be the appropriate treatment:**
    A. Intravenous barbiturate infusion.
    B. Rapid re-warming to 32–34°C.
    C. Intravenous steroid therapy.
    D. Hypoventilation.
    E. Intravenous sodium bicarbonate.

5. **A 65-year-old male patient had open prostatectomy under general anaesthesia. The surgical procedure was complicated, with prolonged anaesthesia for 5 h, and there was a total blood loss of about 2.5 L. Intra-operatively he received 6 units of packed cells and he was transferred to the intensive care unit. In the intensive care unit, the patient was tachycardic and hypotensive. The peak airway pressure was about 30–35 cm H_2O. On chest examination there were bilateral lung crepitations. The most likely cause of his condition is:**
    A. Cardiogenic shock.
    B. Acute myocardial infarction.
    C. Sepsis.
    D. Transfusion-related reaction.
    E. Transfusion-related acute lung injury.

6. **A 35-year-old male is listed for electroconvulsive therapy. He is medically fit but has a family history of allergy to suxamethonium. You are advised by the consultant to use rocuronium and sugammadex. Which of the following statements is true regarding sugammadex?**
    A. Most of the drug is metabolized and excreted by kidney.
    B. Sugammadex binds with rocuronium at the neuromuscular junction.
    C. The drug forms complex with the rocuronium with a ratio of 1:3.
    D. The free plasma concentration of rocuronium increases following complex formation with sugammadex.
    E. It is a modified γ-cyclodextrin with eight side chains and a negatively charged carboxyl group.

7. **As a universal precaution there is a recommendation to use a heat and moisture-exchange filter with each patient. A heat and moisture-exchange filter incorporates a high-efficiency particulate air filter of small size. Which of the following pathogens will pass through the heat and moisture-exchange filter?**
    A. *Pseudomonas aeruginosa.*
    B. *Mycoplasma pneumonia.*
    C. *Mycobacterium tuberculosis.*
    D. *Staphylococcus aureus.*
    E. *Legionella pneumophilia.*

8. **A 70-year-old woman is referred to the pain clinic with severe shooting pains in the upper half of the left side of her face. These are made worse by eating. Physical examination and all investigations are normal. Simple analgesics have not provided effective pain relief. Which of the following would be the initial treatment?**
    A. Carbamazepine.
    B. Topical capsaicin ointment.
    C. Oral morphine.
    D. Transcutaneous nerve stimulation (TENS).
    E. Fluoxetine.

9. **A 70-year-old patient, who had a hip replacement 2 weeks ago, now has dislocated the hip. The patient is on ramipril, simvastatin, aspirin, and dabigatran. Which of the following statements is correct regarding dabigatran?**
    A. The drug is licensed for venous thromboembolism (VTE) prophylaxis in AF patients.
    B. The drug is in its active form.
    C. The drug needs routine coagulation monitoring.
    D. The drug is a direct thrombin inhibitor.
    E. The drug is metabolized in liver and excreted by kidney in inactive form.

10. **An 88-year-old male patient is admitted with fracture of neck of femur for left hip hemiarthroplasty. The patient is a known hypertensive, on atenolol 50 mg and ramipril 5 mg. Following spinal anaesthesia the blood pressure drops to 60/35 mmHg and his heart rate drops from 80 to 60/min. He has received 1.5 L of Hartman's solution. The next step is:**
    A. To transfuse 500 mL crystalloid and recheck the blood pressure every 1–2 min.
    B. To give incremental bolus of 6 mg ephedrine along with the crystalloid.
    C. To position the patient's head downwards and infuse 500 ml crystalloid.
    D. To give 250 ml of gelofusion along with the bolus of 6 mg of ephedrine.
    E. To give 500 mcg metaraminol as bolus, along with the rest of the crystalloid and recheck the blood pressure.

11. **A 50-year-old man with metastatic cancer is listed for intramedullary nailing of a pathological femoral fracture. For the last 3 months he has been on 300 mg/day of oral morphine for cancer-related pain control. What is the most appropriate way to manage his postoperative pain?**
    A. The patient's morphine should be temporarily discontinued during the perioperative period.
    B. This patient has reached the upper limit of opioid and should be reduced before the surgery.
    C. This patient will be tolerant to opioid analgesia—increasing opioid load would lead to addiction and should be avoided.
    D. Routine postoperative patient-controlled morphine would be adequate.
    E. A combination of femoral nerve block and fentanyl patient-controlled analgesia with shorter lock-out and higher bolus would be appropriate.

12. **Twenty-four hours following a normal vaginal delivery a 34-year-old woman is looking drowsy on routine examination. Her heart rate is 110/min and blood pressure is 85/40 mmHg. Her temperature is noted to be 38.9°C. She is treated with 1 L of crystalloid and oral amoxicillin. The midwife is concerned and has asked for an anaesthetic review of the patient. What would be the most appropriate step to follow?**

A. Keep giving fluid until the tachycardia settles.

B. Insert a central venous line to monitor fluids on the ward.

C. Arrange early transfer to an HDU facility.

D. Ask the midwife to do hourly MEWS on the ward.

E. Advise the obstetrician to refer her to the medical team.

13. **A 56-year-old male presents for day-case knee arthroscopy. On the day unit he seems to be slightly confused. Patient is a known alcoholic and had a few admissions to the hospital with upper gastrointestinal bleeding. The last hospital letter shows he was diagnosed with end-stage liver failure. What would be the most appropriate anaesthetic management?**

A. Cancel the case and rearrange as an inpatient procedure.

B. Cancel the patient, as anaesthesia carries high risk and this is not a life-threatening situation.

C. Call the bed manager, arrange an inpatient bed and do the case.

D. Patient would need to be intubated as he is at high risk of aspiration.

E. After the procedure he should be followed up by an alcohol-awareness team.

14. **A 70-year-old man is brought to A&E following a collapse at home. The paramedics gave him 1000 mL of crystalloid and noticed a pulsating swelling in the abdomen. On arrival in A&E his BP is 100/60 mmHg, heart rate is 110/min, and GCS 15/15. The FAST scan was positive and CT scan showed leaking aneurysm. Which of the following is not appropriate management?**

A. Check NIBP in both arms.

B. Good preoperative assessment.

C. Administer IV fluids to restore the BP.

D. Administer IV fluids to aim for a MAP of 90 mmHg.

E. Get blood products as soon as possible.

15. **You are asked to review a 32-year-old woman in the post-delivery ward. Twenty-four hours post forceps delivery, she is complaining of left foot drop. She had a labour epidural for pain relief, which worked very well. On examination she has good power in both legs and there are no other neurological issues. What is the most likely cause?**

A. Epidural haematoma.

B. Dense block from the top up.

C. Epidural abscess.

D. Neuropraxia of the common peroneal nerve from forceps delivery.

E. Spinal cord compression.

16. **A 24-year-old man is brought to A&E following a motorbike accident. On arrival his initial assessment was clear airway, tachypnoeic, tachycardic, and hypotensive. He was immediately given oxygen by mask and intravenous access was secured with two 16-g cannula. He responded to an initial 10 mL/kg fluid bolus. His CT scan shows an unstable spinal fracture at a level of T10. After 10 min his blood pressure dropped again. What is the most likely reason?**
    A. Neurogenic shock.
    B. Septic shock.
    C. Bleeding from an undiagnosed injury.
    D. Allergic reaction.
    E. Sympathetic hyperreflexia.

17. **A 70-year-old patient with coronary artery disease is listed for an elective coronary artery bypass; he has moderate-to-severe left ventricular failure on his most recent echo-cardiogram. During the surgery, after weaning from cardiopulmonary bypass (CPB), there is persistent hypotension with low cardiac index despite the administration of inotropic drugs. What would be the specific management of this condition?**
    A. Correct hypothermia.
    B. Correct electrolyte imbalance.
    C. Insert an intra-aortic balloon pump.
    D. Restart the CPB as soon as possible.
    E. Consider ECMO.

18. **A frail 75-year-old woman was brought to A&E with a Colle's fracture of the left wrist. A junior orthopaedic trainee manipulated the wrist using intravenous regional anaesthesia (Bier's block) with 30 mL of 0.25% levobuvipacaine. Shortly after the cuff was deflated, the patient had symptoms of confusion, seizure, and hypotension, without cardiorespiratory arrest. The most appropriate management would be:**
    A. Follow the ALS guidelines.
    B. Give 10 mg of lorazepam.
    C. Secure the airway.
    D. Give an initial intravenous bolus injection of 20% lipid emulsion 1.5 mL/kg over 1 min.
    E. Refer the patient to intensive care.

19. **A 35-year-old patient was admitted to critical care with pneumonia. He was ventilated and treated with antibiotics. Forty-eight hours post admission his airway pressure is 35 cmH$_2$O and he is on FiO$_2$ of 80% with a PaO$_2$ of 10 kPa. Chest X-ray shows bilateral asymmetrical consolidation. Which of the following criteria fits for acute lung injury?**
    A. Acute onset.
    B. Presence of bilateral infiltrates on chest-X-ray consistent with oedema.
    C. PAWP <18 mmHg or clinical absence of left atrial hypertension.
    D. Hypoxaemia with PaO2 /FiO$_2$ <40 (if PaO$_2$/FiO$_2$ <27, the term ARDS is used).
    E. All of the above answers are criteria for acute lung injury.

20. **A 31-week primigravida presented to A&E complaining of headache and blurred vision. Her blood pressure is 150/109 mmHg and the urine shows proteinuria. Whilst she is waiting to be reviewed by the obstetrician, her blood pressure rises to 157/115 mmHg. What is the next step in the management of the patient?**

    A. Transfer the patient immediately to theatre for emergency LSCS.
    B. Give her a bolus of 100 mg labetalol.
    C. Restrictive fluid therapy.
    D. Load her with 4 g magnesium sulphate and start her on a magnesium sulphate infusion.
    E. Check her FBC and clotting.

21. **A 21-year-old woman is brought to A&E after ingesting 200 g of paracetamol. She is initially managed with N-acetylcysteine and referred to the high-dependency unit. Twenty-four hours later her Glasgow Coma Scale was reduced to 8/15 and her blood results show pH 7.28, PaO_2 12 kPa, $PaCO_2$ 5.1 kPa, HCO_3 16 mmol/L, PT 110 s, and creatinine 210 mmol/L. The appropriate management following intubation should be:**

    A. Early referral to specialist liver centre for liver transplant.
    B. Refer to the haematology team to improve her clotting.
    C. Refer to the psychiatric team before discharging home.
    D. Give her another dose of N-acetylcysteine.
    E. Early haemofiltration to avoid renal failure.

22. **A 28-year-old female patient with a history of asthma arrives in A&E by ambulance. She is short of breath with audible wheeze. She has used her inhalers repeatedly over the last few hours but she has not improved and is unable to talk. On arrival her respiratory rate is 30/min with oxygen saturation of 90%. On arrival she is treated with 10 L of oxygen and nebulized salbutamol 5 mg. 10 min after the treatment her respiratory rate is still 28/min and saturation 91%. The clinical condition has not improved. Arterial gas shows $PaCO_2$ of 9 kPa and PO_2 of 8 kPa. What would be the most appropriate management?**

    A. Nebulized B2-agonist (e.g. salbutamol).
    B. Intravenous corticosteroids for 24 h.
    C. Intravenous magnesium sulphate 2 g slowly.
    D. Intravenous aminophylline 5 mg/kg.
    E. Rapid sequence induction and positive pressure ventilation.

23. **A 65-year-old male is scheduled for elective laryngectomy. He suffers from COPD, coronary artery disease, and had three coronary stents inserted 3 years ago. He smokes 20 cigarettes a day. His nasendoscopy shows a subglottic tumour occupying two-thirds of the airway. He says that he is unable to lie flat and presents with an inspiratory stridor. What is the most appropriate method of induction in this patient?**

    A. He should have an intravenous induction.
    B. He should have gas induction, muscle relaxant, and laryngoscopy.
    C. He should have gas induction and asleep fibreoptic intubation.
    D. He should have an awake fibreoptic intubation and then intravenous induction.
    E. He should have a tracheostomy with local anaesthetic and then general anaesthetic.

24. **A 34-year-old biker had a motorbike accident with open knee injury. He had general anaesthesia for knee washout and ligament repair. He has an arterial tourniquet, inflated at right thigh level. During the operation the blood pressure rose to 180/90 mmHg. Regarding the use of arterial tourniquets, which one of the following statements is most accurate?**

    A. Every 30 min of tourniquet inflation increases the risk of nerve damage by 50%.
    B. Older age is an independent predictor of nerve damage following prolonged tourniquet time.
    C. Ketamine reduces the hypertensive effect of the tourniquet if given perioperatively.
    D. Pain from the surgical site becomes a problem after 1 h of continuous tourniquet inflation, and may cause hypertension.
    E. The use of a tourniquet has no implications for cerebral blood flow.

25. **A 28-year-old woman was brought to A&E following overdose by nasal inhalation of cocaine. Her GCS was 3/15, heart rate was 165/min, blood pressure was 110/60 mmHg, and respiratory rate was 6/min on 15 L of oxygen and oxygen saturation of 94% with Guedels airway and mask ventilation. On arrival she was intermittently convulsing with supraventricular and ventricular tachycardia. Arterial blood gas analysis on arrival showed respiratory and metabolic acidosis. She was immediately intubate and ventilated. What would be the most appropriate next step?**

    A. Treat the convulsions by loading dose infusion of phenytoin 1.2 g (15 mg/kg).
    B. Treat the hypotension by noradrenaline infusion (0.05 mcg/kg/min).
    C. Fluid resuscitation.
    D. Administer initial bolus of lipid emulsion 1.5 mL/kg of 20% followed by infusion.
    E. Correction of respiratory and metabolic acidosis.

26. **A 17-year-old boy is brought to A&E with a reduced level of consciousness and rapid, deep, sighing breathing. On observation, his heart rate is 125/min, blood pressure 120/65 mmHg, respiratory rate 22/min, saturation of 99%, and GCS 13/15. A urine dipstick demonstrates significant ketonuria. The blood gas is as follows: pH 6.89, PO_2 64 kPa, PCO_2 1.6 kPa, HCO_3 4, lactate 2.1, Na^+ 114, K^+ 6.9, glucose 41. What is the most appropriate initial treatment?**

    A. Immediate intubation and ventilation.
    B. Urgent haemofiltration to treat acidosis and hyperkalaemia.
    C. Intravenous bicarbonate slow infusion.
    D. Cautious fluid resuscitation with insulin infusion at 0.1 unit/kg/h until ketonaemia resolves.
    E. Fluid resuscitation with insulin sliding scale adjusted to blood glucose level.

27. **Regarding the nerve supply of the muscles of the larynx, which of the following muscles is supplied by the superior laryngeal nerve?**

    A. Thyroarytenoid.
    B. Posterior cricoarytenoid muscles.
    C. Lateral cricoarytenoids.
    D. Cricothyroid muscle.
    E. Arytenoid muscle.

28. **Regarding the gag reflex, which of the following cranial nerves is the efferent pathway for the gag reflex?**

    A. Cranial nerve XI.
    B. Cranial nerve V.
    C. Cranial nerve VII.
    D. Cranial nerve X.
    E. Cranial nerve IX.

29. **An 11–month-old child is on your list for adenotonsillectomy under general anaesthesia. The routine examination reveals a soft systolic murmur; the rest of the examination is normal. He has no history of shortness of breath. The parents are very anxious. The appropriate action you will take is:**

    A. Proceed with the surgery.
    B. Proceed with the surgery with antibiotic prophylaxis.
    C. Proceed with the surgery and inform paediatric anaesthetist.
    D. Postpone the surgery and refer the patient to GP.
    E. Postpone the surgery and organize urgent echo.

30. **Which statement best describes the correct mechanism of action of the following antiemetics?**

    A. Dexamethasone has been shown to downregulate 5-HT_3 receptors.
    B. Ondansetron is a 5HT_2 receptor antagonist acting in the chemoreceptor trigger zone.
    C. Haloperidol causes central dopaminergic (D2) blockade and post-synaptic GABA antagonism.
    D. Cyclizine is a histamine H1 antagonist at as well as having activity at the muscarinic receptors.
    E. Metoclopramide acts as an atiemetic via 5HT_3 receptors centrally and peripherally.

Single Best Answers—Mini Exam 2

1. **A 24-year-old male fell off a horse and sustained a femoral shaft fracture. The chest X-ray and C-spine were clear. He under went internal fixation of the femoral shaft with intramedullary nail, with blood loss of about a 800 mL. Forty-eight hours later the patient is confused. His respiration is 22/min, blood pressure 80/40 mmHg, oxygen saturation 92%, and temperature 39°C. On examination there are scattered crepitations on the chest with widespread petechial rash noted. What would be the most appropriate next step?**
   A. Immediately alert the orthopaedic team and send blood for investigation.
   B. Transfuse packed red cells and ensure the good circulating blood volume.
   C. Treat with anticoagulation for pulmonary embolism.
   D. Get a CT head scan as patient had a fall from horse.
   E. Transfer the patient to critical care with oxygen for CPAP ventilation and monitoring.

2. **A 28-year-old woman is admitted to the labour ward following prolonged rupture of membrane at 38 weeks of gestation. She is very distressed by labour pains, and is requesting an epidural. On examination she is 6-cm dilated, with temperature of 38.8°C, heart rate of 140/min, and blood pressure of 110/60. She was given paracetamol 1 g orally and 1.2 g of coamoxiclav intravenously. What is the most appropriate course of action?**
   A. Explain the procedure and provide epidural.
   B. It is safe to put the epidural in as she has had antibiotic cover.
   C. Epidural analgesia is contraindicated in this case.
   D. Wait for an hour so the antibiotics may work and then insert the epidural.
   E. Give some fluids first and then insert the epidural.

3. **An 84-year-old woman is admitted with fracture of neck of femur, which she sustained after a fall at her nursing home. She has a history of dementia and ischaemic heart disease and had a coronary bypass 10 years ago. She is on the trauma list for surgical fixation of her hip. In the preoperative visit the anaesthetist noticed that there is an active 'do not attempt resuscitation' form. Regarding the DNAR which of the following statements is correct?**

   A. DNAR form should be respected and the patient should not come to theatre.
   B. DNAR form should be respected and in the event of arrest in theatre CPR should not be undertaken.
   C. DNAR should be cancelled as the patient needs surgery.
   D. DNAR should be reviewed before anaesthesia and surgery.
   E. DNAR form is not valid as the reason for admission is a fracture.

4. **A 45-year-old, 85-kg male is retrieved from a house fire. He has sustained 40% burns with no other injury and is *haemodynami*cally stable. Which of the following is the correct fluid requirement in the first 8 h?**

   A. 800 mL colloid and 3500 mL crystalloid.
   B. 5000 mL crystalloid.
   C. 6800 mL crystalloid.
   D. 13 600 mL crystalloid.
   E. 5000 mL colloid.

5. **A 36-year-old male patient suffering from primary hyperaldoesteronism is scheduled for laparoscopic cholecystectomy. His routine investigation would show:**

   A. High sodium, low potassium, and low hydrogen ions.
   B. High sodium, low potassium, and high hydrogen ions.
   C. Low sodium, low potassium, and high hydrogen ions.
   D. Low sodium, high potassium, and high hydrogen ions.
   E. Low sodium, high potassium, and low hydrogen ions.

6. **A 45-year-old man is undergoing laproscopic cholecystectomy. Following induction in the anaesthetic room he was transferred to the operating table in theatre and the monitor shows heart rate is 150/min. His peak airway pressure is rising. The patient looks flushed and has a feeble pulse. Which of the following would be the most appropriate action in this situation?**

   A. Call for help and check the ventilator.
   B. Call for help and give a bolus of 50 mcg of adrenaline IV.
   C. Call for help and give a bolus of 50 mcg of adrenaline IM.
   D. Call for help and give a bolus of 1 mg of adrenaline IM.
   E. Call for help and give a bolus of 10 mg chlorphenamine and 200 mg hydrocortisone IV.

7. **A 75-year-old woman had a total abdominal hysterectomy for cervical cancer, under general anaesthesia and epidural for pain relief. She is on long-term clopidogrel, which was stopped 7 days before elective surgery. The routine preoperative blood investigations revealed a normal clotting screen. Plasma urea and creatinine were raised, at 9.2 mmol L^{-1} and 112 μmol L^{-1} respectively. Post-operatively, epidural infusion was 10 mL/h of 0.125% bupivacaine. Eight hours postoperatively she has a dense motor block of her right leg. The most appropriate action would be to:**

   A. Remove the epidural catheter and do an MRI.
   B. Stop the epidural and refer her to the neurologist.
   C. Book an urgent MRI and refer to neurosurgeon.
   D. Stop the epidural infusion and reassess the neurology in 2 h.
   E. Change the epidural infusion bag for another of lower concentration.

8. **A 50-year-old man is on your elective list for inguinal hernia repair under general anaesthesia. He had successful cardiac transplant 6 years ago with no problems, and has good exercise tolerance. The ECG showed right bundle branch block, with a rate of 90/min. At anaesthetic induction it would be essential to:**

   A. Ensure adequate preload is maintained.
   B. Avoid nephrotoxic drugs.
   C. Perioperative β-block the patient to avoid risk of ischemia.
   D. Be aware that in the case of bradycardia, atropine would not work.
   E. Be aware that epinephrine will increase the contractility and chronotropy.

9. **A 40-year-old man with myotonic dystrophy is admitted for tonsillectomy to treat his sleep apnoea symptoms. He has no cardiovascular or pulmonary issues, his lung function is normal, and he suffers from type II diabetes, which is well controlled. The best anaesthetic management for this patient would be:**

   A. Patient should be intubated using depolarizing neuromuscular blocking agents.
   B. Patient should be intubated using non-depolarizing neuromuscular blocking agents.
   C. Neuromuscular relaxant should be avoided if possible.
   D. Avoid hypothermia, shivering, and mechanical and electrical stimulation.
   E. Tight control of blood sugar.

10. **A 20-year-old woman is listed for an elective femoral hernia repair. Currently she suffers from indigestion, and 7 months ago she was admitted to critical care with Guillain–Barré syndrome. At the pre-operative visit she is very anxious and would prefer general anaesthesia for the operation. What would be the appropriate method to manage this case?**

   A. Regional anaesthesia with sedation.
   B. General anaesthesia using rapid sequence induction with suxamethonium.
   C. General anaesthesia with modified rapid sequence induction using rocuronium.
   D. General anaesthesia should be avoided for the next 6 months.
   E. General anaesthesia with laryngeal mask airway.

11. **A 58-year-old diabetic patient on insulin is referred to the chronic pain clinic. He complains of severe burning sensations and pain in his foot. His quality of life is very poor and simple analgesia such as paracetamol, NSAIDs, and opioids have been unsuccessful. The first line of treatment would be:**

    A. Pregabalin.
    B. Amitriptyline.
    C. Ketamine.
    D. Methadone.
    E. Duloxetine.

12. **A 29-year-old, on long-term opioids for chronic pain, undergoes exploration of a wound under general anaesthesia. Intra-operatively, intravenous paracetamol, diclofenac, and morphine was administered for pain. In recovery, the patient complains of severe pain. His heart rate is 120/min and blood pressure is 160/85 mmHg. Which of the following would be the most appropriate for management of his pain?**

    A. Intravenous bolus of 10 mg of morphine.
    B. This patient will be tolerant to opioid analgesia—increasing his opioid load in the perioperative period can lead to addiction and should be avoided.
    C. A standard patient-controlled morphine analgesia.
    D. A loading dose of 10 mg morphine followed by morphine infusion in the recovery.
    E. A loading dose of fentanyl 100 mcg followed by patient-controlled fentanyl analgesia regime with a shorter lock-out and possibly with a higher bolus dose.

13. **Pregabalin and gabapentin has been used for multimodal postoperative pain management of acute pain. On which of the following sites does the drug act?**

    A. N-methyl-daspartate receptor.
    B. Aminobutyric acid receptor.
    C. α-2-δ subunit of calcium channel.
    D. Inhibits prostaglandins.
    E. α-2 channel.

14. **A 38-year-old woman was rushed to A&E after indigestion of some unknown tablets. On arrival she is confused and agitated. She has a respiratory rate of 20/min, blood pressure of 130/70 mmHg, and saturation of 95%. The blood gas on arrival was pH 7.50, pO_2 19 kPa, pCO_2 3 kPa, HCO_3 16 mmol/L. Overdose of which of the following drugs will result in such a picture?**

    A. Cocaine.
    B. Ketamine.
    C. Paracetamol.
    D. Aspirin.
    E. 3,4-methylenedioxyethamphetamine.

15. **A 65-year-old male patient had an emergency laprotomy. He was doing well postoperatively, but 24 h postoperatively he is agitated, confused, and vomiting. The surgical registrar has reviewed the patient and there were no surgical issues. The heart rate is 120/min, respiratory rate is 20/min, blood pressure is 180/100 mmHg, and his chest is clear. He has received 5% dextrose to meet his fluid requirements and PCA morphine for pain control. What is the most likely cause?**
    A. Stroke.
    B. Chest infection.
    C. Morphine side effect.
    D. Hyponatremia.
    E. Withdrawal syndrome.

16. **A 30-year-old woman with spina bifida is 34 weeks pregnant. Her MRI showed no tethering of the spinal cord and there are no neurological issues. Her pregnancy has been normal, with no problems. She is very anxious about the pain relief during labour and would like to know the best option. Which of the following would be best management?**
    A. TENS machine.
    B. Pethidine intramuscular.
    C. Epidural.
    D. Entonox.
    E. Combine spinal epidural.

17. **A 4-year-old boy had a fall from swing and has a fractured wrist. He is listed for manipulation under anaesthesia. The young boy is with his father, who has signed the consent form. The mother cannot be contacted. Which is the following is the most correct statement?**
    A. The father cannot give consent in this case.
    B. The child can give consent himself.
    C. The mother does not always have parental responsibility for her child.
    D. Unmarried fathers do not automatically have parental responsibility.
    E. Fathers married to the mother at the time of birth automatically have parental responsibility.

18. **An 8-year-old boy has presented to A&E with severe lower abdominal pain and his left testicle looks ischaemic. He is booked urgently into the emergency theatre for surgical exploration. He is normally fit and well with no anaesthetic issues in the family. He had breakfast 6 hours ago. What would be the appropriate method to anaesthetize him?**
    A. General anaesthesia with laryngeal mask airway.
    B. General anaesthesia and secure the airway with uncuffed tube.
    C. General anaesthesia and secure the airway with cuff tube.
    D. Rapid sequence induction with thiopental and suxamethonium.
    E. Spinal anaesthesia.

19. **A 72-year-old patient underwent vitro-retinal surgery for detached retina under general anaesthesia. The patient has history of hypertension controlled with atenolol. During the operation patient had severe bradycardia, which was successfully treated by atropine 600 mcg. Twenty minutes after arrival in recovery he became very agitated, confused, and restless. His heart rate is 120/min, respiratory rate is 20/min, and blood pressure is 180/110. What would be the most appropriate treatment in recovery?**

   A. Intravenous incremental bolus of morphine 1 mg/mL.
   B. Intravenous incremental propofol 10 mg/mL.
   C. Intravenous labetolol titration with the blood pressure.
   D. Intravenous midazolam.
   E. Intravenous haloperidol.

20. **A 20-year-old man is brought to A&E following a road traffic accident. He is haemodynamically stable and has patent airway. He is on full spinal immobilization and on examination he is found to be paraplegic at the level of T10. Neurological examination confirms the loss of pain and temperature sensation below T10, with preservation of propioception and vibration. Which of the following is the correct diagnosis?**

   A. Central cord syndrome.
   B. Spinal shock syndrome.
   C. Anterior cord syndrome.
   D. Complete cord syndrome.
   E. Brown–Sequard's syndrome.

21. **A 21-year-old man with refractory catatonia presents for electroconvulsive therapy (ECT). Which of the following cardiovascular changes is seen initially during ECT?**

   A. Reactive tachycardia.
   B. Parasympathetic discharge.
   C. Hypertension.
   D. Torsades de pointes.
   E. Ischaemic ST segments.

22. **A 45-year-old male patient is scheduled for left knee arthroscopy as a day-case procedure. He has no significant medical history. He appears to be very apprehensive and has blood pressure of 182/110 mmHg. His ECG shows left ventricular hypertrophy. Repeat blood pressure reading is consistent with the earlier reading. What would be the most appropriate action?**

   A. Request for echocardiogram urgently.
   B. Prescribe temazepam 20 mg as premedication.
   C. Cancel the case, with GP referral.
   D. Continue with the surgery under spinal anaesthesia.
   E. Continue with the surgery with invasive monitoring.

23. **A 48-year-old male patient is undergoing laprotomy for small bowel cancer. He has no other medical conditions. During the procedure the patient's blood pressure is noted to be 240/140 mmHg, with heart rate of 126/min. What would be the most appropriate initial treatment?**

   A. Insert arterial line.
   B. Send urgent urinary vanillyl mandelic acid levels.
   C. Digitalization.
   D. Increase depth of anaesthesia using atracurium, opioid, and volatile.
   E. Give incremental dose of 5 mg/mL labetalol.

24. **A 54-year-old man had scheduled open anterior resection under general anaesthesia with thoracic epidural. The surgery was complicated and lasted for 6 h in Lloyd–Davis position. Following the surgery the patient was transferred to recovery, with thoracic epidural infusion at 8 mL/h of 0.1% bupivacaine. Four hours later the patient complained of bilateral calf pain. On examination patient has decreased mobility and reduced pinprick sensation in all dermatomes below the knees. What is the most likely investigation you would do?**

   A. Ultrasound scan of deep venous system of both legs.
   B. Magnetic resonance imaging of the lumbar spine.
   C. Doppler arterial pulse measurement in both legs.
   D. Nerve conduction study.
   E. Measure the compartment pressure in both the calves.

25. **A 38-year-old man presents to A&E with sore throat and noisy breathing. He also complains of difficulty in swallowing and is unable to lie flat. In sitting position his saliva is drooling. He has marked inspiratory stridor and his temperature is 39.4°C, heart rate 120 /min, BP 140/80 mmHg, and oxygen saturation on room air 89%. You are called to assess the patient in A&E. What is your management plan in this patient?**

   A. The patient should be transferred to the operating theatre for emergency tracheostomy under local anaesthesia.
   B. The patient should be transferred to the anaesthetic room fully monitored for awake fibreoptic intubation under local anaesthesia spray-as-you-go technique followed by transfer to critical care.
   C. Transfer to high-dependency area for monitoring, with intravenous steroids, antibiotics, nebulized adrenaline, and CPAP via face mask.
   D. The patient should be given oral antibiotic, a blood culture taken, and indirect naso-endoscopy performed by an ENT surgeon, with observation in the high dependency unit.
   E. The patient is transferred to anaesthetic room for gas induction, his trachea should be secured by tracheal intubation, with an ENT surgeon present, and he should be transferred to critical care.

26. **A 50-year-old woman is admitted for elective hemi-thyroidectomy. She suffers from rheumatoid arthritis and hypertension. During preoperative assessment she informs you that over the past couple of weeks she has noticed that on extending her neck, her arms feel weak and slightly numb. The next appropriate step in planning her airway management during anaesthesia would be:**

   A. Plan a careful conventional laryngoscopy and intubation, taking care to minimize neck movement.
   B. Plan the use of a flexible laryngeal mask airway and intermittent positive pressure ventilation.
   C. Plan an awake fibreoptic technique for intubation.
   D. Defer the patient for MRI of the neck to look for posterior atlanto-axial subluxation.
   E. Plan an elective tracheostomy prior to induction of anaesthesia.

27. **Pulmonary thromboembolism (PTE) remains a frequently occurring diagnostic problem, with an incidence of approximately 1–2 cases per thousand of population per year. The most common source of symptomatic pulmonary embolus is:**

   A. Iliofemoral vessels.
   B. Superficial veins in calf.
   C. Superficial veins in the thigh.
   D. Veins in the arm.
   E. Deep calf veins.

28. **You are performing an interscalene block on a 52-year-old man for surgery on his shoulder. Using a peripheral nerve stimulator you observe medial movement of the scapula. Which nerve are you stimulating in order to cause this muscular contraction?**

   A. Long thoracic nerve.
   B. Dorsal scapular nerve.
   C. Suprascapular nerve.
   D. Supraclavicular nerve.
   E. Accessory nerve.

29. **A 58-year-old man is undergoing emergency laprotomy for bowel obstruction. He has a past history of hypertension, which is treated with bendroflumethiazide and atenolol. During the operation his heart rate increases from 70/min to 165/min and blood pressure falls to 70/40 mmHg. His blood gases are normal and CVP is 6 cmH$_2$O. Which of the following electrolyte disorders is most likely to contribute to the arrhythmia?**

   A. Serum sodium of 125 mmol/L.
   B. Serum phosphate of 0.50 mmol/L.
   C. Serum potassium 3.5 mmol/L.
   D. Serum magnesium 0.40 mmol/L.
   E. Serum calcium of 2 mmol/L.

30. A 38-year-older Polish builder is scheduled for left shoulder arthroscopy. He does not speak English. What is the best method to consent the patient for the procedure?

A. Provide him with translated material.

B. Call the patient's son, who is 12 years old, but is bilingual.

C. Ask one of the nurses in the ward, who is Polish, to translate.

D. Call a healthcare assistant who can speak fluent Polish.

E. Use a professional telephone translation service.

Single Best Answers—Mini Exam 3

1. **A 53-year-old woman was admitted following a subarachnoid haemorrhage. Two days after her admission, the ALERT team informs you that she is hyponatraemic. On assessment she is not thirsty and is euvolaemic. Her blood test shows plasma sodium 129 mmol/L, urine sodium 29 mmol/L, and plasma osmolality 270 mOsm/kg. What is the most likely diagnosis?**
   A. Iatrogenic hyponatraemia.
   B. Syndrome of inappropriate ADH secretion (SIADH).
   C. Cerebral salt wasting syndrome (CSWS).
   D. Severe dehydration.
   E. Drug-related hyponatraemia.

2. **Concerning the Bain anaesthesia breathing circuit, which of the following is the correct statement?**
   A. Fresh gas flow is along the inner tube.
   B. The minimum length is 2 m.
   C. During controlled ventilation the minimum fresh gas flow is 6 L/min.
   D. End tidal CO_2 concentration cannot be altered by changing the fresh gas flow.
   E. It is a co-axial Mapleson A circuit.

3. **A 36-year-old male had a bike accident and was admitted to critical care with isolated severe head injury. After 24 h his condition is still critical, with no signs of brain stem activity, he is polyuric and his plasma sodium is 154 mmol/L, his condition does not improve despite aggressive fluid therapy. Which of the following is the correct diagnosis and treatment of this condition?**
   A. Diabetes insipidus and small titrated doses of 1-deamino-8-D-arginine vasopressin.
   B. Diabetes insipidus and administration of dextrose saline fluids.
   C. Cerebral salt wasting syndrome (CSWS) and normal saline fluids.
   D. Severe dehydration and oral fluids replacement.
   E. Syndrome of inappropriate ADH secretion (SIADH) and small doses of vasopressin.

4. A 32-year-old pregnant woman is admitted to the labour ward for induction of labour due to reduced foetal movement. She suffers from multiple sclerosis, with her last exacerbation 3 years ago. Her pregnancy had been unremarkable throughout. The CTG shows foetal bradycardia requiring emergency caesarean section (category I). What is the most appropriate method to induce the patient for general anaesthesia?

    A. GA is contraindicated and she should have a spinal.
    B. Rapid sequence using thiopental, suxamethonium, and alfentanil.
    C. Thiopental, rocuronium, and remifentanil.
    D. Modified rapid sequence using thiopental and rocuronium.
    E. Propofol and rocuronium.

5. A 14 year-old boy is brought to A&E following a car accident. He has suffered head injury, with fluctuating level of consciousness. He requires general anaesthesia for urgent CT scan and possible craniotomy. His mother is abroad and his father is an hour's car journey away. What is the most appropriate step regarding consent?

    A. It would be appropriate to proceed with emergency treatment without consent.
    B. Without consent from the mother the proposed treatment is considered battery.
    C. The team can wait for the father to arrive.
    D. Legal advice must be sought urgently before proceeding.
    E. A social worker can sign the consent.

6. A young patient is brought to A&E by the air ambulance and has an isolated head injury with GCS 8/15 at the scene. She is intubated and ventilated with an end tidal CO_2 of 3.1 kPa. Profound hypocarbia should be avoided in traumatic brain injury in order to prevent:

    A. Respiratory alkalosis.
    B. Metabolic acidosis.
    C. Cerebral vasoconstriction with diminished perfusion.
    D. Neurogenic pulmonary oedema.
    E. Shift of the oxyhemoglobin dissociation curve.

7. A 78-year-old male patient was admitted to critical care after emergency repair of abdominal aortic aneurysm. He has been anuric for the last 2 h. Which is the most correct statement pertaining to acute kidney injury?

    A. Perioperative renal failure is a rare complication of major surgery.
    B. Dopamine has been shown to prevent acute renal failure.
    C. Perioperative manitol provides renal protection.
    D. Postoperative renal dysfunction is associated with mortality of up to 60%.
    E. By the nature of the pathophysiolgy, perioperative renal failure is not associated with cardiac dysfunction.

8. A 27-year-old woman is admitted to the labour ward at 40 weeks with early onset labour. Her midwife informs you that the patient is known to suffer from benign intracranial hypertension and her BMI is 35. Which of the following is the best way to manage her?

   A. Avoid any regional anaesthesia.
   B. She could have an epidural but spinal should be avoided.
   C. She could have any regional anaesthesia.
   D. Remifentanil PCA is the best option.
   E. Entonox and opioid IM.

9. A 57-year-old man had laparoscopic cholecystectomy. In recovery his heart rate is 110/min, blood pressure is 210/110 mmHg, and oxygen saturation is 98%. His past medical history includes hypertension treated with enalapril, and he has a BMI of 35. The recovery nurse asks you to review the patient. What would be your next step?

   A. Treat the blood pressure with sublingual nifedipine 5 mg.
   B. Reassure the patient, repeat the blood pressure, and check the pain score.
   C. Reassure the patient and give titrated dose of intravenous morphine.
   D. Give intravenous atenolol, titrating with the blood pressure.
   E. Assess the patient, repeat blood pressure, and then consider titrated dose of 5 mg/mL labetalol.

10. A 59-year-old male is scheduled for left parotidectomy. He has a past medical history of CABG, after which he had an automatic implantable cardioverter-defibrillator (AICD) sited due to recurrent episodes of VT. He has a LVEF of 35%, with trivial mitral regurgitation and cardiomegaly on chest X-ray. With regards to AICD, what would be your first step before induction of anaesthesia?

    A. Check for preoperative electrolyte level.
    B. Ensure only bipolar diathermy is used and prepare the emergency drugs.
    C. Invasive monitoring with transoesophageal echocardiography.
    D. Arrange for magnet along with the resuscitation trolley.
    E. Programmer available to deactivate antitachycardia and defibrillation response and have external pads placed on chest.

11. A 28-year-old primigravida is admitted to the labour ward at 32 weeks' gestation with a mild frontal headache and increasing swelling of her ankles. Her blood pressure is 170/120 mmHg, urine dip stick testing shows 3+ protein, and there is pitting oedema to the mid-calf.
    The most common maternal complication of severe pre-eclampsia is:

    A. Acute renal failure.
    B. Disseminated coagulopathy or HELLP syndrome.
    C. Eclampsia.
    D. Liver failure or haemorrhage.
    E. Pulmonary oedema or aspiration.

12. **A 77-year-old male is admitted to intensive care with an intrabdominal bleed. He has chronic atrial fibrillation, for which he is on long-term warfarin. On admission his INR is 3.5. Which of the following management is most appropriate in this situation?**

    A. Administration of 50 mL/kg fresh frozen plasma.
    B. Administration of intravenous vitamin K 2 mg.
    C. Administration of recombinant factor VIIa.
    D. Replacement of clotting factors II, VII, IX, and X.
    E. Administration of protamine.

13. **Regarding the elimination half-life of a drug, which of the following statements is correct?**

    A. It is half the time taken to totally eliminate the drug from the body.
    B. It is the time taken for the initial plasma concentration to fall by half.
    C. It is used to calculate the maintenance infusion rate of a drug.
    D. It is used for dosing intervals.
    E. It is always a constant in an individual.

14. **On your elective list for general paediatric theatre there is a 5-year-old boy with muscular dystrophy for insertion of PEG. He suffers from recurrent chest infections and the paediatrician thinks he probably silently aspirates overnight. His chest is clear and his oxygen saturation overnight was 97%. The most important reason for monitoring core temperature in the perioperative period is:**

    A. Children with this condition are at risk of hypothermia.
    B. Muscular dystrophies are associated with malignant hyperthermia.
    C. If hypothermia develops the patient can manifest rhabdomyolysis.
    D. If the temperature in recovery is less than 36°C the child has to stay longer in recovery.
    E. Changes in core temperature can affect neuromuscular block.

15. **A 20-year-old builder fractured his radius 2 months ago and was in a synthetic cast for 6 weeks. Despite his fracture healing and his cast being removed, over the last 2 weeks he has been experiencing continuous pain, described as burning, shooting, and aching. He has noticed that the arm fluctuates in colour and temperature, and his arm is weaker than when his cast was removed. What is the possible diagnosis?**

    A. Neuropathic pain.
    B. Complex regional pain syndrome I.
    C. Complex regional pain syndrome II.
    D. Phantom limb pain
    E. Compartment syndrome.

16. **Regarding management of severe venous thromboembolism, vena cava filter insertion is *not* indicated in:**
    A. Severe coagulopathy.
    B. Uncontrollable thromboembolic disease.
    C. Limited life expectancy.
    D. Absolute contraindication to anticoagulation.
    E. Undergoing pulmonary endarterectomy.

17. **A 35-year-old primipara woman had prolonged labour, followed by caesarean section after failure to progress. After the delivery of the baby the estimated blood loss was about 3.5 L. She received 2 L of Hartman's solution, 4 units of packed cells, and 2 units of fresh frozen plasma. The bleeding is still continuing from the wound edges and the uterus. A further two units of packed cells and 2 units of fresh frozen plasma were administered. When is it most appropriate to transfuse recombinant factor VIIa?**
    A. Platelet count 40×10^9/L, pH 7.1, and fibrinogen 0.40 mg/dL.
    B. Platelet count 55×10^9/L, pH 7.2, and fibrinogen 0.50 mg/dL.
    C. Platelet count 35×10^9/L, pH 7.2, and fibrinogen 0.20 mg/dL.
    D. Platelet count 60×10^9/L, pH 7.1, and fibrinogen 0.30 mg /dL.
    E. Platelet count 50×10^9/L, pH 7.2, and fibrinogen 0.30 mg/dL.

18. **A 35-year-old polytrauma patient with multiple fracture is in shock In order to prevent perioperative acute kidney injury, the mean arterial pressure should be maintained at greater than:**
    A. 40 mmHg.
    B. 50 mmHg.
    C. 55 mmHg.
    D. 85 mmHg.
    E. 100 mmHg.

19. **Surgical patients are at risk of developing venous thromboembolism. It is, however, important to recognize that there exist both definable operative procedures and definable groups of patients with significantly higher than normal rates of postoperative thromboembolism. In which of the following conditions is the risk of perioperative thrombosis *not* increased?**
    A. Protein C deficiency.
    B. >40 years old.
    C. Chronic renal failure.
    D. Diabetes mellitus.
    E. Malignancy.

20. **A 38-year-old male patient is admitted to critical care with a chest infection. He is intubated and ventilated. His temperature is 39°C, heart rate 120/min, blood pressure 90/50 mmHg and white cell count 3×10^9/L. The marker of severity in the patient is determined by:**

    A. Anion gap.
    B. Arterial pH.
    C. Base deficit.
    D. Lactate level.
    E. Arterial oxygen (PaO_2).

21. **A 32-year-old 1-week postpartum primigravida presented to A&E with severe frontal headache, nausea, and photophobia. She had had an induced vaginal delivery of a healthy baby boy under labour epidural. She was discharged the day following delivery with no problems having been encountered. She had so far had an uneventful pueperium and was well until this frontal headache began. She had no significant past medical history. Which of the following is the least likely cause?**

    A. Pre-eclampsia.
    B. Central venous sinus thrombosis.
    C. Spinal haematoma.
    D. Postdural puncture headache.
    E. Migraine.

22. **Regarding total parenteral nutrition, the following statements are true except:**

    A. It is indicated where gastrointestinal tract is not functional for >5 days.
    B. It should include glutamine supplementation.
    C. It should not be administered along with enteral nutrition.
    D. Cholestasic liver disease can be caused by intravenous feeding.
    E. It can cause hyperglyceridaemia and acidosis.

23. **With regard to arginine supplementation for nutritional support, all the statements are true except:**

    A. It is associated with reduced mortality in septic patients.
    B. It is a potent antioxidant.
    C. There are beneficial effects on T lymphocyte function.
    D. It increases the formation of nitric oxide.
    E. It can be administered intravenously.

24. **When considering enteral nutrition, which of the following statements is true:**

    A. Gastric residual volumes up to 350 mL are acceptable.
    B. Enteral nutrition can be given continuously A 4-h rest period should always be allowed.
    C. Diarrhoea is uncommon when postpyloric feeding is used.
    D. After insertion of an NG tube, a chest X-ray is mandatory to confirm the tube position.
    E. It is indicated in acute pancreatitis.

25. **A 24-year old man was brought to A&E following of overdose by nasal inhalation of cocaine. Cocaine toxicity causes all of the following except:**
    A. Hyperthermia.
    B. Rhabdomyolysis.
    C. Hyponatraemia.
    D. Seizures.
    E. Tachycardia.

26. **A 28-year-old male farmer presents to A&E with a 2-day history of difficulty in mouth opening, dysphagia, and neck stiffness. He had a laceration of right arm a week ago. Regarding tetanus, which of the following statements is correct?**
    A. Caused by *Clostridia difficile*.
    B. Human tetanus immunoglobulin (HTIG) should be administered on daily basis.
    C. The antibiotic of choice is metronidazole.
    D. β-blocker is used if there is hypertension.
    E. Tetanospasmin releases neurotransmitters from presynaptic vesicles.

27. **A 75-year-old woman had elective aortic valve replacement along with coronary artery bypass (CABG). Prior to closing the sternotomy the surgeon is finding it difficult to achieve haemostasis. Thromboelastography (TEG) shows a prolonged R-time on both the basic and heparinase samples. What treatment will be of most benefit in correcting the coagulopathy?**
    A. Protamine.
    B. Platelets.
    C. Cryoprecipitate.
    D. Fresh frozen plasma.
    E. Aprotinin.

28. **A 42-year-old man is scheduled for repair of umbilical hernia. He weighs 118 kg and is 180 cm tall. His past medical history includes type 2 diabetes and hypertension. His wife reports that he keeps her up at night with his snoring but he has not been investigated for obstructive sleep apnoea (OSA). Which of the following is least likely to suggest a diagnosis of OSA?**
    A. An arterial blood pressure of 140/90 mmHg.
    B. A BMI of 37 kg/m^2.
    C. Age >50.
    D. Neck circumference 37 cm.
    E. Male gender.

29. You are called to A&E to manage the airway of a 21-year-old male motorcyclist who has collided with a car. CT scan of head shows an intracerebral haemorrhage with GCS of 7/15. He is sedated and intubated for the transfer to the regional neurosurgical unit. Just before the transfer you notice his right pupil has increased in diameter. What is least likely to be contributing to his current condition?

    A. An end tidal carbon dioxide of 4.7 kPa.
    B. A PEEP of 10 cmH$_2$O with an FiO_2 of 0.3.
    C. Uncontrolled seizures.
    D. Serum sodium of 152 mmol/L.
    E. Temperature of 38.2°C.

30. A study looking at the efficacy of a new non-steroidal anti-inflammatory drug compares the visual analogue pain scores of patients having day-case knee arthroscopy. One group of patients receives diclofenac as part of a multi-modal analgesic strategy and the other group receives the new drug. What is the appropriate statistical test to assess the significance of the data?

    A. Chi-square test.
    B. Wilcoxon signed-rank test.
    C. Unpaired t-test.
    D. Mann–Whitney test.
    E. Repeated measures ANOVA.

Single Best Answers—Mini Exam 1

1. Answer: B

Local anaesthetic toxicity is less likely considering the duration of the operation. Phrenic nerve palsy is the most likely cause for all the symptoms and signs. The chest X-ray needs to be in inspiratory phase to show the raised diaphragm of left side. Recurrent laryngeal nerve block is a well-known complication after interscalene block, which can cause hoarseness of voice due to ipsilateral paralysis of the vocal cords. The other mentioned complications are possible but are unlikely to be responsible for the symptoms.

Miller, RD (ed). *Miller's Anesthesia*, 7th edn, Churchill Livingstone, 2009: pp. 409, 1640–3.

2. Answer: D

The oculo-cardiac reflex (OCR) can occur secondary to traction on the eye and ocular muscles, resulting in bradycardia. Occasionally it can cause junctional rhythm or asystole. The afferent pathway is ciliary ganglion to ophthalmic division of trigeminal nerve to gasserian ganglion to main trigeminal sensory nucleus fourth ventricle. The efferent pathway is the vagus nerve.

The first step in managing OCR is to releasing the traction on the eye. Persistent bradycardia should be treated with anticholinergic drugs. Intravenous atropine sulphate blocks the peripheral muscarinic receptors at the heart, and release of traction blocks the conduction at ciliary ganglion on the afferent limb of OCR. Atropine or glycopyrrolate can be used to treat this reflex and it can be given prophylactically. Hypoxia, hypercarbia, and light anaesthesia potentiate this reflex and should be avoided. Retrobulbar block does not guarantee attenuation of this reflex.

Karhunen U, Cozanitis DA, Brander P. The oculocardiac reflex in adults. A dose response study of glycopyrrolate and atropine. *Anaesthesia* 1984; 39(6): 524–8.

3. Answer: D

Foot drop can be defined as a significant weakness of ankle and toe. The foot and ankle dorsiflexors include the tibialis anterior, extensor hallucis longus, and extensor digitorum longus. These muscles are supplied by the sciatic nerve. The paresis of sciatic nerve is more like to be due to the insult secondary to the prolonged application of the tourniquet. Pressure injury, ischaemic injury, and DVT are less likely.

Deloughry JL, Griffiths R. Arterial tourniquets. *Contin Educ Anaesth Crit Care Pain* 2009; 9(2): 56–60.

4. Answer: B

Accidental hypothermia exists when the body's core temperature unintentionally drops below 35°C. Hypothermia can be classified arbitrarily as mild (35–32°C), moderate (32–28°C), or severe (<28°C). In a hypothermic patient, the absence of signs of life alone is unreliable for declaring death.

All the principles of prevention, and basic and advanced life support apply to the hypothermic patient. Use the same ventilation and chest compression rates as for a normothermic patient. Hypothermia can cause stiffness of the chest wall, making ventilation and chest compressions more difficult.

There are no reliable predictors for successful resuscitation and there are case reports of survivors with extreme initial physiological derangement. Therefore, resuscitation should be attempted in all drowning victims. During resuscitation, attempts should be made to raise the body temperature of hypothermic patients. A number of rewarming methods exist. Passive rewarming is appropriate for mild hypothermia, but moderate and severe hypothermia will require active external and active internal rewarming, respectively. When return of cardiac output is achieved in the unconscious patient, it is recommended that rewarming is not continued to normothermia, but to 32–34°C.

Carter E, Sinclair R. Drowning. *Contin Educ Anaesth Crit Care Pain* 2011; 11(6): 210–13.

5. Answer: E

The clinical condition presented here is following the transfusion of packed cells. Hence the most likely diagnosis is transfusion-related acute lung injury (TRALI). TRALI is defined as new acute lung injury occurring during or within 6 h after a transfusion, with a clear temporal relationship to the transfusion. Another important concept is that acute lung injuries temporally associated with multiple transfusions can be TRALI because each unit of blood or blood component can carry one or more of the possible causative agents: anti-leukocyte antibody, biologically active substances, and other yet unidentified agents.

Toy P, Popovsky MA, Abraham E, *et al.* National Heart, Lung and Blood Institute Working Group on TRALI. Transfusion-related acute lung injury: definition and review. *Crit Care Med* 2005; 33(4): 721–6.

6. Answer: E

Sugammadex is the first selective relaxant binding agent to reverse neuromuscular blockade. It is a γ-cyclodextrin that forms a tight (1:1) one-to-one complex with rocuronium (vecuronium to a lesser extent), reducing the plasma concentration of the neuromuscular blocking agents and rapidly reversing their effects. It is a modified γ-cyclodextrin with eight side chains and negatively charged carboxyl group to increase the affinity.

Mechanism of action

Sugammadex is unique in the way in which it works. It encapsulates and inactivates rocuronium. The inactive complex follows the elimination kinetics of sugammadex.

Routes of administration/doses

The recommended dose for reversal, 3–5 min after an intubating dose of rocuronium, is 16 mg/kg. Three trials indicated that sugammadex 2 mg/kg (4 mg/kg) produces more rapid recovery from moderate (profound) neuromuscular block than neostigmine -glycopyrrolate.

For more moderate blocks a dose of 2–4 mg/kg is recommended.

Pharmacokinetics

Post intravenous administration, sugammadex demonstrates linear pharmacokinetics.

The inactive complex of rocuronium and sugammadex do not bind to plasma proteins and are primarily excreted unchanged in urine. The elimination half-life is 1.8 h. Renal impairment delays the elimination of sugammadex and its complex with rocuronium.

Uses

Sugammadex is licensed for use in adults to reverse muscle-relaxant effects of rocuronium and vecuronium.

The evidence suggests that there are potential benefits of sugammadex in terms of increased patient safety, increased predictability of recovery from neuromuscular blockade, and more efficient use of theatre time and staff.

Naguib M. Sugammadex: another milestone in clinical neuromuscular pharmacology. *Anesth Analg* 2007; 104: 575–81.

Paton F. Sugammadex compared with neostigmine/glycopyrrolate for routine reversal of neuromuscular block: a systematic review and economic evaluation. *Br J Anaesth* 2010; 105(5): 558–67.

7. Answer: C

A standard heat and moisture exchange filter is tested to 0.3 μm pore size.

The sizes of the organisms are:

- *Pseudomonas aeruginosa*: 1–3 μm
- *Mycoplasma pneumoniae*: 0.15 μm is the smallest.
- *Mycobacterium tuberculosis*: 2–4 μm length, 0.2–0.4 μm wide
- *Staphylococcus aureus*: 0.6 μm diameter
- *Legionella pneumophilia*: 1–3 μm long, 0.5–1.0 μm wide

Vandenbroucke-Grauls KB, Teeuw K, Ballemans K, *et al*. Bacterial and viral removal efficiency, heat and moisture exchange properties of four filtration devices. *J Hosp Infect* 1995; 29(1): 45–56.

Dellamonica N, Boisseau B, Goubaux B, *et al*. Comparison of manufacturers' specifications for 44 types of heat and moisture exchanging filters. *Br J Anaesth* 2004; 93(4): 532–9.

8. Answer: A

Trigeminal neuralgia is an intermittent, usually unilateral, severe neuropathic pain, which can come on spontaneously or by stimulation of the trigger zone. There is an abnormality in the trigeminal sensory system. There is significant female preponderance (2:1). Magnetic resonance imaging is recommended in these patients.

Classification

Type 1 is primary or idiopathic.

Type 2 is secondary to irritation or compression of the trigeminal nerve by tumour or disease, including multiple sclerosis.

Medical treatment

Response to carbamazepine is almost diagnostic of this condition. Gabapentine, baclofen, and sodium valproate have also been used.

Surgical treatment should be considered if secondary causes are detected or medical therapy fails. This includes microvascular decompression (MVD), which has shown to be curative in patients in whom the condition has resulted from vascular compression of the trigeminal nerve. Teflon sponges are placed between dissected blood vessel and neural tissue. Compression is usually caused by a branch of the superior cerebellar artery, which should not be divided. Other procedures include glycerol rhizotomy, percutaneous balloon compression, retrogasserian rhizotomy, and gamma knife radio surgery.

Nurmikko1 TJ, Eldridge PR. Trigeminal neuralgia—pathophysiology, diagnosis and current treatment. *Br J Anaesth* 2001; 87(1): 117–32.

9. Answer: D

Dabigatran is a new oral anticoagulant for prevention of venous thromboembolism. This drug is a specific, competitive, and reversible thrombin inhibitor.

Mechanism of action

Dabigatran is a direct thrombin inhibitor and is used in the form of a pro-drug, dabigatran etexilate. This is metabolized by plasma esterases into active drug, dabigatran. It prolongs APTT, PT, and TT.

The real advantage of the drug is it does not need routine coagulation monitoring. It does not have a specific antidote.

Absorption, distribution, metabolism, and excretion

Dabigatran etexilate has oral bioavailability of about 7%. It is metabolized completely to dabigatran, which is the active form. It has low protein binding and hence is dialysable in emergency situations. It has a half-life of 12–14 h and is predominantly (80%) excreted unchanged in urine.

Contraindications

Contraindications include active bleeding, impaired haemostasis, and hepatic impairment.

Toxicity/side effects

In pooled analyses of the trials the most common side effects were:

- bleeding from the wound and anaemia
- major or minor bleeding—the incidence of such events in studies was similar to enoxaparin sodium

Caution is advised with rifampicin, verapamil, and amiodarone. There are no major drug interactions with atorvastatin or proton pump inhibitors.

Dose

The dose is 110 mg 1–4 h after surgery, then 220 mg once daily for 9 days.

Uses

Dabigatran is currently licensed in the European Union for venous thrombo-embolism prevention in patients undergoing total knee and hip replacement. It is being studied for VTE prophylaxis in AF patients.

Sanford M, Plosker GL. Dabigatran etexilate. *Drugs* 2008, 68(12): 1699–1709.

Eisert WG, Hauel N, Stangier J. Dabigatran: an oral novel potent reversible nonpeptide inhibitor of thrombin. *Arterioscler Thromb Vasc Biol* 2010; 30:1885–89.

British National Formulary, 61st edn. British Medical Association and Royal Pharmaceutical Society of Great Britain, 2011.

10. Answer: E

Central neuraxial block causes reduction of sympathetic outflow, which results in reduction of the sympathetic tone and reduction of the systemic vascular resistance. This is compensated by increase in heart rate and stroke volume; in a group of geriatric patients these are less effective. Furthermore, this patient is on β-blockers and ACE inhibitors, which, along with less compliant ventricles, further compounds the problem for the patient. In the elderly patient hypotension should be treated with cautious use of fluids and vasopressors. Ephedrine is likely to be ineffective in the elderly; α-agonists such as metaraminol or phenylephrine should be used in preference.

Attempts to maintain preload by administering fluids should be limited to 8 mL/kg, given while the block is evolving. Fluid overload is a real risk in this population.

The choice of vasopressor is again open to debate. β-receptor sensitivity is reduced in the elderly, limiting the use of β-agonists such as the mixed α- and β-agonist ephedrine. Pure α-agonists such as metaraminol and phenylephrine, however, produce a response comparable with that seen in the younger adult population.

Murray D, Dodds C. Perioperative care of the elderly. *Contin Educ Anaesth Crit Care Pain* 2004; 4: 193–6.

11. Answer: E

The principles of acute pain management in the patient who is dependent on high-dose opioids represent challenges, as it is difficult to differentiate addiction from dependence and to avoid opioid withdrawal symptoms. It is also difficult to achieve adequate pain management, as tolerance to the effect of postoperative opioids must also be considered.

The aim is to bring acute pain under control. Opioid use in the context of pain/analgesia is unlikely to lead to addiction. Reducing high background opioid doses acutely may precipitate withdrawal. Standard postoperative opioid regimes are unlikely to be adequate for opioid-tolerant patients, who are also less likely to suffer side effects such as respiratory depression. Involvement of a multidisciplinary team will often be necessary to manage behavioural, psychological, psychiatric, and medical problems encountered in this group of patients.

Tolerance is a decrease in sensitivity to opioids resulting in less effect from the same dose. Physical dependence is a physiological phenomenon characterized by a withdrawal reaction when the drug is withdrawn or an antagonist is administered. Addiction is a pattern of drug abuse characterized by compulsive use to experience a psychological effect and to avoid a withdrawal reaction. Pseudoaddiction is iatrogenic drug-seeking behaviour normally due to undertreatment of acute pain by the physician.

Symptoms and signs of withdrawal include yawning, sweating, anxiety, rhinorrhoea, lacrimation, tachycardia, hypertension, diarrhoea, nausea, vomiting, abdominal pain, and cramps. On average, these symptoms peak at 36–72 h after the last dose. Aims of treatment must be provision of analgesia, prevention of opioid withdrawal, and management of abnormal drug-taking behaviour. Non-opioid analgesics such as paracetamol and NSAIDs should be prescribed regularly if possible. Opioid-dependent patients normally fall into one of three groups: opioid addicts, chronic non-cancer pain patients, and cancer pain patients. The principles of management are the same for each group. Non-opioid analgesic drugs (e.g. non-steroidal anti-inflammatory drugs, paracetamol and clonidine) and appropriate regional techniques will have the effect of reducing requirements: an 'opioid-sparing effect'.

This patient, when treated with femoral nerve block along with the patient-controlled fentanyl analgesia, has an added advantage, as a short-acting opioid patient-controlled analgesia regime with a shorter lock-out and higher bolus dose is more appropriate.

Mitra S, Sinatra RS. Perioperative management of acute pain in the opioid-dependent patient. *Anesthesiology* 2004; 101: 212–27.

12. Answer: C

During the 2006–2008 triennium, sepsis was the leading cause of direct maternal death, accounting for 26 direct deaths and with a further 3 deaths classified as 'late direct', particularly those associated with Group A streptococcal infection (GAS).

Most of the deaths occurred in the postpartum period; more than half following lower segment caesarean section. Seven women died from sepsis that developed after vaginal delivery, illustrating how healthy women with uncomplicated pregnancy and delivery can become critically ill and die in a very short time.

Prompt investigation and treatment, particularly immediate intravenous antibiotic treatment and early involvement of senior obstetricians, anaesthetists, and critical care consultants, are crucial.

Current sepsis care bundles call for liberal use of fluids and some sepsis deaths were associated with fluid overload and pulmonary oedema.

Centre for Maternal and Child Enquiries (CMACE). *Saving Mothers' Lives*: reviewing maternal deaths to make motherhood safer: 2006–08. The Eighth Report on Confidential Enquiries into Maternal Deaths in the United Kingdom. *BJOG* 2011; 118(Suppl. 1): 1–203.

13. Answer: B

Patients with end-stage liver disease are at significant risk of mobility and mortality after anaesthesia and surgery. Medical and surgical intervention may exacerbate liver dysfunction and result in life-threatening hepatic failure. End-stage liver disease should constitute a relative contraindication to surgical intervention except for life-threatening situations. Death from liver disease and alcoholism increases by 7% a year.

Vaja R, McNicol L, Sisley I. Anaesthesia for patients with liver disease. *Contin Educ Anaesth Crit Care Pain* 2010; 10(1): 15–19.

14. Answer: C

Ruptured AAA is a surgical emergency and a rapid preoperative evaluation is required. The first response of many anaesthetists confronted with a patient with a ruptured AAA is to administer intravenous fluids to rapidly restore blood pressure to near-normal levels. However, excessive administration of fluids prior to clamping of the aorta will increase bleeding through thrombus dislodgement and dilution of clotting factors. A brief and targeted preoperative assessment should be made. Most patients will have extensive atherosclerotic and smoking-related diseases. Many patients have significant coronary artery disease, which is not always obvious from history and examination. Diabetes, hypertension, and renal impairment are also common. Blood pressure should be checked non-invasively in both arms as there may be brachiocephalic and subclavian artery stenosis. If there is a difference in readings, the higher reading should be use.

Leonard A, Thompson J. Anaesthesia for ruptured abdominal aortic aneurysm. *Cont Educ Anaesth Crit Care Pain* 2008; 8(1): 11–15.

15. Answer: D

Postpartum foot drop is caused by damage to the lumbosacral nerve trunk or, less frequently, the common peroneal nerve. The lumbosacral trunk (L4 and L5) is compressed between the ala of the sacrum and the descending foetal head. It may also occur during a forceps delivery. Typically, it occurs in a mother of short stature with a large baby. The result is a unilateral foot drop, with loss of sensation and/or paraesthesia along the lateral calf and foot. Common peroneal nerve damage may occur due to improper or prolonged positioning during lithotomy, and sensory deficit may be limited to the dorsum of the foot. Nerve-conduction studies are required to identify the site of neural damage with any certainty.

Brooks H, May A. Neurological complications following regional anaesthesia in obstetrics. *Br J Anaesth, CEPD Rev* 2003; 3(4): 111–14.

16. Answer: C

Maintenance of an adequate circulation is essential in spinal cord injury in order to minimize secondary ischaemic damage to the injured cord. Hypotension must be treated promptly with fluid boluses in the first instance. In the polytrauma patient who is hypotensive, hypovolaemia secondary to haemorrhage from concurrent injuries must be excluded according to ATLS principles. Remember that the patient with a high spinal cord injury will not complain of pain from a fractured pelvis or other injuries. Intra-abdominal bleeding is more difficult to diagnose when the abdominal muscles are flaccid.

Neurogenic shock

Hypotension occurs with lesions above T6 due to loss of sympathetic autonomic function and unopposed parasympathetic function. Vasoconstrictor tone is lost and venous pooling occurs. Loss of cardiac accelerator fibres results in bradycardia and patients are unable to increase cardiac output by changes in heart rate. Although the duration of neurogenic shock is variable, recovery tends to be incomplete and postural hypotension can be a persistent problem.

Septic shock is not a acute presentation in trauma patients.

Denton M, McKinlay J. Cervical cord injury and critical care. *Cont Educ Anaesth Crit Care Pain* 2009; 9(3): 82–86.

Veale P, Lamb J. Anaesthesia and acute spinal cord injury. *Br J Anaesth CEPD Rev* 2002; 2(5): 139–43.

17. Answer: C

Intra-arotic balloon pumps (IABP) are used for stabilization of patients with acute myocardial infarction referred for urgent cardiac surgery. IABP support is often initiated in the cardiac catheterization laboratory and continued through the perioperative period. Elective placement is considered in high-risk patients such as those with significant left main stem disease, severe LV dysfunction (ejection fraction <30%), congestive heart failure, cardiomyopathy, chronic renal failure, or cerebrovascular disease. Weaning from cardiopulmonary bypass may be difficult in cases where aortic cross-clamping is prolonged, revascularization is only partially achieved, or preexisting myocardial dysfunction is present. Separation from cardiopulmonary bypass may be marked by hypotension and a low cardiac index despite the administration of inotropic drugs. The use of IABP in this setting decreases LV resistance, increases cardiac output, and increases coronary and systemic perfusion, facilitating the patient's weaning from cardiopulmonary bypass.

Krishna M, Zacharowski K. Principles of intra-aortic balloon pump counter pulsation. *Cont Educ Anaesth Crit Care Pain* 2009; 9(1): 24–28.

18. Answer: D

This lady has local anaesthetic toxicity without cardiorespiratory arrest, as the local anaesthetic used was levo-bupivacaine rather than prilocaine, which is advised for Bier's block as it is less cardiotoxic.

Signs of severe toxicity include:

- sudden alteration in mental status, severe agitation or loss of consciousness, with or without tonic-clonic convulsions.
- cardiovascular collapse: sinus bradycardia, conduction blocks, asystole, and ventricular tachyarrhythmias

Local anaesthetic (LA) toxicity may occur sometime after an initial injection.

Immediate management steps are:

- Stop injecting the LA.
- Call for help.
- Maintain the airway and, if necessary, secure it with a tracheal tube.
- Give 100% oxygen and ensure adequate lung ventilation (hyperventilation may help by increasing plasma pH in the presence of metabolic acidosis).
- Confirm or establish intravenous access.
- Control seizures: give a benzodiazepine, thiopental, or propofol in small incremental doses.

- Assess cardiovascular status throughout.
- Consider drawing blood for analysis, but do not delay definitive treatment to do this.

Without circulatory arrest

Use conventional therapies to treat:

- hypotension
- bradycardia
- tachyarrhythmia.

Consider intravenous lipid emulsion. Give an initial intravenous bolus injection of 20% lipid emulsion 1.5 mL/kg over 1 min followed by an infusion in accordance with the guidelines.

Management of Severe Local Anaesthetic Toxicity. AAGBI Safety Guideline, 2010. http://www.aagbi.org/publications/guidelines.htm.

19. Answer: E

Acute lung injury (ALI) is a condition that is diagnosed clinically and radiologically based on the presence of non-cardiogenic pulmonary oedema and respiratory failure in a critically ill patient.

The diagnostic criteria for ALI are:

- acute onset
- presence of bilateral infiltrates on CXR consistent with oedema
- PAWP <18 mmHg or clinical absence of left atrial hypertension
- hypoxaemia, with PaO_2/FiO_2 < 40 (if PaO_2/FiO_2 < 27, the term ARDS is used).

Mackay A, Al-Haddad M. Acute lung injury and acute respiratory distress syndrome. *Cont Educ Anaesth Crit Care Pain* 2009; 9(5): 152–56.

20. Answer: D

Consider giving intravenous magnesium sulphate to women with severe pre-eclampsia who are in a critical care setting if birth is planned within 24 h. If considering magnesium sulphate treatment, use the following as features of severe preeclampsia:

- severe hypertension and proteinuria or
- mild or moderate hypertension and proteinuria with one or more of the following:
    - symptoms of severe headache
    - problems with vision, such as blurring or flashing before the eyes
    - severe pain just below the ribs or vomiting
    - papilloedema
    - signs of clonus (3 beats)
    - liver tenderness
    - HELLP syndrome
    - platelet count falling to below 100 × 10^9 /L
    - abnormal liver enzymes (ALT or AST rising to above 70 IU/L).

Use the collaborative eclampsia trial regimen for administration of magnesium sulphate:

- loading dose of 4 g should be given intravenously over 5 min, followed by an infusion of 1 g/h maintained for 24 h
- recurrent seizures should be treated with a further dose of 2–4 g given over 5 min.

Hypertension in Pregnancy: the Management of Hypertensive Disorders during Pregnancy. NICE guidelines, August 2010. http://guidance.nice.org.uk/CG107.

21. Answer: A

Paracetamol overdose is a life-threatening occurrence and is likely after ingestion of >10–15 g of paracetamol. Paracetamol is rapidly absorbed and metabolized by conjugation in the liver. Hepatic necrosis occurs due to toxicity of an alkylating metabolite normally removed by conjugation with glutathione. With overdose, glutathione is rapidly depleted and may already be low in cases of starvation, and among alcoholics and those with HIV, thus predisposing these groups to an increased risk of toxicity.

Toxicity is usually asymptomatic for 1–2 days, although laboratory assessment of liver function may become abnormal as early as 18 h after ingestion. Hepatic failure develops after 2–7 days.

Complications

The major complication is hepatic (with or without renal) failure. A rise in prothrombin time, INR, and bilirubin are early warning signs of significant hepatic damage and this should prompt early referral to a specialist centre.

Guidelines for referral to a specialist liver centre

- Arterial pH < 7.3.
- INR > 3 on day 2 or > 4 thereafter.
- Oliguria and/or rising creatinine.
- Altered conscious level.
- Hypoglycaemia.

Guidelines for liver transplantation

- Arterial pH < 7.3.
- All the following:
  - PT > 100, INR > 6.5
  - creatinine > 200 mol/L
  - grade 3–4 encephalopathy.

High lactate levels (> 3.5 mmol/L at 4 h and 12 h) and low factor V levels are also associated with a poor outcome if not transplanted.

Lai WK, Murphy N. Management of acute liver failure. *Contin Educ Anaesth Crit Care Pain* 2004; 4(2): 40–43.

22. Answer: E

Management of asthma

Asthmatics must be managed in a well-monitored area. If clinical features are severe, they should be admitted to an intensive care unit where rapid institution of mechanical ventilation is available. Monitoring should comprise, as a minimum, pulse oximetry, continuous ECG, regular blood pressure measurement, and blood gas analysis. If severe, an intra-arterial cannula with or without central venous access should be inserted.

Treatment is as follows:

1. FiO_2 to maintain SpO_2 in the range 92–98%.
2. Nebulized B₂-agonist (e.g. salbutamol) may be repeated every 2–4 h or, in severe attacks, administered continuously.
3. IV corticosteroids for 24 h, then oral prednisolone. Nebulized ipratropium bromide rarely gives additional benefit and may thicken sputum.
4. IV bronchodilators, e.g. salbutamol, magnesium sulphate.
5. Exclude pneumothorax and lung/lobar collapse with a chest X-ray.
6. Ensure adequate hydration and fluid replacement.
7. Commence antibiotics in accordance with local protocols if there is strong evidence of bacterial chest infection. Green sputum does not necessarily indicate a bacterial infection.

8. If no response to above measures or *in extremis*, consider:
   - IV salbutamol infusion
   - epinephrine SC or by nebulizer
   - mechanical ventilation.

Anecdotal success has been reported with sub-anaesthetic doses of a volatile anaesthetic agent such as isoflurane or sevoflurane, which both calm/sedate and bronchodilate.

Indications for mechanical ventilation are:
   - increasing fatigue
   - respiratory failure—rising $PaCO_2$, falling PaO_2
   - cardiovascular collapse.

Singer M, Webb AR. *Oxford Handbook of Critical Care*, 3rd edn. Oxford University Press, 2009: p. 106.

23. Answer: D

This patient has an airway compromised by a tumour and there is a potential to obstruct the airway after administration of neuromuscular blockers. The intubation would then be extremely difficult as the anatomy is altered by the tumour and it would be narrow.

Seventy two cases reported in the National Audit Project 4: *Major Complications of Airway Management in the United Kingdom* (NAP4) involved an airway problem in association with an acute or chronic disease process in the head, neck, or trachea. Approximately 70% of these cases were associated with obstructive lesions within the airway.

Cook TM, Woodall N, Frerk C. Major Complications of Airway Management in the UK: Results of the Fourth National Audit Project of the Royal College of Anaesthetists and the Difficult Airway Society. Part 1: Anaesthesia. *Br J Anaesth* 2011; 106(5); 617–31.

National Audit Project 4: *Major Complications of Airway Management in the United Kingdom*. Royal College of Anaesthetists, 2011. http://www.rcoa.ac.uk/docs/NAP4_Section2.pdf.

24. Answer: C

Tourniquet is used widely for limb procedures. Complications are rare but can be severe. Most literature recommends a maximum inflation time of 1.5–2 h, followed by break of 10–15 min, which should be used to allow regeneration of muscle ATP. After 15 and 45 min a physiological conduction block affecting both motor and sensory nerve fibres prevents nerve transmission to and from distal to the tourniquet site.

The pain from the tourniquet site itself may be the cause of the 'tourniquet hypertension' seen with increasing duration of tourniquet inflation. This can be treated by use of ketamine (low dose), clonidine, and even topical local anaesthetic cream.

Every 30 min a tourniquet is inflated there is a threefold increase in the incidence of neurological damage. Younger patients are more likely to have neurological damage following prolonged tourniquet time. Pain transmission from distal to the tourniquet will be absent after 1 h. Changes in CO_2 can cause a marked change in cerebral blood flow. Ketamine has been shown to reduce 'tourniquet hypertension'.

Deloughry JL, Griffiths, R. Arterial tourniquets. *Contin Educ Anaesth Crit Care Pain* 2009; 9: 56–60.

25. Answer: D

The patient was presented in a comatose state, suffering from seizures and marked cardiovascularly instability. This requires treating the patient as per the resuscitation guidelines. Hence once initial resuscitation and tracheal intubation have been achieved, the appropriate treatment would be to manage cocaine toxicity. Cocaine is both a local anaesthetic and lipophilic; the appropriate step is immediate administration of lipid emulsion. A 20% lipid emulsion (Intralipid; Frasenius Kabi, Runcorn, UK) is administered intravenously as an initial bolus dose of 1.5 mL/kg (120 mL), followed by an infusion of 15 mL/kg/h (380 ml) over 20 min.

Cocaine poisoning

Modes of action are:

- blocks reuptake of dopamine (causing euphoria, hyperactivity) and norepinephrine (causing vasoconstriction and hypertension); arrhythmias may also result
- blocks Na$^+$ channels, resulting in a local anaesthetic action and myocardial depression
- platelet activation
- mitochondrial dysfunction leading to myocardial depression.

Complications include:

- chest pain related to myocardial ischaemia or infarction, or to coronary artery spasm
- heart failure
- seizures
- cerebrovascular accidents
- pneumothorax
- rhabdomyolysis
- premature labour—abruption
- agitated delirium
- hyperthermia.

Jakkala-Saibaba R, Morgan PG, Morton PL. Treatment of cocaine overdose with lipid emulsion. *Anaesthesia* 2011; 66(12): 1168–70.

Management of Severe Local Anaesthetic Toxicity. AAGBI safety guideline, 2010 http://www.aagbi.org/publications/guidelines.htm.

26. Answer: A

The diagnosis here is severe diabetic ketoacidosis (DKA) with associated acidosis and shortness of breath along with hyperkalaemia. It requires critical care admission with immediate resuscitation and monitoring. The acidosis should be treated by fluid resuscitation and shutting off ketone production. Hyperkalaemia will also be treated by insulin therapy. Rapid fluid resuscitation has a risk of cerebral oedema, hence carefully monitored resuscitation with CVP is appropriate along with insulin therapy. Classical management of DKA focuses on using fluids and insulin to lower elevated blood glucose.

Patients with DKA have a significant fluid deficit and are often water-depleted by up to 100 mL/kg, as well as associated electrolytes deficit. A fixed-rate insulin infusion at 0.1 units/kg is recommended, which will lead to suppression of ketogenesis, reduction of glycosaemia, and correction of electrolyte imbalance.

The aim is to reduce blood ketones by 0.5 mmol/L/h, increase the bicarbonate by 3 mmol/L/h, reduce the blood glucose by 3 mmol/L/h and maintain potassium concentration between 4.0 and 5.0 mmol/L. Insulin is infused at fixed rate of 0.1 U/kg/h. The response to insulin infusion pump is reviewed after 1 h. If blood glucose is not dropping by 5 mmol/h and capillary ketones by 1 mmol/L, the infusion rate is increased by 1 U/h. The increase in insulin infusion rate may be repeated hourly if necessary to achieve reduction in blood glucose and capillary ketones. Monitor blood glucose, capillary ketones, and urine output hourly.

The Management of Diabetic Ketoacidosis in Adults. Joint British Diabetes Societies Inpatient Care Group, 2010. http://www.diabetes.nhs.uk/our_publications/reports_and_guidance/inpatient_and_emergency/.

British Society of Paediatric Endocrinology and Diabetes (BSPED) guidelines. http://www.bsped.org.uk/professional/guidelines/docs/DKAGuideline.

27. Answer: D

The nerve supply of the larynx is derived from the vagus nerve. The nerves are the superior laryngeal nerve and the recurrent laryngeal nerve.

The superior laryngeal nerve arises from the middle of the ganglion nodosum and in its course receives a branch from the superior cervical ganglion of the sympathetic. It descends, by the side of the pharynx, behind the internal carotid artery and, below and anterior to greater cornua of hyoid bone, divides into two branches:

- internal laryngeal nerve supplies mucous membrane down to the vocal cords
- external laryngeal nerve supplies cricothyroid muscle and inferior constrictor muscle of the pharynx.

The recurrent laryngeal nerve:

- supplies all intrinsic laryngeal muscles except the cricothyroid, and the mucous membrane of the larynx below the vocal cords, which is innervated by the external branch of the superior laryngeal nerve
- motor to all intrinsic muscles of larynx and sensory supply below cords.

All the muscles of the larynx, except the cricothyroid muscle, are innervated by the recurrent laryngeal nerve. The cricothyroid muscle is innervated by the superior laryngeal nerve (external branch).

28. Answer: D

The pharyngeal reflex or gag reflex is a reflex contraction of the back of the throat, evoked by touching the soft palate or sometimes the back of the tongue. The gag reflex involves elevation and constriction of the pharynx following stimulation of the posterior pharyngeal wall. The afferent pathway is via the glossopharyngeal nerve (IX), the efferent pathway is via the vagus (X). The clinical relevance of an absent gag reflex is in indicating an airway at risk or as part of brain-stem death testing.

29. Answer: D

This case is not urgent and should be postponed for further investigation by the cardiologist. The parents are very anxious and a full explanation would be very useful via a letter to their GP. In an infant with a murmur, a history of recurrent chest infections, cyanosis, tachypnoea, sweating, feeding difficulties, and failure to thrive is suggestive of pathological heart disease. Most congenital cardiac disease is identified before 3 months of age, but any child under 1 year with a murmur should be referred to a paediatric cardiologist before anaesthesia, even if asymptomatic, as significant lesions can be slow to present.

Bhatia N, Barber N. Dilemmas in the preoperative assessment of children. *Contin Educ Anaesth Crit Care Pain* 2011; 11(6): 214–218.

30. Answer: D

The steroids' mechanism of action is unknown. Ondansetron antagonizes 5HT3 receptors centrally and peripherally; haloperidol causes central dopaminergic (D2) blockade and post-synaptic GABA antagonism; cyclizine is a competitive histamine H_1 antagonist and blocks centrally located H1 receptors and also has some anticholinergic activity at the muscarinic M1, M2, and M3 receptors. The antiemetic effect of metoclopramide seems to be mediated by central dopaminergic (D2) blockade and a decrease in the sensitivity of nerves supplying afferent information to the vomiting centre.

Gwinnu, C. Postoperative nausea and vomiting; In: Allman KG, Wilson IH (eds), *Oxford Handbook of Anaesthesia*. Oxford University Press, Oxford, 2004: p. 1049.

Single Best Answers—Mini Exam 2

1. Answer: E

Fat embolism is commonly seen in patients with major trauma, especially with long bones. The clinical feature described in the question suggests there is embolization of fat and microaggregates of platelets, RBCs, and fibrin in the systemic and pulmonary circulation. Pulmonary damage may result directly from the emboli (infarction) or by a chemical pneumonitis and adult respiratory distress syndrome (ARDS).

The diagnosis is based on clinical presentation of symptoms, which usually appear 1–3 days after injury. Onset is sudden, with presenting symptoms of tachypnea, dyspnoea, and tachycardia. The most significant feature is the potentially severe respiratory effects, which may result in ARDS. Neurologic symptoms may also be present; initial irritability, confusion, and restlessness may progress to delirium or coma. Petechiae appear on the trunk and face and in the axillary folds, conjunctiva and fundi in up to 50% of patients, which helps in diagnosis. Of these symptoms, respiratory insufficiency, central neurologic impairment, and petechial rash are considered major diagnostic criteria, and tachycardia, fever, retinal fat emboli, lipiduria, anaemia, and thrombocytopenia are considered minor diagnostic criteria.

There is no specific therapy for fat embolism syndrome; prevention, early diagnosis, and adequate symptomatic treatment are of paramount importance. Supportive care includes maintenance of adequate oxygenation and ventilation, stable haemodynamics, blood products as clinically indicated, hydration, prophylaxis of deep venous thrombosis and stress-related gastrointestinal bleeding, and nutrition. The goals of pharmacotherapy are to reduce morbidity and prevent complications. Supportive care is the mainstay of therapy for clinically apparent cases of fat embolism syndrome. Mortality is estimated to be 5–15% overall, but most patients will recover fully.

As the patient had no head or chest injury the most appropriate next step would be to transfer the patient to critical care. This will ensure adequate monitoring along with the supportive treatment.

Gupta A, Reilly CS. Fat embolism. *Cont Educ Anaesth Crit Care Pain* 2007; 7(5): 148–51.

2. Answer: C

Signs of infection are contraindications to central neuraxial block.

Relative contraindications are:

- aortic stenosis/mitral stenosis (profound hypotension—sympathetic block)
- previous back surgery (technical difficulty)
- neurological disease (medicolegal)
- systemic sepsis (increased incidence of epidural abscess, meningitis).

Absolute contraindications are:

- local sepsis
- patient refusal
- anticoagulation.

Eldridge J. Obstetric anaesthesia and analgesia. In: Allman KG, Wilson IH, (eds), *Oxford Handbook of Anaesthesia*, 2nd edn. Oxford University Press, 2006: p. 1098.

3. Answer: D

A review of the DNAR decision by the anaesthetist and surgeon with the patient, proxy decision maker, other doctor in charge of the patient's care, and relatives or carers, if indicated, is essential before proceeding with surgery and anaesthesia. Surgery can proceed despite the presence of a DNAR decision if it is in the patient's best interests at that time.

Medical conditions that may require anaesthesia for operative interventions in a patient with a DNAR decision include:

- provision of a support device (e.g. a feeding tube)
- urgent surgery for a condition unrelated to the underlying chronic problem (e.g. acute appendicitis)
- urgent surgery for a condition related to the underlying chronic problem but not believed to be a terminal event (e.g. bowel obstruction)
- procedure to decrease pains (e.g. repair of fractured neck of femur)
- procedure to provide vascular access.

Do Not Attempt Resuscitation (DNAR) Decisions in the Perioperative Period. AAGBI guideline, 2009. http://www.aagbi.org/sites/default/files/DNAR_may09.pdf.

4. Answer: C

A burns patient who has sustained burns over more than 25% of total body surface area (TBSA) produces a marked systemic inflammatory response accompanied by an increase in capillary permeability and generalized oedema. These patients require fluids for both resuscitation and maintenance. Hartmann's solution is the preferred resuscitation fluid. Various formulae have been suggested to calculate the fluid requirements in these patients. A modified Parklands formula is one of most commonly used.

Modified Parklands formula

4 mL/kg/% total body surface area/24 h

The total volume of Hartmann's solution for the first 24 h = 4 mL × 85 × 40 = 13 600 mL. Half the volume is administered in the first 8 h, the rest is delivered over the next 16 h. (Hartmann's solution × bodyweight [kg] × % burn.).

Maintenance fluids are required in addition to the calculated resuscitation fluid. These calculated values are merely an estimate, while the precise volumes required will be guided by urine output (>0.5–1.0 mL/kg) and cardiovascular response.

Mount Vernon formula

The Mount Vernon formula is also used for resuscitation in burns patients:

0.5 × weight in kg × %TBSA (mL) of 4.5 % human albumin in each six periods over 36 h.

Latenser BA. Critical care of the burn patient: the first 48 hours. *Crit Care Med* 2009; 37(10): 2819–26.

Nolan J. The critically ill patient. Burns: early management. In: Allman KG, Wilson IH, (eds), *Oxford Handbook of Anaesthesia*, 2nd edn. Oxford University Press, 2006: Chapter 34.

5. Answer: A

Hyperaldoesteronism is a condition in which excessive aldosterone is secreted by the adrenal gland. This is featured where there are low potassium levels in blood. Clinical features are hypertension, hypokelemia, and alkalosis. Aldosterone is a steroid hormone (mineralocorticoid family) produced by the outer-section (zona glomerulosa) of the adrenal cortex in the adrenal gland, and acts on the distal tubules and collecting ducts of the nephron, the functioning unit of the kidney, to cause the conservation of sodium, secretion of potassium, increased water retention, and increased blood pressure. The overall effect of aldosterone is to increase reabsorption of ions and water in the kidney.

Aldosterone tends to promote Na^+ and water retention, and lower plasma K^+ concentration. Hence excessive aldoesterone secretion leads to excessive renal absorption of sodium in exchange for potassium and increased secretion of hydrogen ions in the collecting duct.

Conn JW. Presidential address. I. Painting background. II. Primary aldosteronism, a new clinical syndrome. *J Lab Clin Med* 1955; 45: 3–17.

Young WF. Primary aldosteronism: renaissance of a syndrome. *Clin Endocrinol (Oxf)* 2007; 66: 607–18.

6. Answer: B

This is a case of anaphylaxis, an acute emergency situation. Anaphylaxis is an IgE-mediated type B hypersensitivity reaction to an antigen, resulting in histamine and serotonin release from mast cells and basophils. The common clinical presentation is cardiovascular collapse, erythema, bronchospasm, oedema, and rash.

Immediate management steps are as follows:

1. Use the ABC approach (airway, breathing and circulation). Team working enables several tasks to be accomplished simultaneously.
2. Remove all potential causative agents (including IV colloids, latex, and chlorhexidine) and maintain anaesthesia, if necessary, with an inhalational agent.
3. Call for help and note the time.
4. Maintain the airway and administer oxygen 100%. Intubate the trachea if necessary and ventilate the lungs with oxygen.
5. Elevate the patient's legs if there is hypotension.
6. If appropriate, start cardiopulmonary resuscitation immediately according to the *Advanced Life Support Guidelines*.
7. Administer adrenaline intravenously. An initial dose of 50 mcg (0.5 mL of 1: 10 000 solution) is appropriate (adult dose). Several doses may be required if there is severe hypotension or bronchospasm.
8. If several doses of adrenaline are required, consider starting an intravenous infusion of adrenaline (adrenaline has a short half-life).
9. Administer saline 0.9% or lactated Ringer's solution at a high rate via an intravenous cannula of an appropriate gauge (large volumes may be required).

Harper NJ, Dixon T, Dugué P, *et al*. Suspected anaphylactic reactions associated with anaesthesia. *Anaesthesia* 2009; 64(2): 199–211. http://www.aagbi.org/sites/default/files/anaphylaxis_2009_0.pdf.

Anaphylaxis Algorithm. UK Resuscitation Council, 2008. http://www.resus.org.uk/pages/anaalgo.pdf.

7. Answer: D

The development of a spinal haematoma is a rare but potentially devastating complication of central neuraxial blockade. Monitoring of sensory and motor block is essential for the early detection of potentially serious complications. The Bromage scale is an accepted tool for the measurement of motor block. An increasing degree of motor weakness usually implies excessive epidural drug administration. However, it can indicate very serious complications including dural penetration of the catheter or the development of an epidural haematoma or abscess. Therefore, it is essential that protocols are in place to manage the scenario of excessive motor block. As a working rule of thumb, some recovery should be seen within 4 h and if this is not seen, further assessment and investigation to exclude major complications is required. Examples of suitable algorithms and specific advice on protocols for this situation are given in the report on the audit of major complications of central neuraxial block performed by the Royal College of Anaesthetists.

An epidural abscess or haematoma can cause severe, permanent neurological damage and must be detected and treated as soon as possible. This diagnosis must be considered if excessive motor block does not resolve rapidly after stopping the epidural infusion. A clear protocol should be in place describing the actions required in this situation, including informing senior anaesthetic staff and immediate availability of suitable imaging and surgical expertise.

Major Complications of Central Neuraxial Block in the UK. Royal College of Anaesthetists, 2009. http://www.rcoa.ac.uk/index.asp?PageID=717.

Best Practice in the Management of Epidural Analgesia in the Hospital Setting. Faculty of Pain Medicine, Royal College of Anaesthetists, Association of Anaesthetists of Great Britain and Ireland, and British Pain Society, 2011. http://www.aagbi.org/sites/default/files/epidural_analgesia_2011.pdf.

Cook TM, Counsell D, Wildsmith JAW. Major complications of central neuraxial block: report on the Third National Audit Project of the Royal College of Anaesthetists. *Br J Anaesth* 2009; 102(2): 179–90.

8. Answer: A

The transplant heart has no autonomic innervations; the resting heart rate is typically 90–100 bpm due to the loss of vagal tone. Normal autonomic system responses are lost (beat-to-beat variation in heart rate, response to Valsalva manoeuvre/carotid sinus massage). Contractility of the heart is close to normal. The transplanted heart should be viewed as permanently denervated. This results in poor tolerance of acute hypovolaemia. An adequate preload must be maintained in a patient with a transplanted heart, as there is a lack of rapid homeostatic adjustments in the heart. Hence wide varation in vascular resistance can produce wide swings in blood pressure, which can be troublesome during anaesthesia.

If pharmacological manipulation is required then direct-acting agents should be used: atropine has no effect on the denervated heart, the effect of ephedrine is reduced and unpredictable, and hydralazine and phenylephrine produce no reflex tachy- or bradycardia in response to their primary action. Adrenaline, noradrenaline, isoprenaline, and β- and α-blockers act as expected.

Direct chronotropic agents should be available in case of bradycardia, as atropine cannot be used. Vagolytic drugs do not work in the denervated heart.

Morgan-Hughes NJ, Hood G. Anaesthesia for a patient with a cardiac transplant. *Cont Educ Anaesth Crit Care Pain* 2002; 2(3): 74–78.

9. Answer: D

Myotonic dystrophy is an autosomal dominant disorder, with an incidence of 2.4–5.5 cases per 100 000 in the UK. The locus for myotonic dystrophy is on chromosome 19. Findings include myotonia (incomplete muscle relaxation, especially the inability to 'let go' after a hand grip), muscle wasting, cardiac abnormalities (conduction defects, cardiomyopathy, structural deformities), respiratory abnormalities (restrictive lung disease and obstructive sleep apnoea), endocrine dysfunction, and intellectual impairment.

Anaesthetic considerations

Factors that may precipitate myotonias must be avoided where possible. These include hypothermia, shivering, and mechanical and electrical stimulation. There may be increased sensitivity to sedatives and analgesics due to the respiratory involvement and therefore these agents should be used judiciously. Depolarizing neuromuscular blocking agents may induce generalized muscular contractures and are therefore not recommended. Non-depolarizing neuromuscular blocking agents are not associated with myotonias, but the use of anti-cholinesterase drugs may precipitate contractures due to the increased sensitivity to acetylcholine. Glucose metabolism may be affected as part of the disease, and therefore levels should be monitored perioperatively. Bulbar muscle weakness may result in aspiration. Conduction defects may require access to pacemaker equipment.

Marsh S, Ross N, Pittard A. Neuromuscular disorders and anaesthesia. Part 2: specific neuromuscular disorders. *Cont Educ Anaesth Crit Care Pain* 2011; 11(4): 115–18.

10. Answer: C

Guillain–Barré syndrome is an immune-mediated polyneuropathy that often follows a viral or bacterial illness within the preceding 4 weeks. The weakness typically ascends from the legs and is symmetrical. Sensory and autoimmune dysfunction can also occur. Ascending weakness can lead to respiratory compromise, requiring prolonged ventilatory support and bulbar dysfunction. The use of depolarizing neuromuscular blocking agents should be avoided even following a long period after recovering from the neurological deficit, as the risk of hyperkalaemic cardiac arrest after depolarizing neuromuscular blocking agents may persist. There may be increased sensitivity to non-depolarizing neuromuscular blocking agents.

Marsh S, Ross N, Pittard A. Neuromuscular disorders and anaesthesia. Part 2: specific neuromuscular disorders. *Cont Educ Anaesth Crit Care Pain* 2011; 11(4): 115–18.

11. Answer: E

The most common symptoms of diabetic neuropathy include pain, burning, tingling, or numbness in the toes or feet, and extreme sensitivity to light touch. The pain may be worst at rest and improve with activity, such as walking. Some people initially have intensely painful feet while others have few or no symptoms.

The first line pharmacological management for diabetic neuropathic pain according to the NICE guideline is duloxetine.

- Class of drug: antidepressant—serotonin/norepinephrine reuptake inhibition.
- Mode of action: 5-HT/NE reuptake inhibition.
- Indications: first-line treatment of diabetic neuropathy.
- Contraindications: hepatic impairment, renal impairment (avoid if GFR < 30 mL/min), pregnancy, breast feeding.

Neuropathic Pain, the Pharmacological Management of Neuropathic Pain in Adults in Non-specialist Settings. NICE guideline, March 2010. http://www.nice.org.uk/CG96.

12. Answer: E

The finding of increased postoperative pain and postoperative opioid consumption in a patient receiving a high rather than low intraoperative opioid dose indicates the possibility of opioid-induced hyperalgesia. Management of postoperative analgesia in patients with opioid dependency is challenging—firstly to differentiate addiction from dependence and avoid opioid withdrawal symptoms, and secondly to achieve adequate pain management, as tolerance to the effect of postoperative opioids must also be considered. Fear of pain can induce requests for increased opioids, which can be mistaken for addiction. Non-opioid analgesic drugs (e.g. non-steroidal anti-inflammatory drugs, paracetamol, and clonidine) and appropriate regional techniques will have the effect of reducing requirements: an 'opioid-sparing effect'.

This patient will require her baseline preoperative opioid dose and a provision made for 'as required' dosing for breakthrough pain. In this scenario, a short-acting opioid patient-controlled analgesia regime with a shorter lock-out and/or a higher bolus dose is more appropriate to her needs.

The opioid-induced hyperalgesia occurs when opioid drugs prescribed for pain relief may paradoxically make the patient more sensitive to painful stimuli.

Tolerance is defined as a reduced effect for an equivalent dose or the requirement of increased doses to attain the same effect. It can occur with strong opioids such as morphine and oxycodone within 1–2 weeks, so in this case a larger dose of opioid will be required to achieve adequate analgesia. Tolerance, however, also develops to some of the side effects of opioids, making patients less likely to suffer from respiratory depression, itching, and nausea than opioid-naive patients, but careful monitoring is still required.

Cancer Pain Management. British Pain Society, London, 2010. http://www.britishpainsociety.org/book_cancer_pain.pdf.

13. Answer: C

Gabapentin (1–[aminomethyl] cyclohexane-acetic acid) is an antiepileptic drug. Recently it has been used in acute pain. There is considerable overlap in their pathophysiology of acute pain. Allodynia and hyperalgesia are cardinal signs and symptoms of neuropathic pain but they are also often present after trauma and surgery. Sensitization of neurones in the dorsal horns, a mechanism in neuropathic pain, has been demonstrated in acute pain models. The persistence of this mechanism may be responsible for the increasingly recognized problem of chronic pain after surgery.

Gabapentin has a high binding affinity for the $\alpha_2\delta$ subunit of the presynaptic voltage-gated calcium channels, which inhibits calcium influx and subsequent release of excitatory neurotransmitters in the pain pathways. It reduces the membrane voltage-gated calcium currents (VGCC channels) in dorsal horn ganglion neurons. It has high affinity for the subunit of the pre-synaptic VGCC channels, which inhibits calcium influx and subsequent release of excitatory neurotransmitters by sensory neurons. It increases serotonin concentrations in the brain. Gabapentin does not affect nociceptive thresholds but has a selective effect on the nociceptive process involving central sensitization. As well as a direct analgesic effect, gabapentin may prevent and/or reverse opioid tolerance.

Editorial II: Gabapentin: a new drug for postoperative pain? Br. J. Anaesth 2006; 96(2): 152–55.

14. Answer: D

The blood gas provides a picture of respiratory alkalosis and metabolic acidosis. This is a typical picture of aspirin overdose. Serious, life-threatening toxicity is likely after ingestion of >7.5 g salicylate with plasma concentrations >350 mg/L (2.5 mmol/L). Aspirin (acetyl salicylic acid) is the most common form ingested.

Symptoms

Common features include vomiting, dehydration, tinnitus, vertigo, deafness, sweating, warm extremities with bounding pulses, increased respiratory rate, and hyperventilation. Some degree of acid–base disturbance is present in most cases. A mixed respiratory alkalosis and metabolic acidosis with normal or high arterial pH (normal or reduced hydrogen ion concentration) is usual in adults. Acidosis may increase salicylate transfer across the blood–brain barrier. Uncommon features include haematemesis, hyperpyrexia, hypoglycaemia, hypokalaemia, thrombocytopaenia, increased INR/PTR, intravascular coagulation, renal failure, and non-cardiac pulmonary oedema. Central nervous system features including confusion, disorientation, coma, and convulsions are less common in adults than in children.

Management

Give activated charcoal if an adult presents within 1 h of ingestion of more than 250 mg/kg. The plasma salicylate concentration should be measured, although the severity of poisoning cannot be determined from this alone and the clinical and biochemical features must be taken into account. Elimination is increased by urinary alkalinization, which is achieved by the administration of 1.26% sodium bicarbonate. The urine pH should be monitored. Correct metabolic acidosis with intravenous 8.4% sodium bicarbonate (first check serum potassium). Forced diuresis should not be used since it does not enhance salicylate excretion and may cause pulmonary oedema. Haemodialysis is the treatment of choice for severe poisoning and should be considered in patients with plasma salicylate concentrations >700 mg/L (5.1 mmol/L), or lower concentrations associated with severe clinical or metabolic features. Patients under 10 years or over 70 have increased risk of salicylate toxicity and may require dialysis at an earlier stage.

Dargan PI, Wallace CI, Jones AL. An evidence based flowchart to guide the management of acute salicylate (aspirin) overdose. *Emerg Med J* 2002; 19: 206–209.

15. Answer: D

Hyponatremia is defined as a serum sodium concentration of <135 mmol/L. Iatrogenic hyponatremia is not uncommon and usually results from the administration of inappropriately hypotonic fluids, often in the postoperative period when ADH levels are raised as part of the stress response. Symptoms and signs of hyponatremia are:

- moderate: lethargy, nausea, vomiting, anorexia, thirst, irritability, headache and muscle weakness/cramps
- severe: hyporeflexia, drowsiness and confusion, seizures, coma and death.

Bradshaw K, Smith M. Disorders of sodium balance after brain injury. *Contin Educ Anaesth Crit Care Pain* 2008; 8(4): 129–33.

16. Answer: E

Combined spinal–epidural is the best option when inserted above the level of the lesion and will cover the lower segments as well.

Spina bifida occulta is part of a spectrum of congenital abnormalities resulting from failed closure of the neural tube. The incidence, ranging from 10–25% of the population, is decreasing due to folate supplementation. Magnetic resonance imaging is mandatory to exclude the presence of a tethered spinal cord, after which it is acceptable to perform regional anaesthesia at a level not affected by the abnormality. This can be achieved with either a combined spinal–epidural, with a low-dose spinal component and either saline or local anaesthetic extension of the block, or an incremental epidural technique.

There is an increased risk of dural puncture with an epidural, due to abnormal supporting ligaments. Excessive cranial spread of epidural local anaesthetic can occur, and due to altered dural permeability and a reduced epidural space, smaller drug volumes are required. An insertion site above the level of the lesion is usually chosen, but there can also be poor caudal spread of local anaesthetic. This can either be overcome by the use of a second epidural catheter placed below the level of the defect or a spinal catheter can be used to manipulate block height, but cautiously, since spinal doses can also be unpredictable. Spina bifida is also associated with difficult intubation and the necessary precautions must be taken if general anaesthesia is indicated.

Griffiths S, Durbridge JA. Anaesthetic implications of neurological disease in pregnancy. *Cont Educ Anaesth Crit Care Pain* 2011; 11(5): 157–61.

17. Answer: E

The Children's Act 1989 and contains a list of key roles, the guiding principle being that of the child's best interests. A mother always has parental responsibility for her child. Fathers married to the mother at the time of birth have parental responsibility. With regard to unmarried fathers the law was changed in the last decade and the change pertains to children born on or after the following dates: 15 April 2002 in Northern Ireland, 1 December 2003 in England and Wales, and 4 May 2006 in Scotland. After these dates, unmarried fathers automatically have parental responsibility, provided they are named on the child's birth certificate. Fathers not named on the birth certificate and all unmarried fathers of children born before these dates do not automatically have parental responsibility and therefore cannot give valid consent to medical treatment. Unmarried fathers without parental responsibility can apply for a court order to give them parental responsibility. Gillick competence applies to older children who are capable of understanding the proposed treatment and its risks.

Williams CA, Perkins R. Consent issues for children: a law unto themselves? *Contin Educ Anaesth Crit Care Pain* 2011; 11(3): 99–103.

18. Answer: D

The acute scrotum is a urological emergency. The differential diagnosis of children presenting with acute scrotal pain includes torsion of the testis, torsion of the appendix testis, or epididymitis/epididymo-orchitis.

Fluid resuscitation may be required before operation and continued during the surgery. Even if the child is fasted, pain and distress may delay gastric emptying, thus a rapid sequence induction is indicated in most cases. LMA should not be considered for such an emergency procedure even though the aspiration risk is minimal as the diagnosis is only provisional.

Gandhi M, Vashisht R. Anaesthesia for paediatric urology. *Contin Educ Anaesth Crit Care Pain* 2010; 10(5): 152–57.

19. Answer: D

Perioperative delirium and long term cognitive disturbance are common and disabling consequences of anaesthesia and surgery in the elderly. The risk of prolonged postoperative cognitive dysfunction (POCD) is 10% following major surgery in patients of more than 60 years of age. Increasing age is a risk factor and the incidence in patients of more than 80 years of age may be as high as one in three. It is a complex condition, with features of dementia and confusional states, which continue after the immediate postoperative period. Disturbance of cerebral perfusion and cellular oxygenation is likely to be a contributory factor. Alterations of central acetylcholine and catecholamine levels as well as central steroid effects from the stress response are thought to play a role.

The patient having vitro-retinal surgery is at high risk of severe bradycardia and the treatment constitutes atropine. Atropine is an anticholinergic drug with side effects including dizziness, nausea, blurred vision, loss of balance, dilated pupils, photophobia, and, in elderly patients, confusion, hallucination, and agitation. Atropine is a tertiary amine, which easily crosses the blood–brain barrier and causes anticholinergic symptoms.

Midazolam is a benzodiazepine. It is a short-acting sedative and also causes anxiolysis. It is good for control of agitation and convulsions.

Haloperidol is an antipsychotic drug used in treatment of delirium, acute psychosis, and in treatment of alcohol and opioid withdrawal.

Propofol may be a good sedative but in the elderly has more side effects.

Coburn M, Fahlenkamp A, Zoremba N, Schaelte G. Postoperative cognitive dysfunction: incidence and prophylaxis. *Anaesthesist* 2010; 59(2): 177–84, Quiz 185.

20. Answer: C

Anterior cord syndrome is characterized by paraplegia and dissociated sensory loss of pain and temperature sensation. Posterior column function (position, vibration, and deep-pressure sense) is preserved. Usually anterior cord syndrome is due to infarction of the cord in the territory supplied by the anterior spinal artery. This syndrome has the poorest prognosis of the incomplete injuries.

Advanced Trauma Life Support for Doctors. 8th edn. American College of Surgeons, 2008.

21. Answer: B

Cardiovascular effects to ECT

The cardiovascular response is secondary to activation of the autonomic nervous system. Beginning with the electrical stimulus, there is an initial parasympathetic discharge lasting 10–15 s. This can result in bradycardia, hypotension, or even asystole. A more prominent sympathetic response follows, during which cardiac arrhythmias occasionally occur. Systolic arterial pressure may increase by 30–40% and heart rate may increase by 20% or more, generally peaking at 3–5 min. Myocardial oxygen consumption, as determined by the rate–pressure product (RPP), therefore increases. RPP increases are more marked with bilateral ECT, in older patients and during hyperventilation-induced hypocapnia. Simultaneously, seizure activity increases tissue oxygen consumption, potentially reducing myocardial oxygen supply. Myocardial ischaemia and infarction can therefore occur, particularly with pre-existing disease. Left ventricular systolic and diastolic function can remain decreased up to 6 h after ECT. Cardiac rupture has also been described.

Uppal V, Dourish J, Macfarlane A. Anaesthesia for electroconvulsive therapy. *Contin Educ Anaesth Crit Care Pain* 2010; 10(6): 192–96.

22. Answer: C

The case is not urgent and the patient is not unwell so he should be referred back to the GP to organise a cardiology referral. The patient concerned has systolic blood pressure >180 mmHg and diastolic is >109 mmHg, with evidence of ECG changes, hence deferring the surgery to allow blood pressure to be controlled and the aetiology investigated is the most appropriate action.

Surgery produces an increase in stress hormones and catecholamine levels. The effect of these increases tachycardia, hypertension, and increased myocardial contractility with increased oxygen demand. In susceptible patients, adverse cardiac events such as myocardial ischemia and arrhythmias can occur.

There is little evidence for an association between admission arterial pressures of <180 mmHg systolic or <110 mmHg diastolic and perioperative cardiovascular complications. A recent meta-analysis of 30 papers involving 12,995 perioperative patients demonstrated an odds ratio for the association between hypertensive disease and cardiovascular complications of 1.35, which is not clinically significant.

Howell SJ, Sear JW, Foex P. Hypertension, hypertensive heart disease and perioperative cardiac risk. *Br J Anaesth* 2004, 92, 570–83.

23. Answer: D

Hypertension is a rise in blood pressure of more than 20% above the preoperative blood pressure.

Intraopertive hypertension may have multifactorial causes. The common causes of intra-operative hypertension are relatively light anaesthesia/pain or pre-existing hypertension, but there are other causes of intra-operative hypertension that must be excluded by the anaesthetist, including hypoxaemia, hypercarbia, unintended administration of a vasopressor, drug interactions, raised intracranial pressure, phaeochomocytoma, volume overload, and a full bladder. The reversible causes should be excluded and anaesthesia deepened with analgesics or anaesthetic agents before using antihypertensives in the acute setting.

Labetalol, a combined α- and β-blocker with a short onset time, for example labetalol, may be titrated intravenously in patients who require supplementary treatment. Sublingual nifedipine should not be used for the treatment of hypertensive emergencies.

The anaesthetist should anticipate the times of high surgical stimulus and increase the depth of anaesthesia. The appropriate management would be to continue ventilation and increase the concentration of volatile anaesthetic or give a further dose of narcotic. Avoid fluid overload and ensure that the patient is oxygenated and ventilated at all times.

24. Answer: E

Compartment syndrome is a serious condition that involves increased pressure in a muscle compartment. It can lead to muscle and nerve damage and problems with blood flow. The Lloyd Davies position was developed to facilitate access to the pelvis for gynaecological, urological, and colorectal procedures. Previous case reports have demonstrated that prolonged adoption (>4 h) of this position has been associated with the development of bilateral compartment syndrome of the calves. All three patients reported here suffered severe bilateral calf pain despite the use of thoracic epidurals. The important clinical feature is the pain in the calves despite the running epidural, which is suggestive of compartment syndrome. Bilateral deep vein thrombosis is highly unlikely. The neurological examination does not suggest spinal cord compression so nerve conduction studies and MRI are not indicated.

Turnbull D, Mills GH. Compartment syndrome associated with the Lloyd Davies position. Three case reports and review of the literature. *Anaesthesia* 2001; 56(10): 980–87.

25. Answer: E

The clinical picture is suggestive of acute upper airway obstruction, probably secondary to acute epiglottitis. The patient with epiglottitis is an airway emergency and the airway needs to be secured by tracheal intubation with intensive antibiotic treatment. The inhalational anaesthesia technique is the safest technique, while any trial with awake fibreoptic intubation is likely to cause laryngeal spasm, which will further compromise the airway.

Maloney E, Meakin GH. Acute stridor in children. *Contin Educ Anaesth Crit Care Pain* 2007; 7(6): 183–86.

26. **Answer: D**

Rheumatoid arthritis is associated with various problems with the airway, including fixed neck deformity, narrowing of cricoarytenoid joint, and involvement of the temporomandibular joint and atlanto-axial subluxation (AAS). AAS can be anterior (80%), posterior (5%), vertical (10–20%), or lateral. Anterior AAS will produce symptoms on neck flexion, while posterior AAS worsens on neck extension with implications for conventional laryngoscopy.

This patient's symptoms are suggestive of posterior AAS and need imaging to diagnose or exclude AAS. She also has an enlarged thyroid, which may in itself compromise her airway. It would not be appropriate to proceed without further imaging.

Fomban F, Thompson JP. Anaesthesia for adult patients with rheumatoid arthritis. *Cont Educ Anaesth Crit Care Pain* 2006: 6(6): 235–39.

27. **Answer: A**

Injury to vessel results in activation of inflammatory process, leading to formation of fibrin network. This may result in formation of a thrombus that occludes blood vessels. The thrombus may detach to reach the right side of the heart and then to the pulmonary vessels, resulting in pulmonary embolus. The pelvic and limb veins are the source of pulmonary emboli. It is rare for the emboli to originate from the veins in the upper limbs. Deep venous thrombosis may be asymptomatic. The veins in the deep calf are usually the site where commencement of the deep venous thrombosis occurs. However, pulmonary emboli are symptomatic when they are large enough to cause obstruction in major pulmonary vessels. The most common site of origin for these is the iliofemoral vein. Thrombi in the superficial vein are less likely to cause pulmonary embolus as compared to the deep vein thrombus.

Pulmonary Embolism. National Heart, Lung, and Blood Institute. http://www.nhlbi.nih.gov/health/dci/Diseases/pe/pe_what.html.

28. **Answer: E**

Medial movement of the shoulder suggests that the trapezius muscle is being activated. This is supplied by the accessory nerve, which runs posterior to the brachial plexus. The needle should be withdrawn and reinserted.

The shoulder is innervated by the cervical and the brachial plexuses. Surgery to the shoulder is a notoriously painful procedure and interscalene brachial plexus block should be considered as the regional technique of choice. At the level of C6, a modified Winnie technique is considered as the most straightforward landmarks technique. The brachial plexus runs within the interscalene groove between scalenus anterior and scalenus medius. Recent developments have seen the introduction of ultrasound-guided peripheral nerve block techniques, and the anatomy of the brachial plexus at the level of the interscalene groove lends itself to visualization using this technique.

Nerve Stimulator Guided Interscalene Brachial Plexus Block. NYSORA, March 2009. http://www.nysora.com/.

29. **Answer: D**

The serum level of 0.40 mmol/L is a significantly low level of magnesium, and furthermore the patient is on a diuretic and also has bowel obstruction. The potassium is low but in comparison to magnesium it is just below the normal level. The more likely the cause of arrhythmia is hypomagnesium. Magnesium is a cofactor in numerous enzymatic reactions in the human body. Magnesium is the fourth most abundant cation in the body and second most important intracellular cation.

Magnesium:

- regulates Na-K-ATPase activity
- regulates K channels activity
- is a natural calcium channel blocking agent.

These properties explain its important place in electrophysiology of myocardial cells and the effects on the tension of smooth muscles, resulting in a vasodilation and a bronchodilation respectively.

The antagonistic effect of magnesium on calcium decreases the presynaptic release of acetylcholine at the neuromuscular junction and the release of epinephrine at the peripheral sympathetic nerves and the adrenals. Magnesium potentiates the effect of non-depolarizing muscle relaxants. Magnesium is required in the biosynthesis of DNA and RNA.

The normal serum level of magnesium is 0.7–1.0 mmol/L and the therapeutic level is 2.0–3.5 mmol/L.

Shechter M, Hod H, Marks N. Beneficial effect of magnesium sulfate in acute myocardial infarction. *Am J Cardiol* 1990; 1(66): 271–74.

30. Answer: E

It is a good practice to use the professional telephone service. The family member or those with limited command of the language should not be used unless it is an emergency situation. This case is a routine operation and requires consent for the operation and interscalene block. In recovery he would also require a professional interpreter to communicate if there is a problem.

Single Best Answers—Mini Exam 3

1. Answer: B

The diagnostic criteria for SIADH are:

- hypotonic hyponatraemia (serum sodium < 135 mmol/L) and serum osmolality < 280 mOsm/kg
- urine osmolality > serum osmolality
- urine sodium concentration > 18 mmol/L
- normal thyroid, adrenal, and renal function
- clinical euvolaemia—absence of peripheral oedema or dehydration.

The most common neurological causes of SIADH are subarachnoid haemorrhage (SAH), traumatic brain injury (TBI), brain tumour, and meningitis/encephalitis. The absence of dehydration in SIADH is very important as this is the key feature differentiating it from CSWS, in which clinical signs of dehydration will always be present. It is important to distinguish between SIADH and CSWS because the treatment of the two conditions is diametrically opposed.

Bradshaw K, Smith M. Disorders of sodium balance after brain injury. *Contin Educ Anaesth Crit Care Pain* 2008; 8(4): 129–33.

Gupta A, Gelb A. *Essentials of Neuroanaesthesia and Neurointensive Care.* Saunders Elsevier, 2008.

2. Answer: A

The Bain circuit is a modification of the Mapleson D system. It is a co-axial system in which the fresh gas flows through a narrow inner tube within the outer corrugated tubing. Essentially, the Bain circuit functions in the same way as the T-piece, except that the tube supplying fresh gas to the patient is located inside the reservoir tube.

The circuit has three phases.

- Inspiration: the patient inspires fresh gas from the outer reservoir tube.
- Expiration: the patient expires into the reservoir tube. Although fresh gas is still flowing into the system at this time, it is wasted, as it is contaminated with expired gas.
- Expiratory pause: fresh gas from the inner tube washes the expired gas out of the reservoir tube, filling it with fresh gas for the next inspiration.

Spontaneous ventilation: normocarbia requires a fresh gas flow of 200–300 mL/kg.

Controlled ventilation: a fresh gas flow of only 70 mL/kg is required to produce normocarbia.

Bain and Spoerel have recommended:

- 2 L/min fresh gas flow in patients <10 kg
- 3.5 L/min fresh gas flow in patients 10–50 kg
- 70 mL/kg fresh gas flow in patients >60 kg.

The recommended tidal volume is 10 mL/kg and respiratory rate is 12–16 breaths/min.

3. Answer: A

Diabetes insipidus is associated with damage to the pituitary gland or hypothalamus, most commonly due to surgery, a tumour, an illness (such as meningitis), inflammation, or a head injury. In some cases the cause is unknown. This damage disrupts the normal production, storage and release of ADH. The incidence of DI can be as high as 35% after traumatic brain injury, when it is associated with more severe injury and increased mortality.

DI results from a failure of ADH release from the hypothalamic–pituitary axis. The ability to concentrate urine is impaired, resulting in the production of large volumes of dilute urine. This inappropriate loss of water leads to an increase in serum sodium and osmolality and a state of clinical dehydration.

There are two aims in the management of DI: replacement and retention of water and replacement of ADH. Conscious patients are able to increase their own water intake and this is often sufficient treatment if the DI is self-limiting. In unconscious patients, fluid replacement is achieved with water administered via a nasogastric tube or IV 5% dextrose. If urine output continues >250 mL/h, synthetic ADH should be administered. This is usually in the form of small titrated doses of 1-deamino-8-D-arginine vasopressin, which can be given intranasally (100–200 mg) or IV (0.4 mg).

Bradshaw K, Smith M. Disorders of sodium balance after brain injury. *Contin Educ Anaesth Crit Care Pain* 2008; 8(4): 129–33.

4. Answer: D

Multiple sclerosis does not contraindicate either regional or general anaesthetic. In this case the foetus has severe bradycardia and GA is the most common practice.

In multiple sclerosis there is up-regulation of nicotinic acetylcholine receptors, and sensitivity to depolarizing neuromuscular blocking agents is increased. Therefore, their administration can result in hyperkalaemia and cardiac arrest. Although this effect may be more significant in patients with a severe neurological deficit, it is advisable to avoid succinylcholine in even mild conditions unless clinically indicated. Rocuronium is now considered an alternative for rapid sequence induction in obstetric anaesthesia.

Opioids—even those with short duration of action—should be avoided unless the maternal condition warrants their use (e.g. to dampen the hypertensive response to intubation in pre-eclampsia).

Griffiths S, Durbridge JA. Anaesthetic implications of neurological disease in pregnancy. *Contin Educ Anaesth Crit Care Pain* 2011; 11(5): 157–61.

5. Answer A

It is clear in this situation that it is in the child's best interests to have appropriate treatment for a head injury as quickly as possible. Using the doctrine of emergency (which assumes a person's consent to medical treatment when he or she is in imminent danger and unable to give informed consent; also known as implied consent), it would be appropriate to proceed with emergency treatment without consent. Best practice would include making sure attempts were being made to contact the child's parents, documentation in the medical records of the reasons for proceeding under the doctrine of emergency, and if possible having a senior colleague confirm and document the decision independently.

Williams CA, Perkins R. Consent issues for children: a law unto themselves? *Contin Educ Anaesth Crit Care Pain* 2011; 11(3): 99–103.

6. Answer C

Ventilation targets in traumatic brain injury include a PaO_2 of 13 kPa and a $PaCO_2$ of 4.0–4.5 kPa. Excessive hyperventilation ($PaCO_2 < 4$ kPa) should be avoided because it has been associated with worsening of cerebral ischaemia secondary to excessive cerebral vasoconstriction.

Gupta A, Gelb A. *Essentials of Neuroanaesthesia and Neurointensive Care.* Saunders Elsevier, 2008.

7. Answer: D

Acute kidney injury is defined when one of the following criteria is met:

- serum creatinine rises by ≥ 26 µmol/L within 48 h *or*
- serum creatinine rises ≥ 1.5-fold from the reference value, which is known *or*
- presumed to have occurred within 1 week *or*
- urine output is < 0.5 mL/kg/h for over 6 consecutive hours.

Acute kidney injury (AKI) occurring around the time of surgery is a common complication of major surgery and is associated with considerable morbidity and mortality. Perioperative AKI accounts for 20–25% of cases of hospital-acquired renal failure. The incidence varies between 1 and 25% depending on the type of surgery and on the definition of renal failure.

At present there is no evidence to suggest that the use of any pharmacological treatment provides perioperative renal protection. The key renal protective strategies include:

- ensuring adequate hydration and renal perfusion
- avoid nephrotoxic agents
- careful glycaemic control
- managing post operative complications promptly and aggressively.

Renal dysfunction after surgery is often associated with multiple organ dysfunction syndrome and may result in a mortality of up to 60%. It is also associated with a high risk of infection, prolonged intensive care unit (ICU) and hospital stay, progression to chronic renal failure (CRF), and dialysis-dependent end-stage renal disease (ESRD). The chance of full recovery from an episode of AKI in the surgical setting is only 15%—many patients progress to develop varying degrees of chronic renal dysfunction.

A number of postoperative complications are known to be associated with renal dysfunction. Prompt diagnosis and management of acute cardiac dysfunction, haemorrhage, sepsis, rhabdomyolysis, and intra-abdominal hypertension are essential to prevent the development of AKI.

Webb ST, Allen JSD. Perioperative renal protection. *Contin Educ Anaesth Crit Care Pain* 2008; 8(5): 176–80.

8. Answer: C

Benign intracranial hypertension is a diagnosis of exclusion described as raised ICP in the absence of an intracranial lesion, hydrocephalus, or infection, and normal cerebrospinal fluid (CSF) composition. The condition is more common in obese women, while symptoms often worsen during pregnancy and improve after delivery. Dural puncture is not contraindicated, but due to the altered CSF circulation, spinal anaesthesia may be unpredictable. There have been reports using combined spinal–epidural anaesthesia and intrathecal catheters for operative delivery, both of which allow augmentation of anaesthesia if required.

Griffiths S, Durbridge JA. Anaesthetic implications of neurological disease in pregnancy. *Contin Educ Anaesth Crit Care Pain* 2011; 11(5): 157–61.

9. Answer: E

Postoperative hypertension can occur due to coughing on emergence of anaesthesia, postoperative pain, bladder distension, or anxiety or due to a residual effect of muscle relaxants. It is also important to remember some patients will be confused and disorientated after anaesthesia and this may worsen blood pressure values. This highlights the importance of the recovery room being a suitably calm environment, with staff trained to anticipate and treat these problems.

The important steps would be to reassess the patient and continue monitoring, which should include ECG, blood pressure, and SpO_2. It is important to treat the reversible causes: first pain and urine retention followed by the treatment of continuing hypertension. Although there is no cut-off value for treatment, a persistently elevated systolic blood pressure reaching 200 mmHg would suggest treatment is appropriate.

This patient is severely hypertensive postoperatively, which may be due to multiple causes. Exclude pain, urinary retention, hypoxia, and anxiety. Repeat the blood pressure measurement if the pressure is persistently high, then consider labetalol 5 mg/mL, which should be titrated to normal blood pressure for that patient. Keep the patient in recovery.

Hypertension: Clinical Management of Primary Hypertension in Adults. NICE guideline, 2011. http://guidance.nice.org.uk/CG127.

10. Answer: E

An automatic implantable cardiac defibrillator is a (AICD) system that consists of a pulse generator and leads, and is used for detection and therapy of tachyarrhythmias. It may provide antitachycardia, antibradycardia pacing, synchronized or nonsynchronized shocks, telemetry, and diagnostic storage. Many devices use adaptive rate pacing to modify the pacing rate for changing metabolic needs. The ICD batteries contain up to 20 000 J of energy. Cardioversion with energy exceeding 2 J results in skeletal and diaphragmatic muscle depolarization and is painful to the conscious patient. High energy discharges of 10–40 J, delivered asynchronously, are used to treat ventricular fibrillation (VF). AICD terminates VF successfully in almost 98% of cases.

For any patient with a pacemaker, it is essential to identify the device so that its response to electrocautery is known. In particular, the backup mode should be determined. If extensive close-proximity electrocautery is required and loss of AV synchrony may compromise the patient haemodynamically (for example, heart failure patients), then it is advisable that a telemetric programmer and an experienced operator is present during surgery.

During surgery, bipolar electrocautery should be used whenever possible; if not, then the anode plate should be positioned as far away from the pacemaker generator as possible. Similarly, the cathode should be kept as far away from the device as possible. the lowest possible amplitude should be used and the operator should apply electrocautery in short bursts rather than continuously.

Careful monitoring of the pulse, pulse oximetry, and arterial pressure is essential during electrocautery, as ECG monitoring can also be affected by interference. For the patient with an implanted defibrillator, facilities for external defibrillation should be available immediately after the device is disabled. If possible, remote pads should be used and applied in a suitable orientation.

Specific postoperative care should include a full telemetric check and re-programming back to the original setting if preoperative re-programming was required. Anti-tachycardia therapies of implantable defibrillators should obviously be re-programmed to their original settings.

Association (ACC/AHA) guidelines also advise that all anti-tachycardia therapy should be disabled before anaesthesia.

Salukhe TV, Dob D, Sutton R. Pacemakers and defibrillators: anaesthetic implications. *Br J Anaesth* 2004; 93(1): 95–104.

11. Answer: B

Pre-eclampsia complicates up to 8% of pregnancies in the developed world. Pre-eclampsia is associated with widespread endothelial dysfunction, leading to placental ischaemia and multi-organ dysfunction. Maternal complications of severe pre-eclampsia include:

- DIC or HELLP syndrome (10–20%)
- pulmonary oedema or aspiration (2–5%)
- abruptio placentae (1–4%)
- acute renal failure (1–5%)
- eclampsia (1%), liver failure or haemorrhage (1%), and rarely stroke and death.

There is an association with long-term cardiovascular disease.

Sibai B, Dekker G, Kupferminc M. Pre-eclampsia. *Lancet* 2005; 365(9461): 785–99.

Steegers EA, von Dadelszen P, Duvekot JJ, Pijnenborg R. Pre-eclampsia. *Lancet* 2010; 376(9741): 631–44.

12. Answer: D

Warfarin is the oral anticoagulant of choice for atrial fibrillation. Nicoumalone and phenindione are licensed in the UK but are potentially more toxic than warfarin and are seldom used. All currently available oral anticoagulants act by antagonizing the effect of vitamin K by preventing the reduction of oxidized vitamin K required for carboxylation of clotting factor precursors, resulting in reduced hepatic production of active coagulation factors II, VII, IX, and X, and hence in prolongation of the prothrombin time and INR. This usually takes 48–72 h to develop fully.

The management of warfarin overdose, following initial resuscitation and stabilization includes administration of prothrombin complex concentrate (PCC), which contains the necessary factors but is expensive. Therefore 15 mL/kg of fresh frozen plasma (FFP) is often administered, but presents a risk of anaphylaxis and transmission of blood-borne pathogens, and is the most common cause of transfusion-related acute lung injury (TRALI). Recombinant factor VIIa (rFVIIa) is increasingly being used in uncontrollable haemorrhage. The Israeli Multidisciplinary Task Force have recommended its use where the platelet count is 50–109/L, pH >7.2, and fibrinogen >0.5; it has been shown to work in oral anticoagulant overdose.

Protamine is used to neutralize the effects of heparin through a physicochemical pH-dependent interaction, but in high doses it has anticoagulant and myocardial depressant action.

Antifibrinolytics, such as tranexamic acid, competitively inhibit activation of plasminogen to plasmin and are thus not helpful in this context.

Vitamin K should also be given but will make reintroduction of warfarin difficult in the short term.

Antithrombotic Therapy. Section 13: Oral Anticoagulants. Scottish Intercollegiate Guidelines Network. http://www.sign.ac.uk/guidelines/fulltext/36/section13.html.

13. Answer: D

The elimination half-life is the time taken for the plasma concentration to drop by half during the elimination phase. The time taken for the initial plasma concentration to fall to half its value is also called as distribution half-life. The removal of a drug from the plasma is known as clearance and the distribution of the drug in the various body tissues is known as the volume of distribution. Both of these pharmacokinetic parameters are important in determining the half-life of a drug. For most of the drugs, initial plasma concentration reduces by the process of distribution or drug uptake by tissues. To maintain steady plasma concentrations, the maintenance infusion rate is determined by the amount of drug that has been eliminated from the body.

The half-life can be determined by giving a single dose, usually intravenously, and then measuring the concentration of the drug in the plasma at regular intervals. The concentration of the drug will reach a peak value in the plasma and will then fall as the drug is broken down and cleared from the blood. This is calculated as:

total amount of drug eliminated = clearance × plasma concentration

Half-life varies between individuals and within the individual depending upon internal homeostasis and organ function.

Calvey TA, Williams NE. Pharmacokinetics. In: *Principles and Practice of Pharmacology for Anaesthetists*, 3rd edn. Blackwell Science, 1997: Chapter 2.

14. Answer: B

Temperature measurement and control is extremely important. Patients with neuromuscular disorders can be vulnerable to both hypo- and hyperthermia. A high index of suspicion should exist for patients with muscular dystrophies and myotonias for concomitant malignant hyperthermia. Unexplained tachycardia with an increase in end-tidal carbon dioxide concentration should alert the anaesthetist to a potential hyperthermic complication, which should be treated aggressively. Hyperthermia may occur due to increased muscle activity seen in myotonias, iatrogenic causes, or malignant hyperthermia.

Marsh S, Ross N, Pittard A. Neuromuscular disorders and anaesthesia. Part 1: generic anaesthetic management. *Cont Educ Anaesth Crit Care Pain* 2011; 11(4): 115–118.

15. Answer: B

In complex regional pain syndrome I (CRPS I) the symptoms are preceded by tissue injury, most commonly limb trauma (absence of nerve injury). Diagnostic criteria for CRPS fall into four categories: sensory, vasomotor, sudomotor, and motor/trophic changes.

The exact pathogenesis of CRPS is unclear. Theories can be divided into peripheral and central mechanisms, with central nervous system abnormality predominating.

Diagnostic criteria

The International Association for the Study of Pain proposed formal diagnostic criteria in 1995.

The diagnostic criteria for CRPS I are as follows.

Following an initiating noxious event:

- spontaneous pain or allodynia/hyperalgesia occurs beyond the territory of a single peripheral nerve and is disproportionate to the inciting event
- there is or has been evidence of oedema, skin blood flow abnormality, or abnormal sudomotor activity in the region of the pain since the inciting event.

The diagnosis is excluded by the existence of conditions that would otherwise account for the degree of pain and dysfunction.

JG Wilson, MG Serpell. Complex regional pain syndrome. *Cont Educ Anaesth Crit Care Pain* 2007; 7(2): 51–54.

16. Answer: A

In patients at high risk of venous thromboembolism (VTE), especially those with cancer, in whom mechanical or pharmacological thromboprophylaxis is not possible, the insertion of a temporary or permanent vena caval filter preoperatively should be considered. The indications for insertion of vena cava filters are:

- uncontrollable thromboembolic disease
- pulmonary endarterectomy for chronic thromboembolic disease

- absolute contraindication for anticoagulation
- limited life expectancy.

Retrievable filters may be used for interim prophylaxis. These devices stay in place for several months.

Surgical patients at increased risk of VTE include those with:

- active bleeding
- acquired bleeding disorders, including acute liver failure
- concurrent use of anticoagulants with INR > 2
- epidural/spinal anaesthesia expected within the next 12 h
- epidural/spinal anaesthesia within the previous 4 h
- acute stroke
- thrombocytopenia (platelets < 75 × 10^9/L)
- uncontrolled systolic hypertension > 230 mmHg
- untreated inherited bleeding disorders.

Venous Thromboembolism: Reducing the Risk. NICE guideline 92, 2010. http://guidance.nice.org.uk/CG92.

Barker RC, Marval P. Venous thromboembolism: risks and prevention. *Cont Educ Anaesth Crit Care Pain* 2011; 11(1): 18–23.

17. Answer: B

Human recombinant factor VIIa is a vitamin-K-dependent protein, which promotes clotting through the extrinsic pathway by forming a complex with tissue factor located on the subendothelial surface of damaged blood vessels. This complex then activates factors IX and X, which go on to generate thrombin. Currently there are several case studies published where factor VIIa has been used in cases of intractable postpartum haemorrhage. In all of the case studies, the factor VII was given as a bolus in doses ranging from 60 to 120 mcg/kg, and effects were seen in as little as 10 min. The major drawbacks of factor VIIa are the short half-life (2 h) and the high cost. Repeat dosing may be necessary in cases of ongoing haemorrhage adding to the already high cost.

Action of rFVIIa is dependant on the presence of adequate numbers of circulating platelets and adequate fibrinogen concentration. Previous reports have shown that the improvements in laboratory markers of DIC, by the administration of blood components prior to the administration of rFVIIa, are associated with a better response to rFVIIa treatment. It is also recognized that correction of acidosis is an important aspect in the success of rFVIIa. Recombinant factor VIIa (rFVIIa) is increasingly being used in uncontrollable haemorrhage. The Israeli Multidisciplinary Task Force have recommended its use where the platelet count is >50 10^9/L, pH >7.2, and fibrinogen >0.50 mg/dL. It has been shown to work in oral anticoagulant overdose.

Mayo A, Misgav M, Kluger Y, *et al.* Recombinant activated factor VII (NovoSeven): addition to replacement therapy in acute, uncontrolled and life-threatening bleeding. *Vox Sang* 2004; 87(1): 34–40.

Martinowitz U, Michaelson M. Israeli Multidisciplinary rFVIIa Task Force. Guidelines for the use of recombinant activated factor VII (rFVIIa) in uncontrolled bleeding: a report by the Israeli Multidisciplinary rFVIIa Task Force. *J Thromb Haemost* 2005; 3(4): 640–48.

18. Answer: D

Acute kidney injury (AKI) is a common clinical problem, is expensive to manage, and is associated with a high mortality. Prompt recognition of the risk factors for AKI, accurate clinical assessment of patients with kidney injury, and avoidance of further nephrotoxic insults can help to prevent or reverse AKI. Normal kidney function depends on having an adequate blood pressure and fluid volume to perfuse the kidneys. The kidney itself must have a sufficient number of intact nephrons (glomeruli and tubules) to achieve normal glomerular filtration and electrolyte balance.

AKI confers independent mortality. Early recognition and intervention are essential. Recognition and resuscitation of the acutely ill patient is essential (NICE CG 50). Even a modest increase in serum creatinine—26.4 μmol/L—is associated with a dramatic impact on the risk of mortality—hence 'acute kidney injury'.

Autoregulation is effective, with a MAP between 85 and 180 mmHg, although 60 mmHg is accepted as adequate during shock resuscitation and perioperative management. Autoregulation is achieved by modulation of afferent arteriolar tone by a local myogenic reflex in the afferent arteriolar wall and tubuloglomerular feedback.

Tang IY, Murray PT. Prevention and treatment of acute renal failure. *Best Prac Res Clin Anaesth* 2004; 18(1): 91–111.

19. Answer: C

Chronic renal failure (CRF) and end-stage renal disease (ESRD) are functional diagnoses characterized by a progressive decrease in glomerular filtration rate (GFR). CRF occurs where GFR has been reduced to 10% of normal function (20 mL/min), and ESRD when GFR falls below 5% (10 mL/min). Patients with CRF have a tendency to excessive bleeding in the peri-operative period. Standard tests of coagulation are usually normal (i.e. prothrombin time, activated partial thromboplastin time, international normalized ratio) and platelet count is within normal limits. However, platelet activity is deranged, with decreased adhesiveness and aggregation, probably caused by inadequate vascular endothelial release of a von Willebrand factor/factor VIII complex which binds to and activates platelets. Chronic renal failure is associated with platelet dysfunction and poor coagulation.

Bombeli T, Spahn DR. Updates in perioperative coagulation: physiology and management of thromboembolism and haemorrhage. *Br J Anaesth* 2004; 93(2): 275–87.

Blann AD, Lip GYH. Venous thromboembolism. *BMJ* 2006; 332: 215–19.

20. Answer: D

Severe sepsis is considered when:

- temperature > 38.3°C or < 36°C
- heart rate > 90 bpm
- respiratory rate of >20/min or $PaCO_2$ < 4.4 kPa.
- white cell count > 12×10^9/L or < 4×10^9/L
- loss of consciousness
- hyperglycemia in non-diabetic.

Hypotension is currently used to define the transition from severe sepsis to septic shock; it is not sufficiently sensitive as a screening tool for tissue perfusion deficits occurring in patients with early sepsis. The use of lactate levels of ≥4 mmol/L as a marker for severe tissue hypoperfusion and therefore as a univariate predictor of mortality is supported by a number of studies. However, anion gap or base deficit are widely used and validated by routine laboratory assessments. In the EGDT study, a normal bicarbonate level or anion gap was observed in 22.2% and 25.0%, respectively, of patients with lactate levels of 4.0–6.9 mmol/L. The combination of a normal serum bicarbonate level and anion gap was observed in 11.1% of these patients. At higher lactate levels, this observation (mixed acid–base disorder) became less common and was not present in any patients with lactate levels of >10 mmol/L, all of whom had marked metabolic acidosis. Early lactate clearance as a surrogate for the resolution of global tissue hypoxia is significantly associated with decreased levels of biomarkers and improvement in organ dysfunction and outcome in severe sepsis and septic shock.

Nguyen HB, Loomba M, Yang JJ, et al. Early lactate clearance is associated with biomarkers of inflammation, coagulation, apoptosis, organ dysfunction and mortality in severe sepsis and septic shock. J Inflamm (Lond) 2010; 28(7): 6.

Page I, Hardy G, Fairfield J, et al. Implementing Surviving Sepsis guidelines in a district general hospital. J R Coll Physicians Edinb 2011; 41(4): 309–15.

Otero RM, Nguyen HB, Huang DT, et al. Early goal-directed therapy in severe sepsis and septic shock revisited: concepts, controversies, and contemporary findings. Chest 2006; 130(5): 1579–95.

21. Answer: E

The cardinal features of PDPH as defined by the International Headache Society are a headache that develops within 7 days of dural puncture and disappears within 14 days. However, PDPH has been reported occurring later and continuing for longer than these times.

Classic features of the headache caused by dural puncture are:

- Headache is often frontal-occipital.
- Most headaches do not develop immediately after dural puncture but 24–48 h after the procedure, with 90% of headaches presenting within 3 days.
- The headache is worse in the upright position and eases when supine.
- Pressure over the abdomen with the woman in the upright position may give transient relief to the headache by raising intracranial pressure secondary to a rise in intrabdominal pressure (Gutsche sign).

Differential diagnosis is as follows:

- Vascular: migraine, cerebral vein thrombosis, cerebral infarction, subdural haematoma subarachnoid haematoma.
- Infective: meningitis, encephalitis.
- Other causes: post-dural puncture headache, pre-eclampsia, tension headache, benign intracranial hypertension, pneumocephalus, lactation headache.

Differential diagnosis is particularly important in the postpartum period; headache or neck/shoulder pain occurs in the first week postpartum in about 40% of women. These headaches are often attributed to dural leak because epidural anaesthesia is very common. Among postpartum headaches, PDPH was the identified cause in a minority of women. When a patient returns to the hospital complaining of headache, the differential diagnosis should be re-evaluated, and the physician should not assume that the patient has a PDPH. Meningitis, central venous sinus thrombosis (CVST), spinal haematoma, cortical/cerebral vein thrombosis, intracranial subdural haematoma, benign intracranial hypertension, migraine, and caffeine-withdrawal headache should all be considered.

The new onset of migraine has been variably reported as occurring in 1% and 10% during pregnancy, usually during the first trimester. During pregnancy, pre-existing migraine improves or disappears in about 60%, has an unchanged frequency in 20%, and an increased frequency in 20%. Improvement often occurs during the second or third trimester.

Headache Classification Subcommittee of the International Headache Society. The International Classificationof Headache Disorders: 2nd edn. Cephalalgia 2004; 24(Suppl 1): 9–160.

Bezov D, Lipton RB. Ashina S. Post-dural puncture headache: Part I Diagnosis, epidemiology, etiology, and pathophysiology. Headache 2010; 50(7): 1144–52.

22. Answer: C

Parenteral nutrition (PN) is the intravenous administration of a solution containing amino acids, glucose, fat, electrolytes, trace elements, and vitamins as treatment for acute or chronic intestinal failure. The National Institute for Clinical Excellence (NICE) recently recommended that PN should be limited to a maximum of 50% of the calculated requirements for the first 48 h after initiation. Although calculated requirements for calorific support using the Schofield method may exceed 2000 kcals per 24 h, it will only rarely be appropriate to deliver such a quantity.

It is mandatory that the PN is properly controlled to avoid hyperglycaemia, hypertriglyceridaemia, uraemia, metabolic acidosis, and electrolyte imbalance.

PN is used in preference to enteral feeding only when the gastrointestinal tract is unavailable or unable to absorb or digest an adequate amount of nutrients on a temporary or permanent basis.

PN should be considered when:

- the gastrointestinal tract is not functioning and it is anticipated that it will remain non-functional for 5 days or longer
- all methods of enteral nutrition have been ruled out
- complete bowel rest is required
- total nutrient requirements cannot be met through the gut alone.

The rationale for glutamine replacement during critical illness is clear, as it is an important fuel for enterocytes and lymphocytes and has a role in nucleotide synthesis. This helps to maintain gut mucosal integrity and cellular immune function.

Simpson F, Doig GS. Parenteral vs. enteral nutrition in the critically ill patient: a meta-analysis of trials using the intention to treat principle. *Intens Care Med* 2005, 31(1): 12–23.

Edmondson WC. Nutritional support in critical care: an update. *Contin Educ Anaesth Crit Care Pain* 2007; 7: 199–202.

23. Answer: B

Critical illness triggers the inflammatory response, leading to a hypermetabolic state. Skeletal muscle is lost as protein is disproportionately used as an energy source. Feeding critically ill patients reduces the rate of muscle loss. Many patients admitted to critical care have pre-existing malnutrition and are less able to tolerate further catabolism.

Arginine supplementation has been shown to be beneficial in cancer patients. In critically ill patients arginine has shown harmful effects by causing haemodynamic instability, immunosuppression, cytotoxicity, and organ dysfunction. In simple terms, increased arginine leads to an increase in the production of nitric oxide (NO), via the constitutive and inducible forms of NO-synthase, which tips the balance from benefit to harm.

At least three studies have confirmed this potential for harm in subgroups of patients with sepsis; significant increases in mortality were demonstrated. Only one study has shown potential benefit and that contained patients with lower Apache II scores and loose definitions of infection. Therefore, arginine supplementation is not recommended for septic ICU patients but, because of its beneficial effects on T lymphocyte function, it has been shown to reduce infective complications in elective general surgical patients. There is no benefit in general ITU/trauma/burns/acute lung injury.

Simpson F, Doig GS. Parenteral vs. enteral nutrition in the critically ill patient: a meta-analysis of trials using the intention to treat principle. *Intens Care Med* 2005, 31(1): 12–23.

Edmondson WC. Nutritional support in critical care: an update. *Contin Educ Anaesth Crit Care Pain* 2007; 7: 199–202.

24. Answer: E

Enteral nutrition (EN) is cheaper and probably safer, but may be associated with significant complications. It may frequently result in under-nutrition unless protocols are used to avoid slow initiation and the too-ready cessation of feeds. Acceptance of gastric residual volumes of 200–250 mL and the early use of pro-kinetics are key elements of such protocols. Head-up tilt of at least 45° should be used whenever possible to facilitate EN. Aspiration is a possible risk with naso-gastric feeding, and post-pyloric tubes have been advocated to reduce this risk.

Even in acute haemorrhagic pancreatitis, the use of EN has been reported as being beneficial and the need for 'pancreatic rest' for such patients has been challenged. The nasogastric route has also been confirmed as being safe and suitable for these patients and, if true pancreatic rest is to be achieved, any tube placed post-pylorically should be sited in the third segment of the jejunum. The nasogastric route has also been confirmed as being safe and suitable for these patients and, if true pancreatic rest is to be achieved, any tube placed post-pylorically should be sited in the third segment of the jejunum. Post-pyloric feeding is also less physiological than gastric feeding because it alters the 'gastric' phase in small bowel motility in response to the administration of feed. This may lead to an increase in the incidence of diarrhoea.

Simpson F, Doig GS. Parenteral vs. enteral nutrition in the critically ill patient: a meta-analysis of trials using the intention to treat principle. *Intens Care Med* 2005, 31(1): 12–23.

Edmondson WC. Nutritional support in critical care: an update. *Contin Educ Anaesth Crit Care Pain* 2007; 7: 199–202.

Atkinson S, Sieffert E, Bihari D. A prospective, randomised, double blind, controlled clinical trial of enteral immunonutrition in the critically ill. *Crit Care Med* 1998; 26: 1164–72.

25. Answer: C

The clinical features of cocaine poisoning are agitation, dilated pupils, excessive sweating, tachycardia, hypertension, and hyperthermia. Other features are seizures, rhabdomyolysis, myocardial infarction, and cardiac arrest.

The mechanism of action of cocaine is:

- blocks reuptake of dopamine (causing euphoria, hyperactivity) and norepinephrine (causing vasoconstriction and hypertension); arrhythmias may also result
- blocks Na^+ channels, resulting in a local anaesthetic action and myocardial depression
- platelet activation
- mitochondrial dysfunction leading to myocardial depression.

The common complications are:

- chest pain secondary to
  - ◆ myocardial ischaemia
  - ◆ infarction
  - ◆ coronary artery spasm
- heart failure
- seizures
- cerebrovascular accidents
- pneumothorax
- rhabdomyolysis
- premature labour or abruption
- agitated delirium, hyperthermia.

Singer M, Webb AR. Poisoning. In: *Oxford Handbook of Critical Care*, 3rd edn. Oxford University Press, 2009: Chapter 30.

26. Answer: C

Tetanus is caused by a gram-positive bacillus, *Clostridium tetani*, which is commonly found in soil, but may also be isolated from animal or human faeces. It is a motile, spore-forming, obligate anaerobe. Spores are not destroyed by boiling but are eliminated by autoclaving at 120°C for 15 min (at 1 atm pressure). Tetanus is usually diagnosed clinically as the bacterium is rarely cultured. Tetanus is a disease mediated by the neurotoxins released by the bacteria.

In the UK there is a good vaccination programme, hence it is rare, although it is occasionally seen in high-risk groups such as intravenous drug users.

Tetanus toxin (tetanospasmin) binds to the neuromuscular junction and transport to the cell body occurs retrogradely, with subsequent trans-synaptic spread to adjacent motor and autonomic nerves. The primary targets are inhibitory pathways (glycine and GABAergic pathways) leading to increased muscle tone and rigidity. Tetanospasmin disables release of neurotransmitter from presynaptic vesicles Disinhibited autonomic nervous system activity is seen, resulting in cardiovascular instability.

The management requires involvement of critical care staff, microbiologists and surgeons, with a view to:

- assessing the patient's airway, breathing, and circulation
- neutralizing circulating toxin: passive immunization
- eradicating the source of the toxin: extensive debridement, antibiotics
- minimizing effects of bound toxins
- general supportive care.

Human tetanus immunoglobulin neutralizes free-circulating neurotoxin, but does not affect toxins already fixed to nerve terminals; it does not need to be repeated. Recovery from a tetanus infection does not confer immunity.

Metronidazole and surgical debridement are effective at reducing the bacterial toxin load. Muscle spasms can be treated with benzodiazepine and opioids. Sedation, clonidine, and magnesium have all been used with some success to control this instability. ⊠-blocker use is associated with cardiovascular collapse, pulmonary oedema, and death.

Taylor AM. Tetanus. *Contin Educ Anaesth Crit Care Pain* 2006; 6: 101–4.

Cook TM, Protheroe RT, Handel JM. Tetanus: a review of the literature. *Br J Anaesth* 2001; 87: 477–87.

Beeching NJ, Crowcroft NS. Tetanus in injecting drug users. *BMJ* 2005; 330(7485): 208–209.

27. Answer: D

Thromboelastography (TEG) measures whole-blood viscoelastic changes associated with fibrin polymerization. Its ability to generate information about coagulation factor activity and platelet function within 10–20 min make it a reliable test for monitoring coagulation during and after CPB.

R-time (or reaction time) is the time from the initiation of the TEG until the amplitude of the trace reaches 2 mm, corresponding to initial fibrin formation. The *R*-time is functionally related to plasma clotting and inhibitor factor activity.

Features of *R*-time are:

- Normal range: 15–30 mm (whole blood), 10–14 mm (celite activated); 8–12 mm (kaolin activated).
- Prolonged by anticoagulants, factor deficiencies, and severe hypofibrinogenaemia.
- Reduced by hypercoagulable conditions.

A prolonged *R*-time on TEG suggests the presence of heparin or clotting factor deficiency. The defect failed to correct with the addition of heparinise, suggesting that excess heparin is not the culprit and the appropriate management is to give fresh frozen plasma.

Mackay JH, Arrowsmith JE. Coagulopathy during cardiopulmonary bypass. In: Mackay JH, Arrowsmith JE (eds), *Core Topics in Cardiac Anaesthesia*. Cambridge University Press, Cambridge, 2004: pp. 269–70.

28. Answer: D

Patients with obstructive sleep apnoea (OSA) are at an increased risk of perioperative complications. The diagnosis of OSA can often be established based on clinical history and examination alone.

Predisposing conditions combined with a history of snoring, restless sleep, headaches, and daytime sleepiness should alert to the possibility of OSAS.

The STOP-BANG (S, snoring; T, tiredness; O, observed apnoea; P, high blood pressure; B, BMI > 35; A, age > 50; N, neck circumference > 40 cm; G, male gender) score has been shown to be a useful screening tool for OSA during pre-operative assessment.

In the STOP-BANG questionnaire:

- Yes to more than three questions indicates high risk of OSA.
- Yes to fewer than three questions indicates low risk of OSA.

When the STOP-BANG is positive it is normally followed by a sleep study incorporating polysomnography (PSG), which will establish the extent and severity of OSA. PSG examinations include recordings of heart rhythm (ECG), electroencephalography (EEG), eye movements, and electromyography.

Martinez G, Faber P. Obstructive sleep apnoea. *Contin Educ Anaesth Crit Care Pain* 2011; 11(1): 5–8.

29. Answer: D

The unilaterally enlarged right pupil in the context of traumatic brain injury suggests raised ICP. Hypercarbia, excessive PEEP, seizures, and pyrexia can contribute to raised ICP. Whilst hyponatraemia can contribute to raised ICP, hypernatraemia will not.

Management involves:

- ensuring normal oxygen and normocapnia (PaO_2 >11 kPa, $PaCO_2$ 4.5–5 kPa), with tracheal intubation and ventilatory support where required
- treating precipitating factors such as fits, pyrexia, and electrolyte abnormalities
- treating raised ICP with:
  - ◆ raised head
  - ◆ mannitol 0.5 mg/kg IV over 15 min, repeating at 4-hourly intervals depending on cerebral perfusion pressure (CPP) measurements and/or clinical signs of deterioration, and stopping when plasma osmolality reaches 310–320 mOsm/kg
  - ◆ hyperventilation (if pupillary dilatation/clinical picture merits)
- monitoring ICP if appropriate (e.g. trauma).

Godsiff LS, Matta BF. Intensive care management of intra-cranial haemorrhage. In: Matta BF, Menon DK, Turner JM (eds), *Textbook of Neuroanaesthesia and Critical Care*. Greenwich Medical Media, 2000: p. 334.

30. Answer: D

Visual analogue scores are classified as ordinal data. Of the options, only B and D are used for ordinal data, with option B used for paired data. The data in the question is unpaired, with two separate groups of patients.

Kiff K, Spoors C. Training *in Anaesthesia: The Essential Curriculum*. Oxford University Press, 2010: pp. 566–67.

INDEX

Key: ■ denotes question, ■ denotes answer

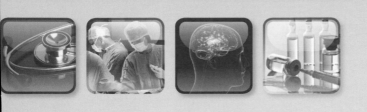
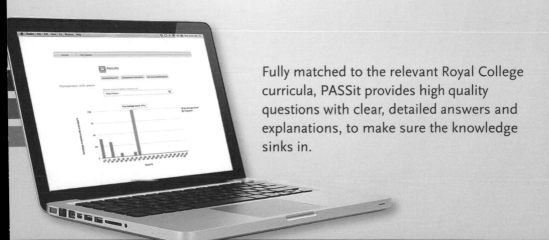

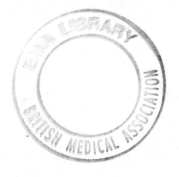